Emergent Vascular Access

James H. Paxton

Editor

Emergent Vascular Access

A Guide for Healthcare Professionals

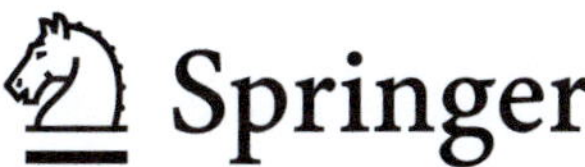

Editor
James H. Paxton
Department of Emergency Medicine
Wayne State University School of Medicine
Detroit, MI
USA

ISBN 978-3-030-77179-9   ISBN 978-3-030-77177-5   (eBook)
https://doi.org/10.1007/978-3-030-77177-5

This Springer imprint is published by the registered company Springer Nature Switzerland AG
The registered company address is: Gewerbestrasse 11, 6330 Cham, Switzerland

Preface

Emergency care providers are accustomed to figuring things out for themselves. Whether at "home" in the prehospital arena, emergency department, inpatient wards, or the intensive care unit, healthcare providers who work with critically-ill patients face austere circumstances and unexpected challenges every day. When time is limited, care must be provided even in the absence of information. This lack of real-time information underscores the importance of being prepared for a wide variety of circumstances. Providers learn from their own successes and failures in obtaining vascular access, as well as those of their colleagues and mentors. But an overreliance on anecdotal evidence and apprentice-style learning can leave gaps in one's training. Although most providers will pick up what they need to know as they advance in their careers, better formalized training in emergent vascular access techniques is needed. Emergency care providers should not have to figure it out for themselves.

Vascular access is an essential component in the treatment of unstable patients across a wide spectrum of disease, and techniques for establishing vascular access are included in most clinical medical textbooks. But medical textbooks are typically written for a broad audience, with a general scope of content intended to capture an entire medical specialty or discipline between its covers. Those of us who treat critically-ill patients under emergent conditions inherently understand that what we do every day is different than what is done for stable patients in a controlled environment. Yet, even within our own disciplines, the techniques and thought processes espoused in medical textbooks often fail to relate to the urgency and chaos that characterizes patient management in the acute care setting.

We need our own resources, our own educational materials, and our own research to inform the practice of establishing emergent vascular access. Traditionally, those who provide emergent vascular access have been obliged to scavenge practice tips from a confusing array of often-contradictory resources, including medical textbooks, blogs, and podcasts. It is time for us to centralize these resources into a coherent, targeted educational curriculum. This book is intended to begin this process of consolidating resources across the spectrum of nursing, critical care, and prehospital and emergency medicine texts into a single reference that may help to inform the practice of providing emergent vascular access. This book is not a primer, as it also includes many advanced concepts. But it is not a truly comprehensive reference, as no single resource can hope to inform the great diversity of practice seen in the modern healthcare environment. New evidence emerges almost daily in our field. Clinical practice defies our efforts to inform providers on every eventuality. However, we hope that this guide will serve as a starting-off point for those whose daily clinical duties involve establishing emergent vascular access for critically-ill patients. It is the first of what we hope will be many future references to educate and advance the field of emergent vascular access.

This textbook is intended to be of value to both the novice and advanced provider. It includes expert opinion as well as evidence-based guidance on vascular access device selection, including the potential advantages and disadvantages of various techniques. However, no book can replace our greatest educational tool: clinical experience. Guidelines and policies on vascular access are constantly being released and updated, and providers must know which practices represent standard of care in their own local healthcare environment. Providers should use their own clinical judgment in interpreting the guidance provided in this book. New evidence must be carefully weighed in the context of contemporary practice, and clinical decisions should continue to be made utilizing the best available evidence. However, great effort has been made to justify the suggestions made in this book using modern references from the medical literature. As conflicting evidence may exist, these recommendations should be considered in the clinical and historical context within which they are delivered. Despite these limitations, this reference will provide at least a rudimentary understanding of the basic principles underlying our chosen practice.

Chapter 1 offers a definition for "emergent vascular access," recognizing the importance of timing and acuity when considering vascular access selection. This discussion sets the stage for the rest of the book.

Chapter 2 introduces the reader to the physics and physiology of vascular access. Many of the factors that influence our decision-making regarding device and site selection relate to basic human physiology and anatomy. Thus, an understanding of the scientific principles underlying vascular access technologies is key.

Chapter 3 relates to landmark-based peripheral intravenous (i.e., "peripheral IV") line placement. This remains the "gold-standard" technique against which all other techniques are measured. Practical advice and tips to improve the likelihood of successful peripheral IV insertion are provided.

Chapter 4 builds upon the previous chapter with special attention to the use of ultrasound guidance in identifying target vessels and facilitating peripheral IV insertion. The use of ultrasound guidance for peripheral line placement has dramatically changed practice, but this approach requires specific training and an understanding of its limitations.

Chapter 5 describes the historical landmark-based approach to central venous catheter (i.e., "central line") insertion at various sites. Although most major guidelines now recommend the use of ultrasound guidance for central line placement, emergent conditions may still necessitate landmark-based methods in specific circumstances. Providers should be aware of these techniques and be confident in their performance for those rare circumstances in which an ultrasound-guided approach is not feasible.

Chapter 6 builds upon the previous chapter by describing how ultrasound-guidance can be used to facilitate and confirm central venous catheter placement. The use of ultrasound guidance for central line placement has led to substantial improvements in the safety and first-attempt success rates for certain central venous access techniques. However, these benefits are best realized when providers are familiar with the pitfalls and potential limitations of this approach.

Chapter 7 discusses intraosseous catheter placement, including the most commonly-seen devices encountered by emergency care providers. Intraosseous cannulation represents an under-utilized approach to indirect venous access, and is associated with certain advantages and disadvantages when compared to direct peripheral venous access techniques. Considerations relating to device and site selection are described, including limitations of this often life-saving technique.

Chapter 8 incorporates information from the previous chapters into a targeted discussion relating to pediatric vascular access. Children present providers with very different vascular access challenges than adults, including differences in anatomy, compliance, and complication risks. Providers should be aware of these differences and incorporate them into their decision-making process when managing critically-ill children, infants, and neonates.

Chapter 9 addresses emergent vascular access in cardiac arrest, including evidence from the medical literature and recent guidelines. In many ways, managing cardiac arrest is the ultimate challenge for vascular access providers. Delays in establishing vascular access for cardiac arrest victims are simply unacceptable, as the inability to rapidly infuse resuscitative medications may reduce a patient's likelihood of survival with good neurologic outcomes.

Chapter 10 provides a multi-faceted clinical context for "difficult vascular access" (DVA), a concept which has been inconsistently dealt with in the existing literature. This is an area of increasing research activity, as modern humans are living longer with a greater burden of chronic disease. Patients with DVA may test our competence and our patience, but learning how to care for them properly can make us better providers for all our patients.

Chapter 11 tackles decision-making in providing emergent vascular access, which is (and should be) a deeply-personalized subject. No single resource can fully elucidate this process, but a systematic approach may be helpful. Factors affecting decision-making are discussed, and examples of algorithms including appropriate references are provided.

Chapter 12 provides insight into the future of emergent vascular access, including techniques and technologies that are just beginning to influence our practice. Although traditional methods and devices will likely be around for a long while, new adjuncts and techniques are available and needed.

Chapter 13 addresses our patients' arterial access needs. Most of this book is committed to (direct or indirect) venous access, as it is far more common than arterial access in clinical practice. Although some of the underlying principles of cannulation are common to both arterial and venous access, many differences exist and deserve special attention.

Throughout this book, you will find illustrative examples and helpful references for those who wish to read more about a specific topic. Each of the authors has been carefully selected for his or her expertise in the area, including healthcare professionals from a wide variety of backgrounds. Each chapter provides a mix of basic and advanced concepts, with the aim of providing valuable content for providers of all experiential levels. We hope and expect that every reader will find something of value in each chapter, regardless of their previous training and experience.

Detroit, MI, USA   James H. Paxton

Contents

Contributors

Abdallah A. Ajani, MD, FACEP Department of Emergency Medicine, University of Massachusetts Medical Center, Worchester, MA, USA

Andrew J. Butki, DO Department of Emergency Medicine, Ascension Michigan St. John Hospital, Detroit, MI, USA

Department of Emergency Medicine, McLaren Oakland Hospital, Pontiac, MI, USA

James G. Chirackal, DO Michigan State University College of Human Medicine, East Lansing, MI, USA

Call G. Coddington, DO Michigan State University College of Osteopathic Medicine, East Lansing, MI, USA

Nicholas J. Corsi Wayne State University School of Medicine, Detroit, MI, USA

Chrystal T. Eichenlaub, BSN, RN Detroit, MI, USA

Jeffrey M. Eichenlaub, BSN, RN Detroit, MI, USA

Theodore Falcon Department of Emergency Medicine, Wayne State University, Nursing Development & Research, Henry Ford Health System, Detroit, MI, USA

Mark J. Favot, MD Department of Emergency Medicine, Wayne State University School of Medicine, Detroit, MI, USA

Kinza Ijaz, MD Department of Internal Medicine, Detroit Medical Center, Detroit, MI, USA

Catalina Kenney, EMT-P Wayne State University School of Medicine, Detroit, MI, USA

Lyudmila Khait, MS, MD Department of Emergency Medicine, Wayne State University School of Medicine, Detroit, MI, USA

Alexandra Lemieux, MD Wayne State University School of Medicine, Detroit, MI, USA

Megan A. MacKenzie, BS Wayne State University School of Medicine, Detroit, MI, USA

Adrienne N. Malik, MD Department of Emergency Medicine, Kansas University Medical Center, Kansas City, KS, USA

Sarah Meram, MS Department of Emergency Medicine, Wayne State University School of Medicine, Detroit, MI, USA

Brendan F. Mullan, BS Wayne State University School of Medicine, Detroit, MI, USA

Jennifer R. Noble, MD Department of Pediatrics, Division of Pediatric Emergency Medicine, Children's Hospital of Michigan, Detroit, MI, USA

James H. Paxton, MD, MBA Department of Emergency Medicine, Wayne State University School of Medicine, Detroit, MI, USA

Michael P. Petrovich, MD Department of Emergency Medicine, Adventist Health, Portland, OR, USA

Eugene B. Rozen, MD Department of Emergency Medicine, Wayne State University School of Medicine, Detroit, MI, USA

Jordan Schneider, MD Department of Pediatrics, Division of Critical Care Medicine, Children's Hospital of Michigan, Detroit, MI, USA

Jessica M. Shuck, BA Department of Emergency Medicine, Wayne State University, Detroit, MI, USA

Bethanie Ann Szydlowski, RN, VA-BC Medline Industries, Inc., Mundelein, IL, USA

Abbreviations

ABG	Arterial blood gas
AC	Antecubital
ACEP	American College of Emergency Physicians
ACLS	Advanced cardiac life support
ACS	American College of Surgeons
AHA	American Heart Association
AHRQ	Agency for Healthcare Research and Quality
AP	Anterior-posterior
AS	Accelerated Seldinger
ASIS	Anterior superior iliac spine
ATLS	Advanced trauma life support
AV	Arteriovenous
AVA	Association for Vascular Access
AVF	Arteriovenous fistula
AVG	Arteriovenous graft
AX	Axillary
BC	Brachiocephalic
BIG	Bone injection gun
BMI	Body mass index
CA	Cardiac arrest
CA	Carotid artery
CCA	Common carotid artery
CDC	Centers for Disease Control and Prevention
CFA	Common femoral artery
CHG	Chlorhexidine gluconate
CKD	Chronic kidney disease
CLABSI	Central line-associated bloodstream infection
cm	Centimeters
CoN	Catheter over needle
CPR	Cardiopulmonary resuscitation
CRBSI	Catheter-related bloodstream infection
CRT	Catheter-related thrombosis
CT	Computed tomography
CV	Central venous

CVAD	Central venous access device
CVC	Central venous catheter
CVR	Catheter-to-vein ratio
DBP	Diastolic blood pressure
DFA	Deep femoral artery
DH	Dorsal hand
DS	Direct Seldinger
DVA	Difficult vascular access
DVT	Deep vein thrombosis
ECG	Electrocardiogram
ED	Emergency department
EDTA	Ethylenediaminetetraacetic acid
EJ	External jugular
EMLA	Eutectic mixture of lidocaine and prilocaine
EMS	Emergency medical services
ENA	Emergency Nurses Association
ESD	Engineered stabilization device
ESRD	End-stage renal disease
FDA	Food and Drug Administration
FEM	Femoral
FIND	Fast intelligent needle delivery
Fr	French
gtt	Drops
HHS	Department of Health and Human Services
ICA	Internal carotid artery
ICU	Intensive care unit
IJ	Internal jugular
IM	Intramuscular
IN	Intranasal
INR	International normalized ratio
INS	Infusion Nurses Society
IO	Intraosseous
IV	Intravenous
IVC	Inferior vena cava
LED	Light-emitting diode
LPC	Long peripheral catheter
MAC	Multi-access catheter
MAGIC	Michigan Appropriateness Guide for Intravenous Catheters
MAP	Mean arterial pressure
mL	Milliliters
MLC	Midline catheter
mm	Millimeters
mOsm	Milliosmoles
mRSS	Modified Rodnan Skin Score
MS	Modified Seldinger

NIR	Near-infrared
OHCA	Out-of-hospital cardiac arrest
OR	Operating room
PA	Pulmonary artery
PaCO2	Partial pressure of carbon dioxide
PALS	Pediatric Advanced Life Support
PaO2	Partial pressure of oxygen
PEA	Pulseless electrical activity
PEBA	Polyether-block-amide
PFA	Profunda femoris artery
PHIO	Proximal humerus intraosseous
PICC	Peripherally inserted central catheter
PIV	Peripheral intravenous
PIVC	Peripheral intravenous catheter
PO	Per os (by mouth)
PR	Per rectum
PT	Prothrombin time
PTFE	Polytetrafluoroethylene
PTIO	Proximal tibial intraosseous
PTT	Partial thromboplastin time
PTX	Pneumothorax
PUD	Portable ultrasound device
PUR	Polyurethane
PVC	Polyvinyl chloride
pVT	Pulseless ventricular tachycardia
RA	Right atrium
RBC	Red blood cell
ROSC	Return of spontaneous circulation
RSI	Rapid sequence induction
SBP	Systolic blood pressure
SC	Subclavian
SCM	Sternocleidomastoid
ScvO2	Central venous oxygen saturation
SD	Standard deviation
SFA	Superficial femoral artery
SHEA	Society for Healthcare Epidemiology of America
SL	Sublingual
SQ	Subcutaneous
ST	Sternal
SVC	Superior vena cava
TALON	Tactically Advanced Lifesaving Intraosseous Needle
TdP	*Torsades de pointes*
TLC	Triple-lumen catheter
UAC	Umbilical artery catheterization
US	Ultrasound

USG	Ultrasound-guided
US-PIV	Ultrasound-guided peripheral intravenous
UVC	Umbilical vein catheterization
VAD	Vascular access device
VASD	Vascular access support device
VBG	Venous blood gas
VF	Ventricular fibrillation
VHP	Vessel health and preservation
VP	Ventriculoperitoneal
VT	Ventricular tachycardia

What Is Emergent Vascular Access? 1

James H. Paxton

Introduction

According to the US Centers for Disease Control (CDC), Americans logged approximately 136.9 million visits to the emergency department (ED) in 2015, with about 12.3 million (7.4%) visits resulting in a hospital admission [1]. According to these same figures, 31.3 million patients (23%) receive intravenous (IV) fluids, and 752,000 patients (0.6%) require central venous catheter (CVC) placement annually in the United States [1]. Although these figures do not address the acuity of line placement, they do reflect the reality that many patients require immediate vascular access in the ED to treat their presenting medical condition. But the ED is not the only place that "crash" lines are placed. Paramedics and Emergency Medical Technicians (EMTs) commonly establish venous access in the prehospital environment, often in more austere environments and under greater time constraints than other providers. Rapid response teams are often called to beds on the inpatient floors to help stabilize crashing patients, many of whom have inadequate vascular access and require immediate intervention. In fact, most physicians, nurses, and technicians who provide direct clinical care to patients will be called upon at some point to establish venous access under emergent conditions. Unfortunately, it is not always clear how decision-making can and should be different during emergent line placement, as compared to the low-acuity line placement techniques that are universally taught to health professionals. Scores of authoritative organizations have published extensive guidelines on how vascular access devices (VADs) should be placed, managed, and removed. But few of these guidelines address the thought processes that clinical care providers utilize when making decisions about VAD placement, or

J. H. Paxton (✉)
Department of Emergency Medicine, Wayne State University School of Medicine, Detroit, MI, USA
e-mail: james.paxton@wayne.edu

© Springer Nature Switzerland AG 2021
J. H. Paxton (ed.), *Emergent Vascular Access*,
https://doi.org/10.1007/978-3-030-77177-5_1

offer any useful insight into how providers should approach the emergent patient's vascular access needs differently than those of other patients.

In the real world, providers are expected to determine the acuity of a patient's condition, including the degree of a patient's need for vascular access, on their own. No single resource can hope to teach providers everything that they need to know about VAD placement, or account for every potential set of clinical conditions. A wide range of VADs, including *peripheral intravenous* (PIV) catheters, *intraosseous* (IO) catheters, and *central venous catheters* (CVCs), are readily available to providers in the ED and other acute care settings, but very little guidance is typically offered to clinicians in their selection of the appropriate VAD for a patient's presenting medical condition. Consequently, clinicians must often rely upon their own understanding of VADs when selecting the most appropriate approach for their patients. This can lead to great variability in clinical practice, thereby promoting great variability in VAD appropriateness.

Schools of medicine and nursing do spend time instructing physicians and nurses on the proper placement of VADs, including indications and techniques recommended for VAD placement in a generic acute care setting. However, very little time is spent in these curricula explaining the rationale and decision-making behind the decision to select a specific VAD for specific patient presentations. In many ways, *the provider's choice of VAD dictates the care that is subsequently available to a patient.* Infusions of various medications and fluids are often required in the care of emergent patients, but the provider's ability to effectively provide these interventions can be easily undermined by inadequate or otherwise inappropriate vascular access. This underscores the importance of making the right decisions about VAD selection and placement technique as early as possible in the care episode. Bad vascular access decisions can delay or even prevent the provision of necessary intravenous therapies. In order to make the *right* decisions, providers must understand how clinical conditions can and should influence their VAD choices.

Recognition of the need for "emergent" vascular access carries with it many implications for the provider, as well as the patient. The goals of care served by establishing vascular access will vary according to the patient's presenting condition and other factors. However, this book is designed to be of greatest use to the provider who requires immediate vascular access for their patient, to facilitate a wide range of anticipated interventions. The concepts in this book will be most relevant when vascular access is needed "emergently," in other words, to *provide some intervention for a patient that must be administered as soon as possible.* Whether this intervention is the administration of intravenous fluid, pain medication, vasopressors, antibiotics, or other medications, it is understood in this context that the intervention is expected to convey some time-dependent benefit to the patient that is less valuable (or perhaps futile) if it is delayed.

In general terms, an "emergency" may be defined as an unexpected but potentially dangerous situation requiring immediate action. Thus, an emergent condition should be both serious and requiring immediate intervention. In other words, emergent vascular access must be both: 1) *required to correct a serious problem; and 2) immediately necessary.* What constitutes a "serious" medical problem is subject to provider interpretation, as is the acuity of the need for intervention. Consequently, declaration of the need for "emergent vascular access" is predicated upon several inter-related factors:

- The provider's perception of the seriousness of the patient's presenting medical condition.
- The patient's actual medical condition, including the presence of hemodynamic instability or other evidence of risk to "life or limb".
- The availability and anticipated efficacy of immediate interventions to correct or treat the presenting condition.
- The risks of delayed intervention, including the risks of reduced efficacy and futility.

In other words, whether vascular access is considered "emergent" or not *depends upon a combination of patient-, provider-, and intervention-specific factors.* In this book, we assume that the patient's underlying medical condition is agreed to be serious (i.e., life- or limb-threatening), and that the intervention to be provided is considered to be time-critical.

Throughout this book, we will discuss factors contributing to a provider's decision on which VAD and insertion site is appropriate under various clinical conditions. We will also provide "tips and tricks" to improve the likelihood that the provider will successfully achieve the vascular access solution that they are attempting. The experienced clinician (whether MD, RN, paramedic, EMT, or other) will undoubtedly recognize many of the clinical vascular access scenarios presented in this book. It is our hope that both the casual and careful reader of this text will gain additional skills augmenting their ability to provide immediate and appropriate vascular access to patients experiencing an emergent medical condition.

The provision of emergent vascular access is a poorly-defined aspect of medical care, and those individuals charged with the task of providing it often go unrecognized in their efforts. Medical textbooks spend a great deal of time describing the interventions required to treat emergent medical conditions, without adequate attention paid to the vascular access methods by which these therapies are achieved. In this book, we hope to correct some of these oversights.

That said, reading this book will not transform the novice into an expert vascular access provider overnight. Skill acquisition in this area requires confidence, insight, and experience (including past successes and failures), which must be gained through clinical practice. The medical information provided in this book will supplement, but not replace, expert knowledge and training. As with all medical training, the information in this book should be viewed with a critical eye towards continuous improvement. Emergent vascular access is a constantly changing field, with new strategies and approaches constantly being developed. That said, much can learned from the insight that this book's authors have gleaned from years (sometimes decades) of experience providing emergent vascular access. We hope you enjoy it, and maybe learn a thing or two.

Reference

1. Rui P, Kang K. National Hospital Ambulatory Medical Care Survey: 2015 Emergency Department Summary Tables. Available from: http://www.cdc.gov/nchs/data/ahcd/nhamcs_emergency/2015_ed_web_tables.pdf.

The Physiology and Physics of Vascular Access

2

James H. Paxton and Megan A. MacKenzie

Introduction

Vascular access, for purposes of clinical care, refers to access to the anatomic system of veins and arteries that serve as conduits for the flow of blood through the human body. Of course, most healthcare providers are focused upon accessing the *venous* system for the infusion of fluids and medications for the emergent management of their patients. Consequently, most of the attention paid to this topic is related to venous access.

Vascular access is an essential first step in the care of many patients in the emergency department and inpatient wards. Although many other routes exist for the introduction of fluids and medications into the vascular system, including the oral, subdermal, subcutaneous, intramuscular, rectal, and endotracheal routes, the intravascular approach is often the fastest and most efficacious route available for the infusion of fluids and medications required for the emergent management of critically ill patients. Consequently, an understanding of the cardiovascular system and its routes of ingress is indispensable to the emergent vascular access provider.

J. H. Paxton (✉)
Department of Emergency Medicine, Wayne State University School of Medicine, Detroit, MI, USA
e-mail: james.paxton@wayne.edu

M. A. MacKenzie
Wayne State University School of Medicine, Detroit, MI, USA
e-mail: megan.mackenzie2@med.wayne.edu

© Springer Nature Switzerland AG 2021
J. H. Paxton (ed.), *Emergent Vascular Access*,
https://doi.org/10.1007/978-3-030-77177-5_2

Anatomy of the Cardiovascular System

It is generally understood that the cardiovascular system consists of both arterial and venous channels, which can be accessed by clinicians for myriad purposes. Clinically, access to the arterial system allows providers the ability to monitor the arterial blood supply for measurements and blood samples that provide insight into the patient's arterial blood pressure, carbon dioxide tension, and oxygenation. While these measurements and samples may provide information pertaining to the patient's relative concentrations of oxygen and carbon dioxide and may also provide insight into the patient's arterial blood pressure, arterial cannulation is not generally of great use for the infusion of therapeutic interventions. Venous cannulation, on the other hand, is of great use to the clinician as a route by which fluids and medications can be introduced to the systemic circulation. With the routine use of central venous punctures, a thorough knowledge of anatomy is required by the physician to reduce complications.

Human medicine has developed over thousands of years, with common vascular access points predicated upon many generations of medical providers and their collective decisions relating to the best site for venous and arterial cannulation. In general, medical providers have come to select cannula insertion points that are superficial and easily accessible. In the last few decades, the use of prosthetic arterio-venous graft (AVG) and central venous catheters (CVCs) has allowed physicians to choose the most beneficial method of vascular access for their patients. Patients with a variety of conditions, such as those on hemodialysis, are now experiencing higher life expectancy and quality of life with these methods [1]. At the same time, all medical specialties including vascular surgeons, emergency medicine physicians, and members of the dialysis staff benefit from these options in providing care. A well-planned procedure, along with an acute awareness of both the surface anatomy and underlying vascular structures, can allow for precise procedures and minimal trauma.

The Arterial System

By definition, the *arterial system* carries blood away from the heart. While this blood is usually oxygenated, the pulmonary arteries provide an exception to this rule by carrying deoxygenated blood from the heart to the lungs. However, for purposes of peripheral artery cannulation and blood sampling, it can be assumed that arterial blood should be more highly oxygenated than blood sampled from the venous system.

Vascular systems (including the arterial and venous systems) may be considered analogous to a "tree," with the largest vessels (e.g., aorta) forming the trunk of the tree and the branches becoming progressively smaller as one approaches the periphery of the tree. Figure 2.1 demonstrates this analogy.

The network of arteries forming the arterial "tree" originates from the large elastic arteries (e.g., the aorta and its major branches), which divide into medium muscular arteries, thence to small arteries, arterioles, and the capillary beds. In the

Fig. 2.1 The human
vascular system

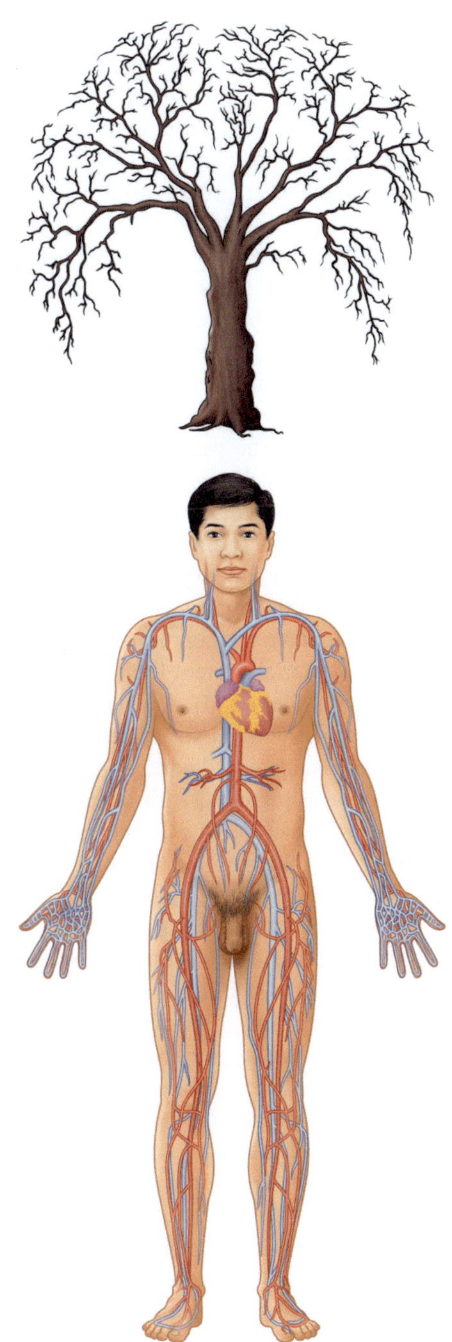

capillary beds, the blood passes through the peripheral tissues, off-loads a portion of its oxygen content, and is then picked up by the post-capillary venules. Once the blood has entered the venules, it may be taken up into the venous system, ultimately returning to the heart to begin the cycle again.

Elastin is a protein found in the extracellular matrix, which allows tissues to return to their original form after being stretched – so-called reversible elasticity [2]. Elastic fibers are formed only during early human development and childhood, and are gradually degraded in the aging process. The aorta and major central vessels have a substantial amount of elastin in their composition, which allows "smoothening of the discontinuous blood flow and pressure" generated by the heart's pumping function [3]. Smaller arteries, near the periphery of the arterial tree, have much less elastin than the central vessels. This allows them to vasodilate or vasoconstrict more easily and rapidly than the larger vessels, in response to changes in the systemic blood pressure. The variation in size of these arteries is important in pathology, as each class of vessel is predisposed to particular types of disease. Importantly, elastin is lost with the aging process, resulting in a host of cardiovascular maladies with advanced age, including hypertension, atherosclerosis, arterial calcification, and aortic dissection / aneurysm formation.

Because of the high pressures applied to the arterial system by the heart's pumping, arteries have thicker, more muscular walls than their venous counterparts. This makes the arterial system less prone to collapse than the venous system in the setting of hypovolemia [4]. Arteries and arterioles are also highly responsive to circulating catecholamines and other vasoactive substances, especially as mediated by the alpha-1 and beta-2 adrenergic receptors. The smallest members of the arterial tree are the capillaries, with walls composed of only a single layer of endothelial cells surrounded by the basal lamina. Nutrients, gases, water, and solutes are exchanged in the capillary beds. Selective perfusion of the capillary beds is determined by the degree of dilation or constriction of the arterioles, enabling the body to react quickly to a variety of clinical conditions [4].

Arterial cannulation is often performed emergently when arterial blood sampling is required, or to facilitate continuous blood pressure monitoring. Pressure waveforms from arterial lines can allow the clinician to detect sudden changes in blood pressure that may require a timely intervention. The radial and femoral arteries are the two arteries that are most frequently cannulated for such purposes. Other arteries, such as the brachial artery, tend to have a higher risk of complications due to the lack of collateral blood flow and the risk of distal extremity ischemia [4]. The carotid artery is another large and superficial artery, but it is not often used for arterial monitoring due to concerns about embolization events to the brain and the risk of hematoma formation with subsequent airway impingement [4].

The *radial artery* access site is located on the radial side of the distal forearm, with minimal overlying soft tissue. It can be traced along the lateral aspect of the forearm through the anatomic snuff box and is palpable at the distal radius. Luckily, less anatomic variation is found in the distal forearm, where cannulation is typically performed. This site is the most used for access both in adults and pediatrics and is quite useful for blood sampling and preoperative period information [5]. This artery is often easily accessible in the operating room and is not adjacent to clinically important nerves.

The *femoral artery* is found in the so-called femoral triangle and is easily palpable in even the most obese patients. It is sufficiently proximal to approximate central blood pressure, but remains quite distal to the heart. The femoral artery is generally larger than most other available arteries, and therefore it is often a viable target for arterial line placement even when other vessels (e.g., the radial or ulnar arteries) cannot be cannulated. When accessing the femoral artery, bleeding risk is increased in relation to the radial artery due to the greater diameter of the femoral vessel [5]. A femoral approach may also increase the risk of catheter-related infection in the perineum [6].

In emergent situations, critically ill patients require arterial lines to monitor blood pressure and obtain blood samples for blood gases. Once the catheter is inserted into the radial artery, a transducer system will continuously infuse a 0.9% sodium chloride solution under pressure. The arterial pressure is sensed by the transducer and then converts that signal into a waveform, reflecting the pressure generated by the left ventricle during systole. This bedside monitoring system allows for easier interpretation of a patient's vitals [6]. Even in the event of decreased or near-absent pulse, a reliable measurement of arterial blood pressure can still be measured.

The human arterial system is depicted in Fig. 2.2.

The Venous System

Central venous sites that are frequently selected for cannulation include the internal jugular vein, the subclavian vein, and the femoral vein. More peripheral sites include the external jugular vein; the brachial and cephalic veins of the forearm; and the distal veins of the wrist, hand, and fingers. In general, the peripheral veins of the lower extremities are not selected for venous cannulation, due to their greater distance from the central venous circulation.

The veins of the human body are generally thin-walled vessels with very little smooth muscle. This allows veins to collapse and expand easily to accomodate changes in intraluminal pressure. Rapid expansion or contraction of the vessels can occur in response to changes in fluid status; this ability to accomodate large volumes of fluid infusion rapidly can be advantageous when treating patients with profound hypovolemia. Additionally, veins contain the largest percentage of blood in the cardiovascular system, called the unstressed volume. The walls of the veins contain alpha-1 adrenergic receptors, which contract the veins and reduce their unstressed volume. However, the extreme collapsibility of the venous system also presents a challenge to clinicians. For example, patients can present with extreme intravascular depletion, causing their collapsed veins to become very poor targets for cannulation.

The peripheral venous system is generally divided by the superficial fascia into a superficial system, and a deep system. Blood from the superficial system drains to the deep system by way of the perforating veins. The venous system performs two main tasks: (1) returning blood to the heart; and, (2) storing blood that is not immediately needed. This second task is facilitated by the elasticity of the venous system. In general, veins are 30 times more compliant than arteries, although vascular

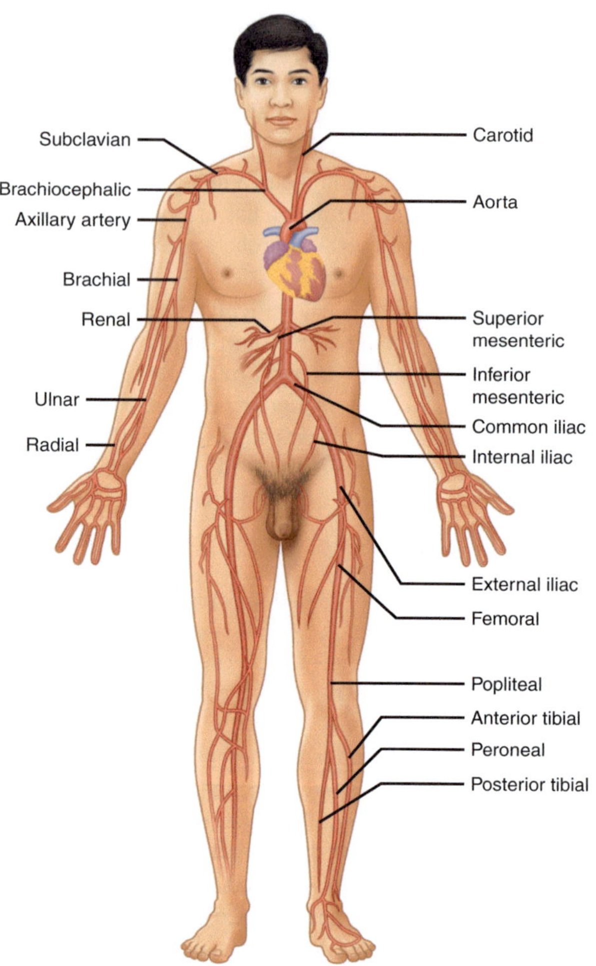

Fig. 2.2 The human arterial system

compliance can increase under certain conditions such as pregnancy and nitroglycerin administration [7]. Consequently, veins can accommodate changes in blood volume and can serve as a beneficial route of medication and fluid administration.

Despite this elastic property, venous obstruction can still occur, with partial or complete occlusion of the lumen. Such luminal occlusions are characteristic of deep vein thrombosis. Over 100 years ago, Virchow proposed that venous thrombosis could be caused by venous stasis, changes in vessel walls, or changes in blood components [8]. These venous thrombi are composed of fibrin and red blood cells. In preparation for a long-term venous access, it is important to support normal cardiac output and decrease the risk of venous thrombosis. Today, we know that high levels of some coagulation factors and defects in anticoagulants can also contribute to this risk. Due to the multitude of factors that can contribute to thrombosis, it is important to keep a patient's age, sex, and cardiovascular health in mind during cannulation.

A depiction of the human venous system is provided in Fig. 2.3.

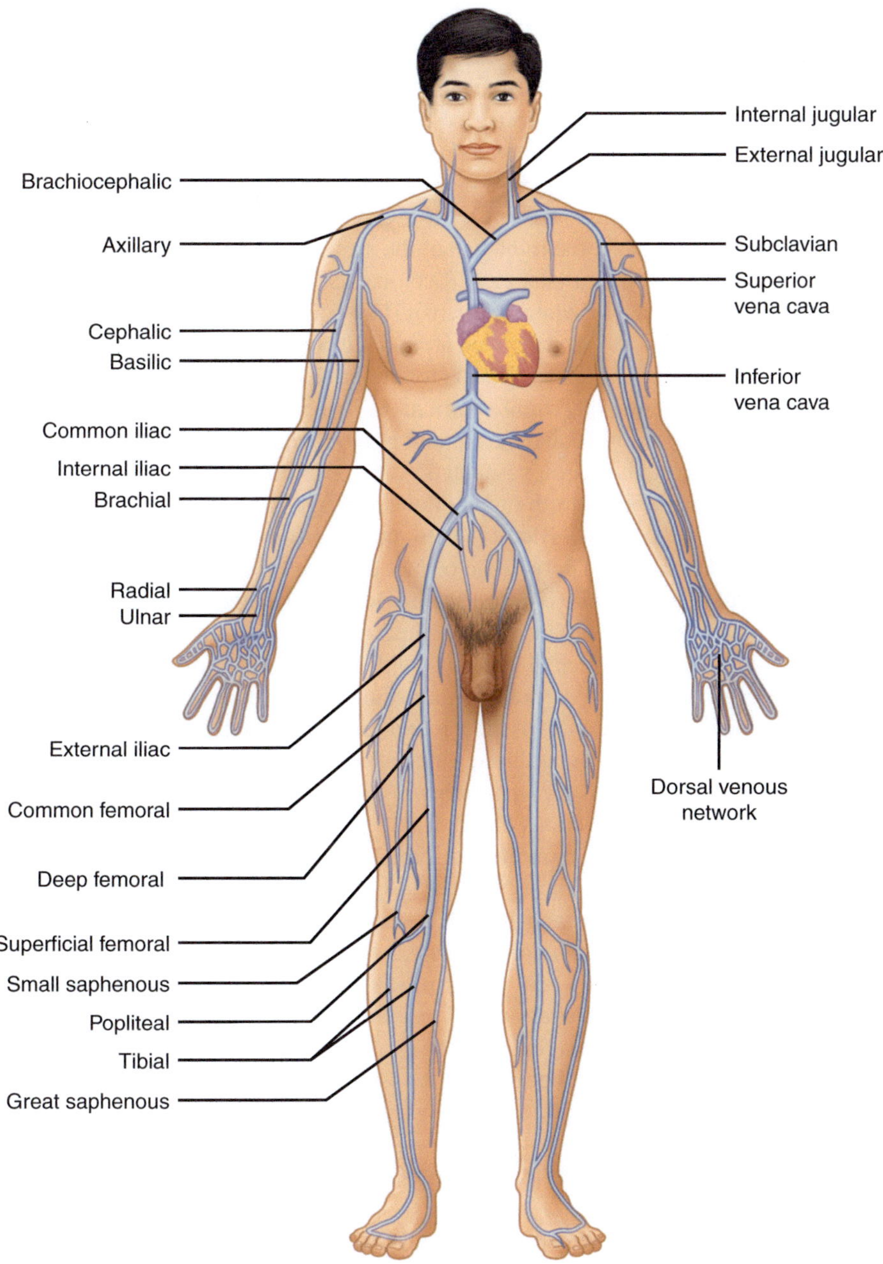

Fig. 2.3 The human venous system

Cardiovascular Physiology

The cardiovascular system is involved in numerous homeostatic functions that are governed by the laws of physics and restricted by human anatomy. This system is important in regulating arterial blood pressure, delivering hormones to target sites, and in adjusting to physiologic states such as disease, trauma, or exercise. The left and right heart have different functions: the left heart and its associated vessels are called the, **systemic circulation**, while the right side of the system is collectively called the ***pulmonary circulation***. The four chambers (two on each side) of the heart function like rooms in a house, and are separated by valves (like doors). Blood is pushed from one chamber to another before it is circulated around the body. Furthermore, the two sides of the heart are arranged in series, allowing for the cardiac output of the left ventricle to equal the cardiac output of the right ventricle. In its normal steady state, the cardiac output from the heart should equal the amount of blood returned to the heart.

One can think of the cardiovascular system as a complete circuit within the body. Oxygenated blood from the lungs flows through the *left atrium* into the *left ventricle* via the *mitral valve*. Blood is then ejected from the left ventricle into the *aorta* via the *aortic valve*. The volume of blood ejected from the left ventricle per unit time is called the *cardiac output*. The blood is distributed throughout the arterial system and to various organs. Unlike the heart in isolation, the organ systems are arranged in parallel, which allows for the distribution of cardiac output to vary among the organ systems. For example, muscles will require more energy during intense aerobic exercise in order to meet increased metabolic demand. At the end of the circuit, the blood is collected in the veins and is returned to the right side of the heart. Since the pressure in the *vena cava* is higher than in the *right atrium*, the atrium can fill with mixed venous blood. This is termed "venous return to the right atrium," which equals cardiac output from the left ventricle. Eventually, this blood flows into the *right ventricle* through the *tricuspid valve* and is ejected into the *pulmonary artery* to become oxygenated once again. The cycle then repeats again.

The anatomy of the human cardiovascular system is depicted in Fig. 2.4. The circulatory system is depicted here with arrows representing blood circulation in the body. Blood takes many parallel paths from the left to the right heart. It can flow through arrangements in parallel and series paths, and even mix deoxygenated blood with oxygenated blood bound for the systemic arteries.

Other Physiological Considerations

Aging brings with it many physiological and morphological changes that can alter cardiovascular function. As life expectancy around the world increases, pathological conditions and age-related illnesses have become more prevalent. Vascular aging leads to an overall senescence of the vascular endothelium [9]. Functionally, the arteries become more calcified, and lose their elasticity, contributing to overall reduction in arterial compliance. Therefore, elderly patients require special considerations in the placement of VADs, especially in emergency situations.

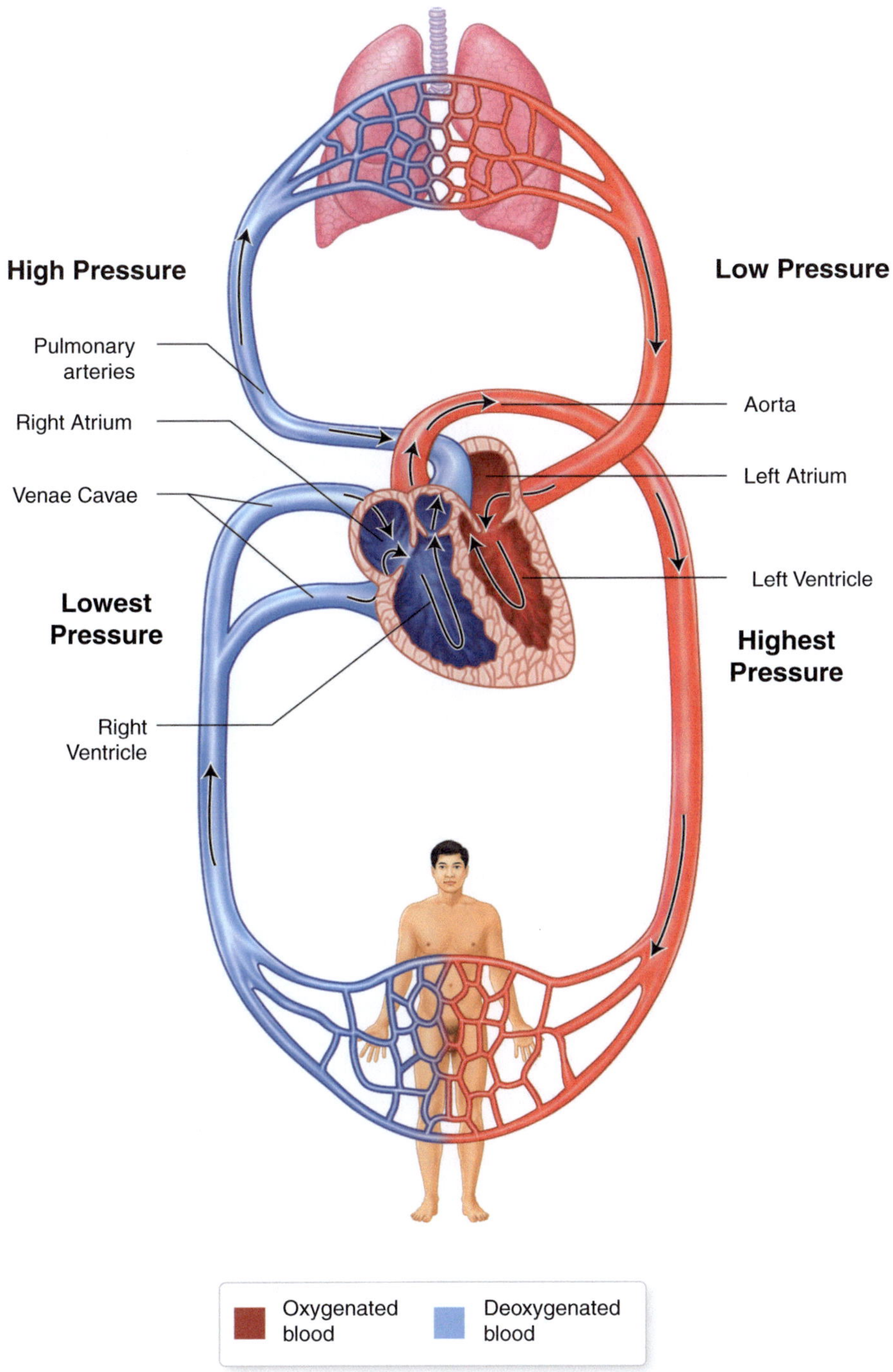

Fig. 2.4 The human cardiovascular system

Another point of consideration relates to vascular access during *pregnancy*. Pregnancy is a dynamic process full of adaptive changes to accommodate for fetal growth and development. In the systemic vasculature and kidneys, vasodilation occurs as early as 5 weeks' gestation [10]. A characteristic decrease in blood pressure typically occurs early in pregnancy, while total blood volume, plasma, and red blood cell mass increase significantly. Chronic venous insufficiency is common during the third trimester, and venous thromboembolism affects pregnant women nearly five times more than non-pregnant women [11]. Thus, for pregnant patients, clinicians should choose the smallest and least invasive device, with the fewest lumens possible, to minimize the risk of thrombotic events.

The *skeletal system* should also be considered in terms of the anatomy and physiology of vascular access. Long bones are richly vascular, with a dynamic circulation. These bones can accept large volumes of fluid and transport drugs to the central circulation. Within the bone cavity, medullary venous sinusoids drain into a central venous channel. These sinusoids accept fluids and drugs during IO infusion. The medullary cavity itself is rigid and capable of accepting these infusions even during times of profound shock or cardiopulmonary arrest [12].

The Physics of Flow

Understanding the laws of physics as they apply to the cardiovascular system allows for better vascular access placement techniques. Blood flow throughout the body is measured as the rate of blood displacement per unit time. As previously discussed, the blood vessels of the body vary in terms of diameter, cross-sectional area, and elasticity. As a simplified relationship, the velocity of flow can be considered by the equation $v = Q/A$. Here, v (velocity of blood flow in cm/s) is equal to Q (flow in mL/s) multiplied by A (cross-sectional area in cm^2). Nutrient exchange is optimized across the capillary wall in part because of the low velocity of blood flow within the capillary beds.

The success of intravenous cannulation depends heavily upon pressure gradients. The *Law of Laplace* has important consequences beyond basic physiology and is directly related to the pulmonary system and vascular access (Fig. 2.5). According to *Laplace's equation*, the tension (T) in a hollow cylinder (e.g., blood vessel) is directly proportional to the cylinder's radius (r) and the pressure (p) across the wall caused by the flow inside, according to the equation: $T = p \times r$ [13]. Though oversimplified, this equation illustrates how tiny, thin-walled capillaries can withstand surprisingly large pressures because of their tiny radii.

Vascular phenomena are further explained by *Poiseuille's Law*, which states that the flow (Q) of fluid through a cylinder is determined by the viscosity (η) of the fluid, the pressure gradient across the tubing (P), and the length (L) and radius (r) of the cylinder as: $Q = (\pi P r^4 / 8 \eta L)$ (Fig. 2.6). If one considers the vascular access device as a cylinder, it becomes quickly apparent that the rate of flow through a catheter is improved by increasing the pressure gradient (e.g., pressure bags), increasing the radius of the catheter (e.g., selecting a larger-bore catheter), decreasing viscosity of the infused fluid (e.g., saline versus blood), or decreasing catheter

Fig. 2.5 The Law of Laplace

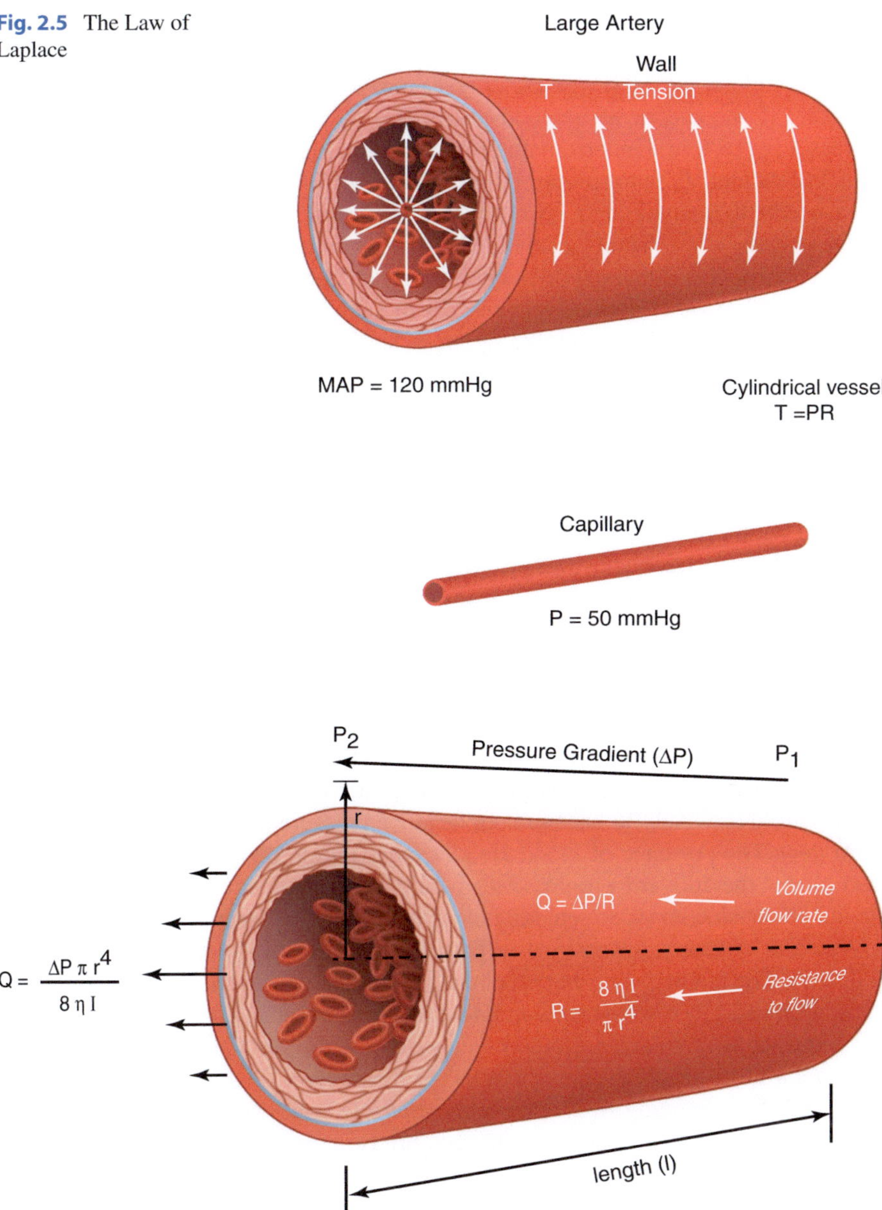

Fig. 2.6 The Law of Poiseuille

length [14]. Put simply, the physics of flow through cannulae inserted into human blood vessels depends primarily upon the intraluminal radius and length of the catheter. In general, fatter and shorter catheters produce greater flow rates. This law does include a few assumptions, such as (1) assuming laminar flow, (2) assuming the fluid is in a steady state, and (3) assuming the fluid is viscous so that neighboring fluid sheets create frictional forces. This powerful relationship shows that when the radius of a blood vessel decreases, its resistance increases by the fourth-power. For example, if the radius of a blood vessel decreases by one-half, the resistance increases by 16-fold. Understanding these basic fluid mechanics can optimize vascular access and allow for proper IV transfusion – from choosing the appropriately sized needle to maintaining a good flow rate of fluids.

Of course, other factors can influence the rate of forward flow that can be achieved through a catheter. For example, valves within the veins produce increased resistance to forward flow, and the presence of venous valves will diminish the realized flow rate from that predicted by these laws of physics. Some vascular flow regions may also be subject to increased turbulence (due to odd angles or the presence of vascular branches) and other forces resulting from the pumping action of the heart, or external forces such as extrinsic pressure from the surrounding soft tissues. A patient's intravascular hydration status will also affect the fluid flow rate. Dehydration increases blood viscosity, but hypovolemia also lowers intraluminal pressure within the venous system, reducing resistance to flow. While arterial systems do generally have a positive pressure, venous systems typically have a negative pressure which will tend to pull fluid into the vasculature. Vasomotor tone, which can alter the ability of a vessel to accommodate increased blood volume, also affects intraluminal blood pressure and the intrinsic resistance to flow into the target vessel.

Consequently, a patient's hydration status, as well as the vasomotor tone dictated by the type and degree of circulating adrenergic hormones, will alter the realized flow rate through a cannula that can be achieved by the provider. The radius of the target vessel is also an important determinant of resistance and flow, since larger vessels are more likely to have greater negative pressure and less resistance to forward flow. The presence of blood clots or other intraluminal barriers to flow may also hinder the forward progression of fluids and medications. All these factors should be considered when selecting the appropriate cannula and target vessel.

Vascular anatomy is arranged in both *in-series* and *in-parallel* configurations (Fig. 2.7). The relative contribution of each segment (e.g., arterioles and capillaries) to the total resistance across the system determines how changes in resistance within a specific segment will affect total resistance across the vascular system. Within the human cardiovascular system, arteriolar segments have the highest relative resistance and thus changing resistance in the arteriole segment will exert the greatest possible effect on total resistance. In fact, arterioles and arteries constitute about 70% of the total vascular resistance through most organs [15]. The total resistance (R_{Total}) to flow across a bed of four hypothetical arterioles arranged in a parallel fashion (as depicted in Fig 2.7) can be related to the resistance of the individual arterioles by the equation: $1/R_{Total} = 1/R_1 + 1/R_2 + 1/R_3 + 1/R_4$.

Human blood flow is generally laminar. However, under "high-flow" conditions (such as in the ascending aorta), or in the presence of stenosis and partial vascular obstruction, blood flow can become quite turbulent. The *Reynolds number* is a dimensionless value that offers a means of measuring this degree of turbulence. The *Reynolds number formula* is expressed by: $R_e = \rho V L / \mu$, where ρ = density of the

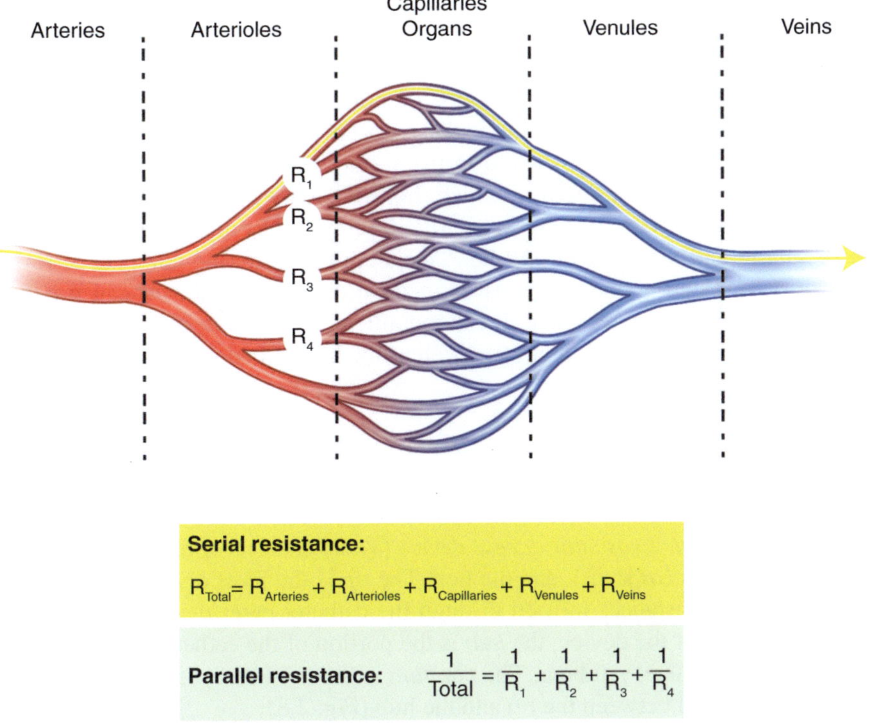

Fig. 2.7 Intravascular resistance to blood flow

fluid, V = velocity of the fluid, μ = viscosity of fluid, and L = length of the fluid [15]. When $R_e < 2000$, flow is considered laminar. If $R_e > 4000$, flow is considered turbulent. Clinically, the Reynolds number can be increased by decreasing blood viscosity, increasing the velocity of blood flow, or narrowing the blood vessel [15]. Thrombi (i.e., intraluminal blood clots) can narrow the diameter of a blood vessel, increasing the Reynolds number.

Clinically, *Korotkoff sounds* (produced by turbulent blood flow) are used in the measurement of blood pressure. Although these sounds are very low frequency (25–50 Hz), they are audible in a quiet room. Low-flow states will diminish the intensity of Korotkoff sounds, creating a tendency to underestimate the systolic blood pressure for patients in low blood-flow states.

The *viscosity* of blood is also important. The word "viscosity" derives from the Latin *viscum*, meaning "thick glue." Viscosity is the material property relating viscous stresses in a material to the rate of change of deformation. Put simply, the viscosity of a fluid is how well it resists deformation at a given rate. Hematocrit values, plasma fibrinogen, and erythrocyte deformability are the most important factors affecting blood viscosity [12]. Intraluminal resistance increases directly with increased viscosity of the material being infused through the IV catheter. For example, medications, fluids, and blood all flow more slowly when they are cold, due to increased viscosity. Warming fluid before infusion not only prevents iatrogenic hypothermia but also increases the rate of infusion by decreasing the fluid's viscosity.

When assessing sources of resistance to flow, providers should consider the length of the tubing connecting the catheter to the source of medication or fluid (e.g., the bag). Although pressurized infusion may help to increase rates of flow, excessively long IV tubing will diminish this advantage by increasing total resistance within the delivery system. Similarly, different types of connectors between the IV tubing and the catheter will be associated with differing amounts of resistance to flow. Hand-syringing fluids or medications into a catheter can produce much higher infusion rates than other modalities, due to both the short distance between the syringe and the catheter as well as the high infusion pressure generated by the syringe itself.

Vascular Access Devices

In its simplest form, a *vascular access device (VAD)* consists of three components: the tip, the cannula (or shaft), and the hub. The *tip* is the most distal portion of the catheter, where substances infused through the catheter enter the target vessel. At the proximal end of the device, the *hub* is the portion of the catheter that interfaces and connects with the IV tubing. The *cannula* is that middle cylindrical portion of the catheter located between the tip and the hub (Fig. 2.8).

In general, the *radius* and *length* of the cannula are the primary determinants of flow through a catheter. Providers (unlike physicists) generally describe the radius of a catheter using the diameter, which is equal to twice the radius. One system of describing the *intraluminal* diameter of a catheter is the *"gauge" system* developed for wire sizing in the nineteenth century by Peter Stubs. The gauge system operates on a descending scale, as opposed to the French scale, which ascends [16]. In other words, wider catheters have a smaller gauge.

The *"French" scale* (a.k.a., Charrière's system) describes the size of a catheter by its *outer* diameter. Each increment of the French scale equals 0.33 mm. Whether dealing with a single-lumen or a multi-lumen catheter, the French system can still be used. However, a catheter's French size does *not* specify the intraluminal diameter of the catheter. For this reason, the gauge of a catheter is much more important in predicting flow rates than the catheter's French size. A comparison of the measurements associated with standard peripheral intravenous (PIV) catheters is provided in Table 2.1.

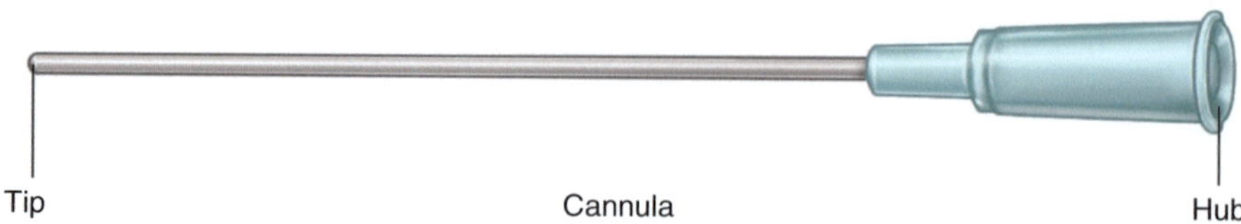

Fig. 2.8 Components of a generic vascular catheter

Table 2.1 Comparison of gauge and French measurement systems

Gauge	Width (mm)	French equivalent (Fr)
26	0.7	1.5
24	0.8	2
22	0.9	2.5
20	1.1	3
18	1.3	4
16	1.7	5
14	2.2	6

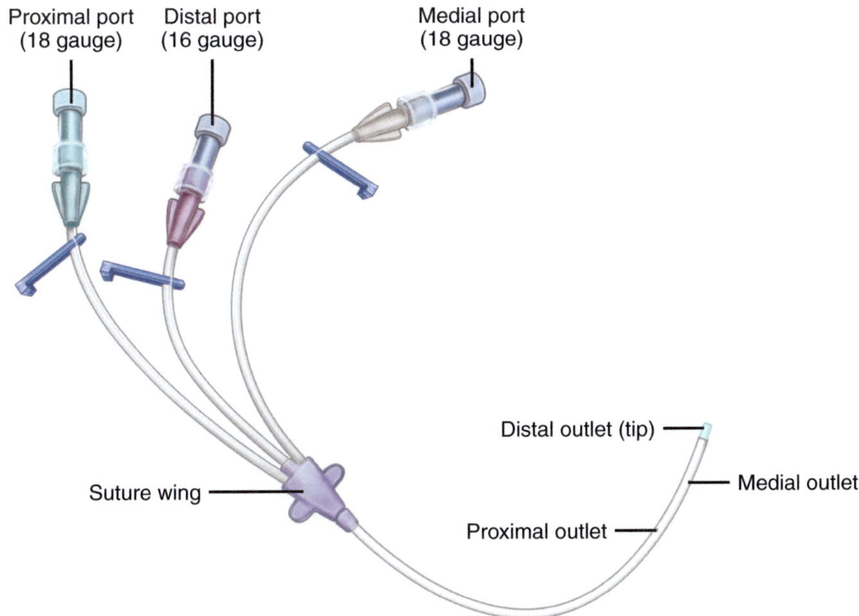

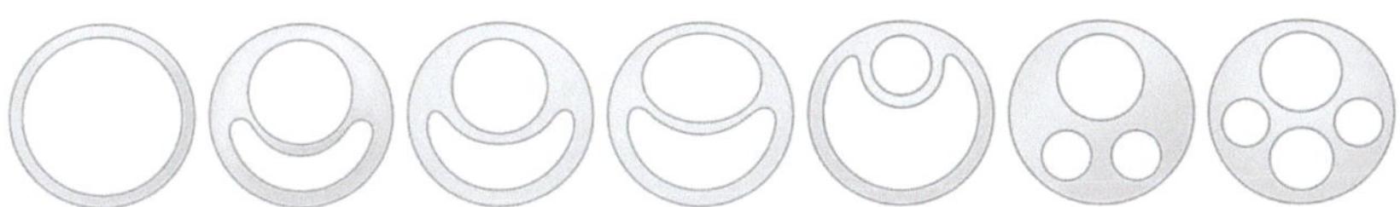

Fig. 2.9 Components of a generic CVC, including cross-sectional depiction of various lumen configurations

The distinction between a catheter's gauge and French size is especially important when assessing the performance of a multi-lumen catheter, such as the standard triple-lumen central venous catheter (CVC). While the French size (i.e., outer diameter) determines how much space the catheter will occupy within the target vessel, it is the gauge (i.e., intraluminal diameter) that predicts resistance to flow through the device. This can become especially complicated when using multi-lumen CVC lines, since each lumen has its own hub and outlet into the vessel, as well as its own length and gauge (including the associated resistance to flow). Figure 2.9 demonstrates the components of a generic CVC, including examples of commonly encountered variations in luminal size and shape.

Conclusion

In this chapter, we have discussed some of the fundamental concepts of vascular physics and physiology relevant to providers in selecting and placing vascular access devices. We have explored the anatomy of the cardiovascular system and how arteries and veins contribute to the vascular tree. We traced the path of blood through the circulatory system and discussed the various properties of the vessels in this circuit, considering human physiology in relation to vessel structure and function. We further discussed the changes in vascular physiology with regard to aging, pregnancy, and the influence of the skeletal system. We also related several fundamental laws of physics governing blood flow. Finally, we have described the components of a vascular access device and considered their variations in size and shape. By better understanding vascular physics and physiology, providers can be more equipped to select the proper location and appropriate vascular access device for safe and effective cannulation of a target vein.

Key Concepts
- A basic understanding of the physics and physiology of the human vascular system provides many important insights to successfully placing venous access devices.
- The human cardiovascular system contains both arterial and venous channels, allowing for numerous sites for cannulation, each with its own relative advantages and disadvantages.
- Physiological changes such as aging, elasticity of vessels, pregnancy, and metabolism all influence the placement of venous access devices.
- Certain laws of physics, such as The Law of Laplace, Poiseuille's Law, and Reynolds number should all be understood and considered by providers when assessing sites for vascular access.
- Vascular access devices consist of three basic components: tip, cannula, and hub.
- When selecting the appropriate venous access catheter, providers must consider multiple device characteristics, including the catheter's gauge and French size.

References

1. Santoro D, Benedetto F, Mondello P, et al. Vascular access for hemodialysis: current perspectives. Int J Nephrol Renovasc Dis. 2014;7:281–94.
2. Cocciolone AJ, Hawes JZ, Staiculescu MC, et al. Elastin, arterial mechanics, and cardiovascular disease. Am J Physiol Heart Circ Physiol. 2018;315(2):H189–205.
3. Fhayli WB, Boëté Q, Harki O, et al. Rise and fall of elastic fibers from development to aging. Consequences on arterial structure-function and therapeutical perspectives. Matrix Biol. 2019;84:41–56.
4. Costanzo LS. Cardiovascular physiology. 4th ed. [Internet] In: Cicalese B, Schmitt W, ed. Philadelphia, PA: Saunders/Elsevier: 117–188. Cited 2019 October 9. Available from: https://www.elsevier.com/books/physiology/costanzo/978-1-4160-6216-5.
5. Hager HH, Burns B. Radial artery cannulation. StatPearls website. Treasure Island, FL: StatPearls Publishing, 2019. Cited 2019 October 9. Available from: https://www.ncbi.nlm.nih.gov/books/NBK482242/.
6. Lakhal K, Robert-Edan V. Invasive monitoring of blood pressure: a radiant future for brachial artery as an alternative to radial artery catheterisation? J Thorac Dis. 2017;9(12):4812–6.
7. Gelman S. Venous function and central venous pressure: a physiologic story. Anesthesiology. 2008;108(4):735–48.
8. Esmon CT. Basic mechanisms and pathogenesis of venous thrombosis. Blood Rev. 2009;23(5):225–9.
9. Mikael LR, Paiva AMG, Gomes MM, et al. Vascular aging and arterial stiffness. Arq Bras Cardiol. 2017;109(3):253–8.
10. Sanghavi M, Rutherford JD. Cardiovascular physiology of pregnancy. Circulation. 2014;130(12):1003–8.
11. DiMuzio P. Know the danger signs of CVI and VTE in pregnant patients. Vascular.org. Published March 1, 2018. [Internet] Cited 2019 December 9. Available from: https://vascular.org/news-advocacy/know-danger-signs-cvi-and-vte-pregnant-patients.
12. Sarkar D, Philbeck T. The use of multiple intraosseous catheters in combat casualty resuscitation. Mil Med. 2009;174(2):106–8.
13. Schmidt-Nielsen K. Animal physiology: adaptation and environment. 5th ed. Cambridge, MA: Cambridge University Press; 1997. Cited 2019 December 9. Available from: https://trove.nla.gov.au/work/9710227?q&sort=holdings+desc&_=1588256212853&versionId=46514901.
14. Wilson WC, Grande CM, Hoyt DB. Trauma: emergency resuscitation. Perioperative anesthesia, surgical management. New York, NY: CRC Press; 2007. [Internet] Cited 2019 December 9. Available from: https://cirugiatraumaponiente.files.wordpress.com/2010/07/trauma-critical-care-volume-1.pdf.
15. Klabunde RE. Cardiovascular physiology concepts. Hagerstown, MD: Lippincott Williams & Wilkins; 2012. Cited 2019 December 9. Available from: https://www.academia.edu/34670778/Cardiovascular_Physiology_Concepts_Klabunde.pdf.
16. Ahn W, Bahk JH, Lim YJ. The 'gauge' system for the medical use. Anesthes Analg. 2002;95(4):1125.

Landmark-Based Peripheral Intravenous Catheters

Jeffrey M. Eichenlaub, Chrystal T. Eichenlaub,
Jessica M. Shuck, and James H. Paxton

Introduction

Peripheral intravenous (PIV) catheters are the most common lines placed by providers treating emergent patients. Because of this, the landmark-based PIV line is often considered to be the "gold standard" by which other vascular access attempts are measured. We feel that mastery of the landmark-based PIV insertion is essential for all providers who wish to provide venous access for patients under emergent conditions.

As described in Chap. 2, the venous system is composed of both central and peripheral veins. Peripheral veins emanate from the central veins, much like the branches of a tree. Access to these peripheral veins may be compromised by factors reducing blood flow to the extremities, including the human body's normal response to hypotension. Because peripheral veins have a less pronounced vasomotor response to circulating adrenergic factors, due to their relative lack of smooth muscle as compared to arterial vessels, they are likely to be collapsed in states of low intravascular volume.

Under emergent conditions, when hypovolemia and hypotension are likely present, blood flow to the lower extremities may be inordinately compromised [1]. Although blood flow to the upper extremities may also be somewhat compromised under such conditions, we suggest that the optimal peripheral veins to target in the

J. M. Eichenlaub · C. T. Eichenlaub
Detroit, MI, USA

J. M. Shuck
Department of Emergency Medicine, Wayne State University, Detroit, MI, USA
e-mail: jmshuck@med.wayne.edu

J. H. Paxton (✉)
Department of Emergency Medicine, Wayne State University School of Medicine,
Detroit, MI, USA
e-mail: james.paxton@wayne.edu

© Springer Nature Switzerland AG 2021
J. H. Paxton (ed.), *Emergent Vascular Access*,
https://doi.org/10.1007/978-3-030-77177-5_3

unstable patient are in the upper extremities. Thus, the peripheral veins of greatest interest to the emergent provider will be found in the neck, torso, and upper extremities.

Peripheral Intravenous Catheter Design

Peripheral intravenous catheters have traditionally been composed of polytetrafluoroethylene (PTFE), specifically Teflon® materials, although superior materials have recently been introduced into the market. The polyurethane biomaterial Vialon® appears to possess a substantially higher tensile strength than traditional materials [2], and clinical studies have shown reduced incidence of phlebitis and longer dwell times when compared to Teflon® [3, 4].

The parts of a generic PIV catheter include the *hub, cannula,* and *tip.* Infused substances enter the catheter at the hub end, travel through the cannula, and egress from the catheter tip into the vessel lumen (Fig. 3.1).

As described in Chap. 2, the *radius* and *length* of the cannula are the primary determinants of flow through a catheter. In general, wider and shorter catheters provide less resistance to flow and are therefore capable of higher flow rates (typically measured in milliliters/minute). The radius of the catheter is reflected by the *gauge* of the PIV catheter, which is a measure of the internal (i.e., intraluminal) cross-sectional diameter of the cannula. The most common gauges of PIV catheter are listed below in Table 3.1, along with their usual characteristics. Differently gauged PIV catheters typically have differently colored hubs, to aid in easy identification during clinical use. The gauge number is *inversely* related to the diameter of the cannula and usually

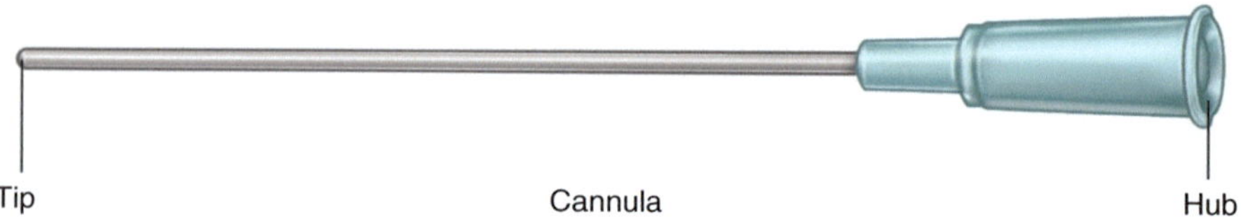

Fig. 3.1 Components of a PIV catheter

Table 3.1 Characteristics of common PIV gauges [5–8]

Gauge	Hub color	Cannula width (mm)	Cannula length (mm)	Gravity flow rate (mL/min)
26	Purple	0.7	19	~10–15
24	Yellow	0.8	19	~20
22	Blue	0.9	25	~22–50
20	Pink	1.1	32	~60–80
18	Green	1.3	32–45	~80–120
16	Gray	1.7	45	~150–240
14	Orange	2.2	45	~240–300

also inversely related to catheter length. In other words, larger gauge catheters have a smaller internal diameter and usually have a shorter cannula length. It should be noted that the approximate flow rates provided in Table 3.1 are for *in vitro* water infusion with gravity and would be expected to be slower for more viscous substances (e.g., blood, albumin) and faster with pressure bag application [5–8].

In the emergent setting, an 18- or 20-gauge PIV catheter is generally preferred, to permit efficient fluid volume infusion. Keep in mind that larger-diameter PIV catheters may inordinately occlude venous flow around the catheter, while smaller-diameter PIV catheters may provide inadequate flow rates.

Another consideration with larger-gauge (e.g., 14-, 16-, and 18-gauge) PIV catheters is the *rigidity* of these cannulae. Since they are thicker and less flexible, these catheters may perform better in areas characterized by thick or severely scarred soft tissues. When targeting an insertion site demonstrating extensive scarring, the provider should weigh this potential advantage against the need to use the smallest-gauge PIV catheter adequate for the patient's needs. When first learning techniques for PIV access, a familiarity with the larger catheter gauges is important. Once placement of the larger devices has been perfected, use of the smaller catheters will come easily. Providers should feel confident in their ability to place a large-gauge PIV in the emergent patient. When limitations due to smaller vessels or suboptimal location are encountered, the smaller-gauge devices can be a fallback for life-saving measures. Whatever the choice, any access is better than no access under emergent conditions.

Although some variation exists in the design and safety features present in modern devices, a generic safety PIV catheter would include certain features: *activation button, safety barrel, flashback chamber, projection finger grip, PIV cannula* (i.e., catheter) *with push-off tab and colored hub*, and the *guidance needle*. The activation button will cause retraction of the guidance needle after penetration of the target vessel has occurred, which leads to retraction of the needle into the *safety chamber*. This chamber shrouds the needle once it has been retracted, to reduce the risk of inadvertent provider injury following cannulation. The *guidance needle* is located at the interior of the catheter and includes a beveled tip which is used to penetrate the target vessel. Once the tip of the needle has entered the vessel, blood will be seen entering the *flashback chamber* (in larger catheters), although larger-gauge (i.e., smaller diameter) catheters may not have a flashback chamber, so blood may instead be seen entering the catheter lumen after successful penetration of the vessel. The *projection grip* is a prominence of the catheter-needle complex which promotes optimal control of the complex during needle insertion, while the *push-off tab* (a part of the catheter itself) gives the provider a point of traction on the catheter for advancing the catheter over the guidance needle during cannulation. Some catheters (especially those used for pediatric patients) may have "wings" emanating from each side of the hub which promote more stable anchoring of the catheter once it has been properly inserted. The cannula usually has a tapered tip, which promotes minimal injury to the target vessel with insertion. Because modern PIV catheters are tapered at the tip, it is not recommended to trim PIV catheters before placement, as this will remove the tapering at the tip and will increase the risk of vascular injury during insertion attempts. Figure 3.2 illustrates these features of modern safety PIV catheters.

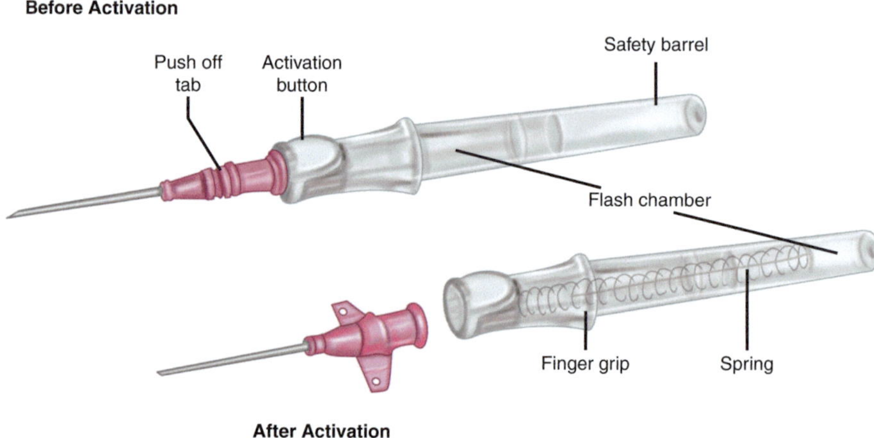

Fig. 3.2 Components of a generic PIV safety catheter

Fig. 3.3 Standard and extended-length short 18-gauge PIV catheters

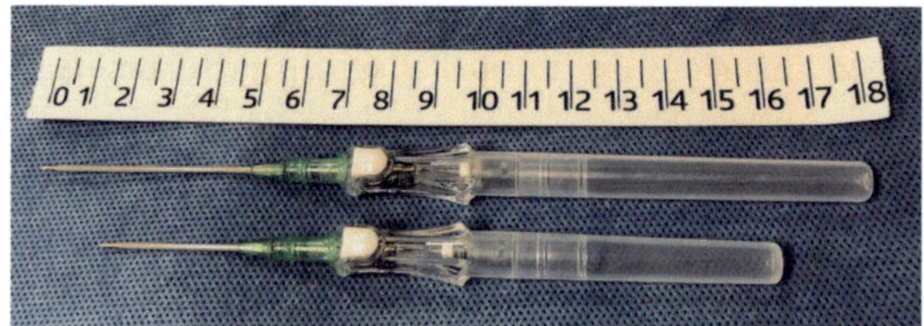

In addition to standard "short" PIV catheters, extended-length standard PIV catheters are also available. These longer catheters may be utilized for US-guided techniques or for cannulation of deeper veins, such as the *external jugular (EJ) vein*. It should be noted that the cannula length is not equivalent to the entire catheter length, as the cannula length only refers to the length of the portion of the catheter that is deep to the skin surface with placement, and does not include the length of the hub. For example, Fig. 3.3 shows a standard 18-gauge 30-mm (1.16-inch) short PIV safety catheter compared to the extended-length version of the same catheter, which features a 48-mm (1.88-inch) cannula. The only difference between these catheters is the length of the cannula and safety barrel.

Technique for Landmark-Based PIV Placement

In general, the steps required for placement of a peripheral intravenous catheter should be similar regardless of the specific catheter and location selected. These steps include:

1. Provider preparation
2. Insertion site selection

3. Tourniquet application
4. Site targeting and sterilization
5. Puncture of targeted vessel and tourniquet release
6. Confirmation of back flow
7. Needle retraction and vein occlusion
8. Heplock/infusion tubing attachment
9. Catheter flushing
10. Dressing application
11. Catheter stabilization
12. Assessment of catheter infusion

1. *Provider preparation* includes attention to standard antiseptic techniques. Providers must wash hands with warm water and soap prior to PIV insertion and wear appropriately fitted gloves. The provider should also adequately confirm the patient's identity and consider any patient preferences or contraindications for PIV insertion sites. Relative site contraindications for PIV placement are discussed later in this chapter. When possible, the risks and benefits of PIV insertion should be reviewed with the patient, and the patient should be made aware of the need and indication for PIV insertion. Emergency providers should remember that PIV attempts will likely be uncomfortable to the sensate patient. Patients should reasonably expect the provider to establish PIV access quickly, with minimal patient discomfort, and they may also have personal preferences about the location or type of PIV insertion that should be attempted. Of course, it is not always possible to accommodate all patient requests, especially if the patient's preferred access site or device would not be adequate for the type and level of care required. The provider should carefully assess the patient's therapeutic needs with PIV insertion and determine the appropriate gauge of PIV likely to be required for adequate patient care.

Provider comfort and safety are of paramount importance. Providers should assume that all patients have an infectious disease and avoid splash exposure to blood. When preparing to place a PIV, the emergency care provider must guard against needlesticks and awkward angles, by positioning the targeted venous access site at a level of comfort for the provider, so that the provider will not be strained during the cannulation attempt. The provider should sit down, when possible, and remain as close as possible to the patient. Ideally, PIV insertions should be attempted with the target site near the provider's waist level. In the ED or hospital setting, providers should ensure that the bed rail opposite to the access attempt is up before elevating the bed, and providers should never leave a bed raised when stepping away from the patient. Patients can sustain serious injuries with a fall from the bed if left unattended. If patients are uncooperative or disoriented, providers should obtain help from other healthcare providers in restraining the patient to avoid injury to the provider and the patient during the vascular access attempt.

During this phase of preparation, the provider should gather any needed equipment for PIV insertion, including sterile 2×2-inch sterile gauze, a transparent

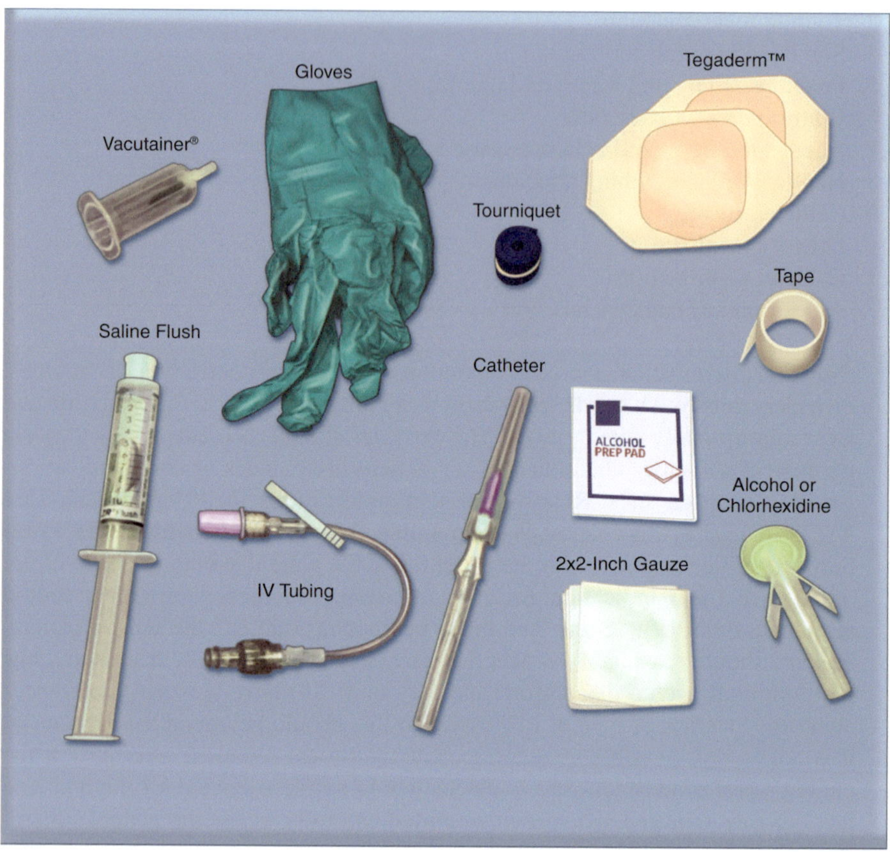

Fig. 3.4 Supplies required for PIV catheter insertion

semipermeable dressing, IV extension tubing, a prefilled normal saline flush syringe, an elastic tourniquet, a 70% alcohol wipe or chlorhexidine antiseptic swab, and clear 1-inch transpore tape. These supplies should be brought to the patient's bedside and made easily accessible prior to initiation of the PIV insertion attempt. Figure 3.4 shows the supplies needed to perform PIV insertion.

2. *Insertion site selection* should be guided by the patient's medical condition and a thorough examination of the patient. When high-volume infusion is needed, providers should seek to target the largest, most proximal veins available, especially those in the AC fossa or the EJ vein. On the other hand, if a smaller-caliber vein is adequate, it is best to start distally on the extremity, since a blown proximal vein may limit options more distally. If attempts on distal sites fail, the provider can always move more proximally.

Once the target vein has been selected, the vein should be palpated to identify sclerosed or hardened veins (which may be suboptimal), or areas where venous valves are located (which may feel like "bulges" in the vein). The provider must feel that cannulation is likely possible before attempted catheter insertion. This phase of preparation is especially important and should be given adequate time to complete, given the great importance of target vein selection to ultimate cannulation success. Once the desired target vein has been identified, providers should optimize their chance of success by ensuring proper patient positioning and ensuring adequate lighting of the area targeted for insertion. Considerations for proper selection of a target vein will be discussed later in this chapter.

3. *Tourniquet application* is generally applied 10–15 cm proximal to the desired insertion site and is intended to engorge the target vein to facilitate easy cannulation. Once the target vein has been cannulated, the tourniquet should be released immediately. In general, tourniquet placement should be above the elbow. However, in certain patients it may be desirable to place the tourniquet below the level of the elbow, especially if there is a significant amount of adipose tissue on the upper arm. Excessive adipose tissue may prevent the tourniquet from achieving its goal of restricting venous blood flow. The location of tourniquet placement should be informed by the amount of adipose tissue identified at the site at which the tourniquet is applied. For extremely fragile veins, it may be best to avoid the use of a tourniquet at all, to minimize the risk of a "blown" vessel.

Although elastic latex tourniquets are most commonly used for this purpose, an adequately inflated manual blood pressure cuff can provide similar vein engorgement. The use of two elastic tourniquets (spaced at least one inch apart) may offer additional benefit, but conflicting evidence exists. If the single tourniquet is adequately tightened, the one-tourniquet approach should be sufficient. Tourniquets should not be left tightened for more than 60 seconds, to prevent ischemic injury and pain through reduced perfusion of the distal extremity. If necessary, apply the tourniquet to identify the target vein, and then release the tourniquet while preparing for insertion and reapply the tourniquet(s) when ready to cannulate. Dependent positioning of the extremity will also aid in vein engorgement by leveraging the effects of gravity on venous return. Tapping or slapping the PIV site should be avoided, as this can cause trauma to the area, although vigorous rubbing or firm palpation of the target veins can create the same vein engorgement without such deleterious effects. Palpation should be done with the non-dominant hand. If the vein "rolls," the dominant hand will be occupied by the PIV cannula, so it is most efficient to be able to palpate with the non-dominant hand while redirecting the catheter with the dominant hand.

"Fist-pumping" by the patient may engorge the vein but can also lead to *pseudohyperkalemia* (i.e., falsely elevated potassium level on serum testing), so this practice should be avoided.

4. *Site targeting and sterilization* are the next steps in PIV insertion. Sterilization is performed with a 70% alcohol wipe or chlorhexidine antiseptic swab for at least 30 seconds, to reduce the risk of iatrogenic contamination of the PIV insertion

site by native skin flora. The recommended cleansing technique is in an abrasive "back and forth" and "up and down" motion for 30 seconds along the path of the target vein, not in a circular motion from the inside-out at the target site. It is important to allow the skin at the target site to completely dry after application of a sterilizing agent, and the provider should not touch the targeted insertion site again after the area has been sterilized.

5. *Puncture of the targeted vessel* can be attempted after the insertion site has been identified and adequately sterilized. The PIV catheter should be gripped firmly in the dominant ("active") hand with the middle finger and thumb placed on each side of the catheter hub, as illustrated in Fig. 3.5. The pointing finger of the dominant hand (when using the one-hand technique) should be left available to advance the catheter once the vessel has been cannulated. The provider's non-dominant ("free") hand is used to apply skin traction 4–5 cm distal to the insertion site, thereby stabilizing the vein and insertion site. Care should be taken to avoid contaminating the insertion site during this step. Improper free hand positioning while providing traction can obstruct needle insertion or place the provider at increased risk for needlestick injury. For example, placement of the non-dominant thumb too close to the insertion site may force an inappropriately large angle of insertion during the PIV attempt, as depicted in Fig. 3.6.

The needle should puncture the skin with its bevel facing upward (i.e., pointed toward the ceiling), usually at an angle of 15 to 20 degrees relative to the plane of

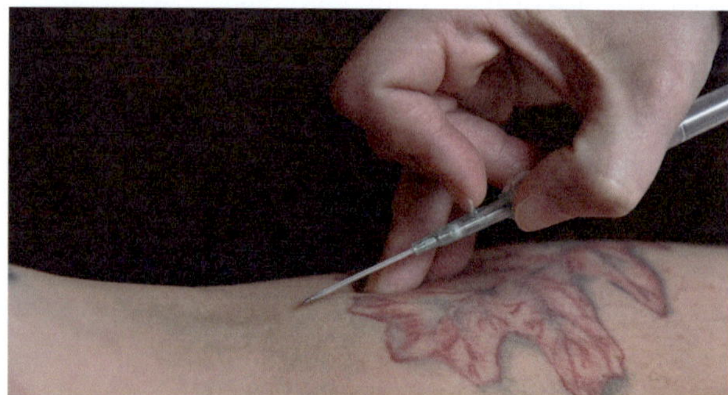

Fig. 3.5 Dominant hand position with PIV insertion. (*Image courtesy of Jeffrey Eichenlaub RN*)

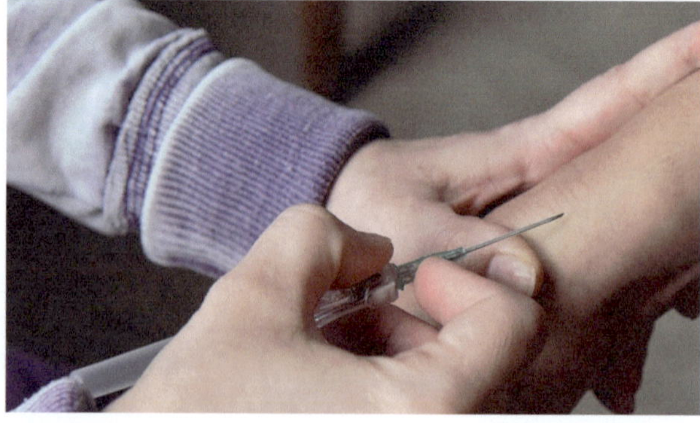

Fig. 3.6 Improper non-dominant thumb interference with PIV insertion. (*Image courtesy of Jeffrey Eichenlaub RN*)

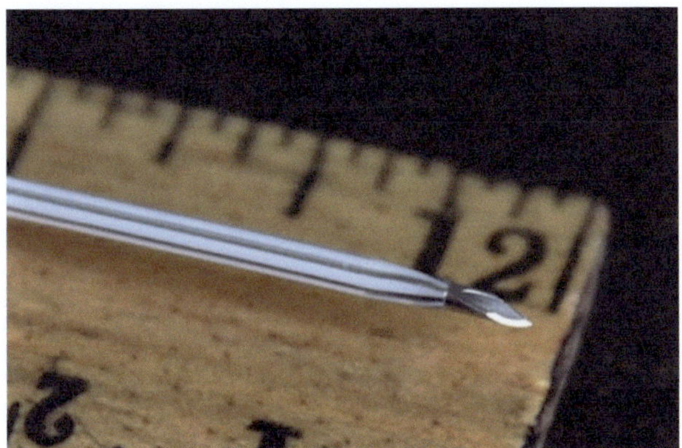

Fig. 3.7 Recommended "bevel-up" needle positioning

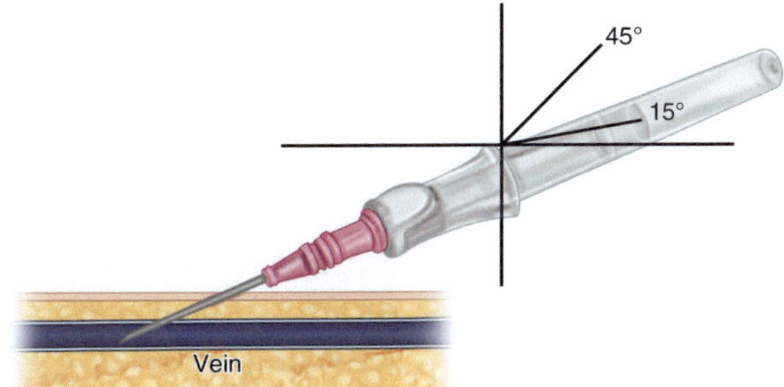

Fig. 3.8 Recommended PIV needle insertion angles during skin puncture

the extremity. Proper bevel placement is depicted in Fig. 3.7. The range of insertion angles typically used is depicted in Fig. 3.8. In general, the angle of insertion should be kept at 15 and 30 degrees relative to the projected plane of the target vessel, as depicted in Fig. 3.8. When deciding upon a skin puncture angle, *the lower the angle, the better*. Excessive angles of insertion (especially those above 45 degrees) risk injury to the vessel wall (Fig. 3.9). As illustrated in Fig. 3.9, excessive angles of insertion for the PIV catheter are more likely to lead to unintentional penetration of the deep wall of the vein, leading to inability to cannulate the vessel and increased likelihood of extravasation and line failure. Of course, the precise angle of skin puncture used (normally ranging from near-zero to 35 degrees) will depend upon limb positioning and the presence of nearby anatomical structures, as well as the predicted fragility and depth of the target vessel. Deeper veins (e.g., AC fossa, or when utilizing ultrasound for guidance) will require a greater angle of insertion, while tortuous, fragile, or superficial (e.g., hand or forearm) veins often require a shallower angle of insertion (Fig. 3.10).

Emergency care providers should ensure that the direction of insertion for the PIV catheter points proximally toward the heart. If a PIV catheter is placed "backward" (i.e., directed away from the heart), the placement will be associated with increased risk of infiltration and/or extravasation.

Fig. 3.9 Improper
(excessive) insertion angle
for skin puncture

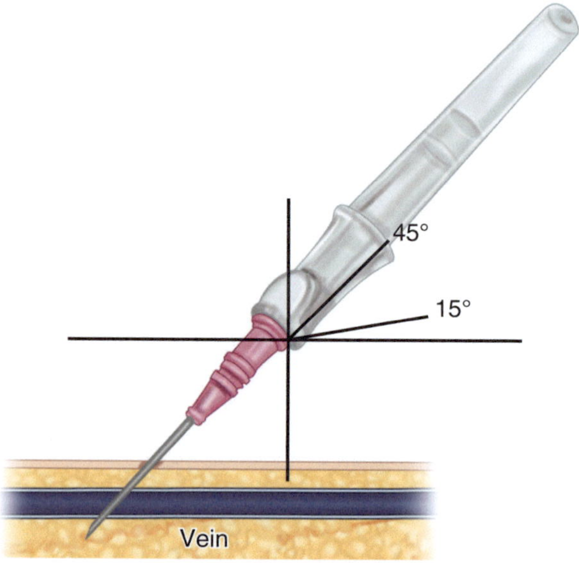

Fig. 3.10 Angle of
insertion utilized with PIV
insertion at the level of the
forearm. (*Image courtesy
of Jeffrey Eichenlaub RN*)

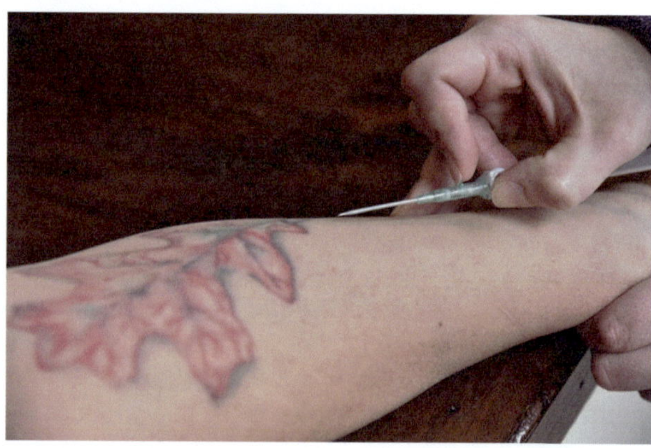

Both one-handed and two-handed PIV insertion techniques can be utilized, primarily distinguished by which hand is used to advance the PIV catheter after cannulation. Hand positioning with these techniques is illustrated in Figs. 3.11 and 3.12.

The one-handed method is usually preferred, as it frees the non-dominant hand to provide continued traction and stabilization of the targeted insertion site during the access attempt. The non-dominant hand is then available for immediate occlusion of the vein just proximal to the insertion site, while the needle is retracted and heplock is picked up and connected to the hub. The two-handed technique will be suboptimal when patient movement or other environmental factors make stabilization of the insertion site difficult. The experienced emergency care provider should be comfortable with utilizing either the one-handed or two-handed approach, as conditions warrant.

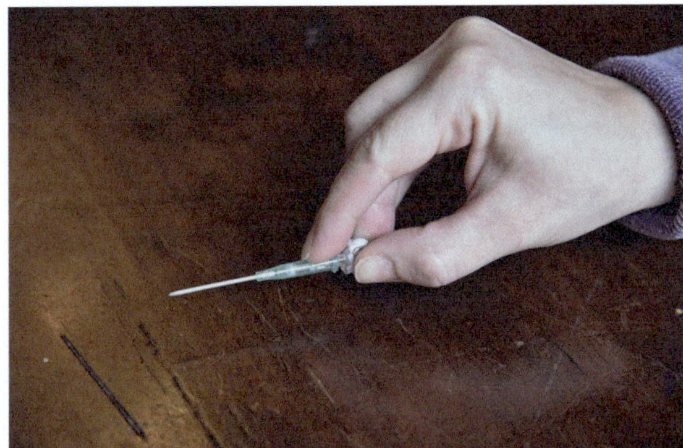

Fig. 3.11 One-handed PIV insertion technique. (*Image courtesy of Jeffrey Eichenlaub RN*)

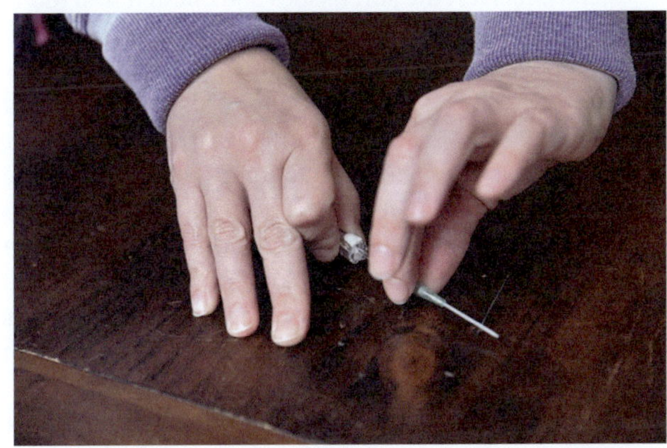

Fig. 3.12 Two-handed PIV insertion technique. (*Image courtesy of Jeffrey Eichenlaub RN*)

When opening the catheter, it is best to break the seal between the catheter and needle hub so that the index finger of the dominant hand can freely move the tip. While inserting the needle tip, the provider must hold the PIV catheter securely and be guarded against any movement or disruption by the patient. The speed of insertion will depend upon the depth of the targeted vessel, as patient movement can substantially disrupt the access attempt. In general, deeper vessels should be cannulated as fluidly and swiftly as possible, while more superficial or delicate veins may benefit from a slower, more deliberate insertion.

While the PIV catheter is still loaded on one guidance needle, a small (1–2 mm) distance exists between the beveled tip of the needle and the distal tip of the PIV catheter. This relationship is illustrated in Fig. 3.7. When cannulating the vein, the provider must advance the needle-catheter complex just far enough so that the catheter tip is in the lumen, but not so far that the bevel is poked through the opposite side of the vessel. This provides only a small margin of error for the provider when targeting small-caliber veins.

Nursing textbooks and guidelines describe the "direct" and "indirect" methods for PIV insertion [9]. The distinction between these two methods is the number of steps required and the aspect of the vein that is punctured. With the *direct method*, the provider punctures the skin and the superficial aspect of the vein at the same time. Thus, the cannula exits the superficial aspect of the vein, adjacent to the skin surface. With the *indirect method*, the provider first punctures the skin adjacent to the vein and then redirects and punctures the side of the vein. Thus, the cannula exits the side of the vein. The angle of skin puncture (relative to the plane of the vein) should be approximately 30 to 40 degrees using either method [9].

6. *Confirmation of back flow* will be obtained immediately after cannulation and release of the tourniquet, as blood should flow out from the properly placed PIV catheter and directly into the flash chamber. The provider may also feel a "popping" sensation, associated with a sudden change in resistance, once the needle tip has penetrated the vessel. This loss of resistance suggests that the tip of the needle has left the soft tissues and entered into the vessel lumen, as blood is less dense than the surrounding tissues and offers less resistance. Once this "flash" of blood has been observed, the angle of insertion should be dropped immediately by a few degrees. Failure to drop the angle of further insertion after this initial flash will increase the risk of penetrating the opposite vessel wall, leading to extravasation and line failure, or may spear the catheter on the beveled tip of the needle leading to catheter damage. After dropping the angle of insertion, the needle-catheter complex is advanced another 1–2 millimeters, just enough to ensure that the tip of the PIV catheter remains within the lumen of the target vein. If this forward movement is met with resistance, the catheter tip is likely not in the lumen of the target vessel. If this resistance is encountered, the provider should not attempt to advance the needle tip further into the vessel. The provider should either retract the needle tip 1–2 millimeters (if the tip is believed to be too deep) or advance it 1–2 mm further (if considered too shallow) and then re-attempt cannulation. Once the provider believes that the tip of the needle is within the vessel lumen, the index finger of the dominant hand (if using the one-handed technique) is then used to carefully advance the PIV catheter into the lumen of the vessel. When cannulation is successful, venous blood should be noted to flow freely from the catheter.

7. *Needle retraction and vein occlusion* should be performed once the provider has confirmed adequate intraluminal catheter placement through observed continued blood flow through the catheter following insertion. In this step, the provider retracts (i.e., decannulates) the needle from within the catheter and applies firm pressure to the skin just proximal to the insertion site with the index finger of the non-dominant hand to occlude the venous lumen and reduce further blood flow from the catheter. This will facilitate connection of the IV extension apparatus to the hub of the PIV catheter.

8. *Heplock/infusion tubing attachment* is performed after the catheter has been placed and is believed to be in good position without suspicion for misplacement. Continued blood flow from the catheter hub may be an indicator of good positioning within the vessel lumen. Care should be taken to avoid touching the hub or connector portion of the infusion tubing with the gloved hand, as this

may contaminate the catheter with skin flora. It is also important to stabilize the catheter during attachment of the infusion tubing, to avoid inadvertent dislodgement of the catheter during this step.

9. *Catheter flushing* is performed once the catheter has been adequately positioned and the needle has been retracted. The provider should flush the catheter with a prefilled 3-mL or 10-mL normal saline flush to confirm that immediate extravasation of the infused saline into the tissues surrounding the target vein does not occur. If the vein has been properly cannulated, catheter flushing should be painless, without swelling or extravasation of the adjacent soft tissues. However, the vein just proximal to the insertion site will normally blanch and cool slightly due to infusion of the saline solution. If swelling of the soft tissues in this area is observed, the vein is likely ruptured and the placement attempt failed. Further infusion will likely yield extravasation of the infused materials and should be discontinued. Once extravasation has been observed, future attempts at more distal sites on the same extremity should be avoided. However, if the catheter appears to be in good position within the vein, without evidence of extravasation, the catheter should be deemed well-seated and useable for subsequent infusion.

10. *Dressing placement* should be performed immediately after appropriate cannulation of the target vein has been confirmed. Dressing application is usually achieved by placing a transparent sterile semipermeable dressing (e.g., Tegaderm™) over the insertion site, with the center of the dressing located over the insertion site. This dressing shields the insertion site from subsequent bacterial infection, maintaining a waterproof barrier that will also allow oxygen to penetrate for appropriate skin health and wound healing. When the patient is diaphoretic, a sterile absorptive gauze dressing should be applied to the site until the diaphoresis is resolved. If the dressing becomes moist, loose, or soiled, it should be replaced immediately. Certain liquid adhesives (e.g., Mastisol® or tincture of benzoin) can help maintain dressing integrity while providing an additional adhesive property. When using liquid adhesives, the provider should ensure that the liquid adhesive has completely dried after application before applying the overlying dressings. It is worth noting that these liquid adhesives may be more commonly utilized in the ICU setting or with PICC and midline catheters but can be utilized with PIV catheters.

11. *Catheter stabilization* is a critical final step in the placement of PIV catheters. The intention of PIV catheter stabilization is to reduce movement at the insertion site, to prevent inadvertent dislodgement of the catheter. An engineered stabilization device (ESD), placed subcutaneously or topically after PIV placement, is recommended to reduce these risks [9]. Cyanoacrylate tissue adhesives (e.g., Dermabond® or Histoacryl® or ESDs (e.g., "wings") incorporated into the catheter hub are the standard recommended measures for catheter stabilization.

12. *Assessment of catheter infusion* should be performed immediately after insertion of the catheter and intermittently following catheter insertion. *Drip rates* can be used to estimate fluid flow rates. Drip chambers come in two types:

Table 3.2 Drip volumes according to drip set utilized [10]

Drip set	Drip volume (mL/gtt)
Macro (10 gtt/mL)	0.10
Macro (12 gtt/mL)	0.0833
Macro (15 gtt/mL)	0.0666
Macro (20 gtt/mL)	0.05
Micro (60 gtt/mL)	0.0166

macro drip sets (ranging from 10 to 20 drips (gtt)/mL) or micro drip sets (60 drips (gtt) / mL). By counting the number of drips in the chamber over one minute, one may estimate the corresponding infusion flow rate according to the following formula:

$$\text{Flow Rate}\left(\text{mL / min}\right) = \text{Drip Rate}\left(gtt \text{ / min}\right) \times \text{Drip Volume}\left(\text{mL / } gtt\right)$$

In this formula, the Drip Volume has a constant value, which is determined by the type of drip set utilized. The corresponding Drip Volume (mL / gtt) values needed for this calculation are found in Table 3.2.

Providers should periodically observe the drip rate in the IV tubing chamber to determine whether the infusion rate is appropriate. If the provider observes that the drip rate is lower than expected, the catheter and infusion tubing should be inspected to determine whether the IV line is clamped and/or kinked. Catheters located at joint creases (e.g., the AC fossa) may be at higher risk of catheter kinkage with occlusion due to joint flexion, and providers should advise the patient to extend the joint if drip rates are observed to be lower than expected values.

Common Peripheral Vein Targets

We recommend that emergency care providers seek "any port in a storm" when attempting to establish vascular access in the "crashing" patient. Even the most tenuous and hard-fought PIV may have value to critically ill patient under the right clinical conditions. However, there are certain "ports" that are more likely to be available to the emergency care provider than others. The wise clinician will know where to look for these "go-to" access points and should assess the usual and optimal sites first, before deciding to pursue a suboptimal site. Deeper and more proximal veins are usually of larger caliber, providing a larger target for cannulation as well as improved rate of flow, when compared to smaller and more superficial veins. However, deeper veins may also be difficult to visualize and may increase the risk of complications including line placement failure. Thus, an optimal target for landmark-based venous cannulation would be an adequately sized vein that is also identifiable from the skin's surface. Optimal insertion sites should also offer few impediments to access, provide adequate blood return, be able to withstand high infusion pressures, and be associated with minimal risk of complications from line placement and infusion.

It is critically important when selecting a peripheral target vein to consider (1) whether the selected site is likely to last the full course of the patient's expected therapy and (2) whether the selected site likely exposes the patient to an excessive risk of complications.

The Antecubital (AC) Fossa

The most common sites for PIV access in the emergent setting are located within the antecubital (AC) fossa, which is positioned anterior to the elbow joint. Optimal target veins in this area, also known as the cubital fossa, include the *median cubital, basilic,* and *accessory cephalic veins.* These veins are illustrated in Fig. 3.13.

The *median cubital vein* is the largest and most accessible vein for cannulation within the antecubital fossa. As a result, it is often the "go-to" site for PIV insertion at the AC fossa. The *basilic vein* is the next largest but is usually the "last resort" due to concerns about injuring the underlying *brachial artery* and *median nerve.* The *accessory cephalic vein* is smaller, more challenging to secure, but remains an often-accessed vein.

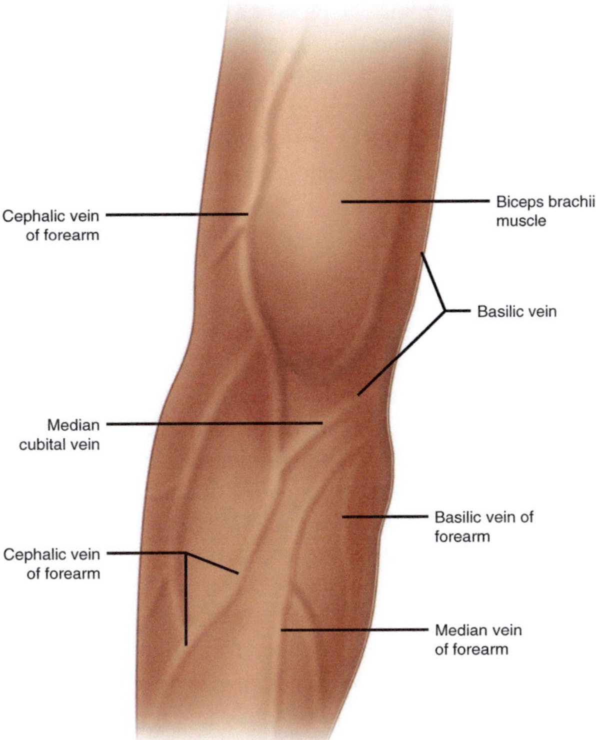

Fig. 3.13 Veins of the antecubital fossa

Although the AC fossa is a commonly utilized site for emergent PIV insertion, there are several disadvantages to the use of veins in this region. Proximity of the brachial artery and median nerve (just deep to the basilic vein) complicates cannulation with the risk of injury to these structures. In addition, flexion at the elbow may cause kinking of the PIV catheter, which will ultimately inhibit forward flow through the catheter. Patients with a PIV inserted at the AC fossa should be instructed to keep their elbow extended as much as possible during venous infusions, which may be both uncomfortable to the patient and difficult to maintain during prolonged infusions. Once inserted, the PIV catheter can compress the median nerve, causing pain that worsens with elbow flexion.

The Upper Arm

If a PIV insertion site cannot be identified at the AC fossa, landmark-based cannulation of an upper arm vein may still be possible. Proximal to the elbow, the provider may be able to visualize and palpate the *basilic vein* or an accessory vein in the upper arm. These veins are large and have the same desirability for cannulation as the AC region. Unlike more distal peripheral targets, upper arm veins are usually straight, out of the way, and not very positional with patient movement. However, access to these veins can present a challenge to novice providers due to the angle for insertion required and increased mobility of the veins. The *brachial vein* may present itself in select patients, but this vein is not always visible on surface landmarking. If the brachial vein is not readily visible, blind placement should not be attempted, due to the poor reliability of this technique and high risk of iatrogenic injury to the underlying nerves and arteries.

The Forearm

Distal to the AC fossa, the most commonly accessed veins are the *basilic, cephalic,* and *median veins,* all of which should be accessible on the ventral side of the forearm. The basilic and median veins are located on the medial aspect of the forearm, while the cephalic vein is generally located more laterally. Understanding that proximal veins are likely larger in diameter and therefore preferable for cannulation, providers should seek to cannulate the most proximal vein that presents itself to the provider. The search for a suitable vein should start proximally (i.e., in the upper arm or near to the AC fossa) with attention turned distally once more proximal veins have been deemed inaccessible. The commonly accessed veins of the forearm are illustrated in Fig. 3.14.

The *basilic vein* is located on the medial aspect of the forearm. This vein is often easily visualized and palpated but can be difficult to access. When it travels over a bony prominence, it will be mobile and require firm securement to access. When it travels over the length of the arm, it is more flexible and may require unique positioning to access. One approach to accessing the basilic vein is depicted in Fig. 3.15.

Fig. 3.14 Peripheral veins of the forearm

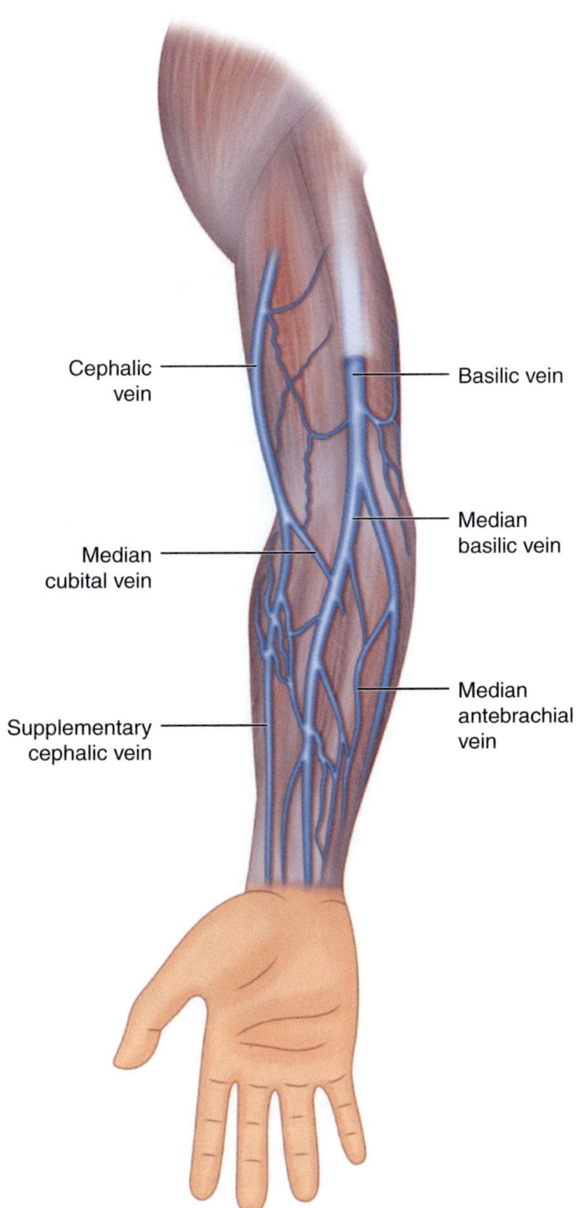

Note that the patient's elbow is flexed and the provider is situated on the medial and inferior aspect of the forearm.

The *supplementary cephalic vein* is an often-accessed forearm vein that is large, straight, and situated at an optimal anatomic insertion site. This is the "go-to" vein in most trauma resuscitations, as a large (e.g., 14- or 16-gauge) PIV catheter can

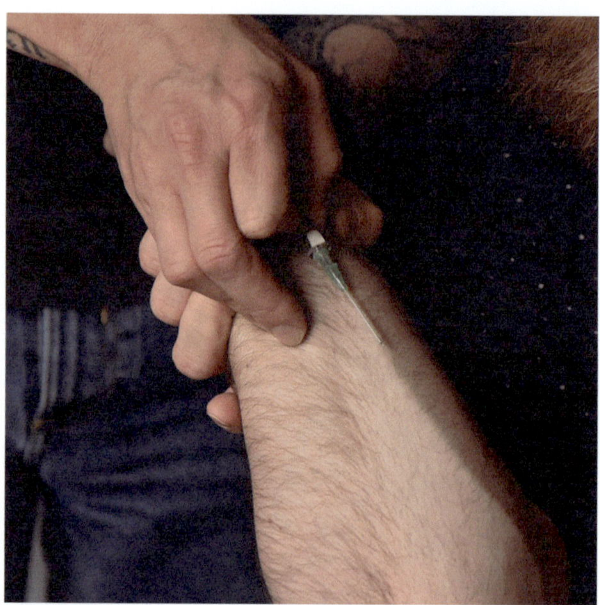

Fig. 3.15 Approach to accessing the basilic vein. (*Image courtesy of Jeffrey Eichenlaub RN*)

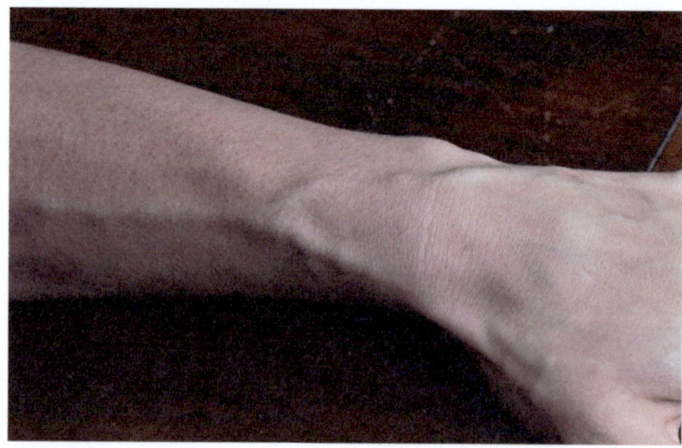

Fig. 3.16 View of the cephalic vein. (*Image courtesy of Jeffrey Eichenlaub RN*)

often be accommodated, providing high infusion rates. The most common site selected for insertion is just proximal to the wrist joint, on the lateral aspect of the dorsal forearm. This vein must be accessed at a lower angle relative to the plane of the arm when compared to more proximal veins and requires stable securement. An example of the cephalic vein is provided in Fig. 3.16.

The Hand and Wrist

If forearm and AC fossa veins are not available, the next areas to consider are the hand and wrist. The hand is generally not an optimal area for emergent PIV placement, as these veins are usually more tortuous, have smaller diameter, and have

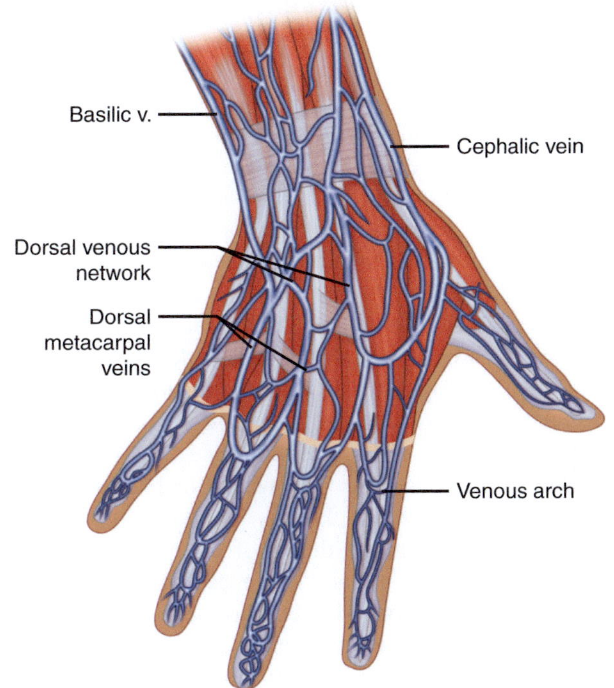

Fig. 3.17 Peripheral venous network of the hand

more valves than the proximal veins of the upper extremity. These smaller veins can be problematic when medications must be infused quickly or may be caustic to the soft tissues. Valves in these small veins may obstruct forward advancement of the catheter. Placing a PIV in the hand also prevents blood draws from being performed proximal to the site when IV fluids are being infused, due to dilution of the venous blood sample with infusates. Furthermore, intravenous contrast injection and other testing may not be able to be delivered through PIVs distal to the wrist due to concern with extravasation of caustic infusates. An illustration of the venous network of the hand is provided in Fig. 3.17.

The most commonly accessed hand veins are the *cephalic, dorsal metacarpal, and palmar metacarpal veins*. The dorsal digital veins arise from the adjacent sides of the fingers to form three *dorsal metacarpal veins*, terminating in a dorsal venous network opposite the middle of the metacarpus. These veins are a popular site for peripheral venous cannulation because they tend to be prominent veins which are easily accessible and do not lie over a point of flexion, so cannulation is usually not too uncomfortable for the patient. Veins in the fingers can be used, but require a smaller-gauge PIV catheter, and are usually accessed as a last resort. Veins of the anterior wrist can also be accessed, with the same limitations as digital veins.

The use of veins located on the ventral (palmar) aspect of the wrist, as well as the cephalic vein at the level of the wrist, is not generally recommended due to increased risk of nerve and/or vascular injury [9].

The External Jugular Vein

When veins of the upper extremities are inaccessible, the external jugular (EJ) vein should be considered for cannulation. The EJ vein usually extends between the angle of the mandible and the midpoint of the clavicle, as depicted in Fig. 3.18. The EJ vein is separated from the carotid artery and other vital structures by the sterno-cleidomastoid muscle (SCM), but iatrogenic injury to the vital structures of the neck (e.g., trachea, lungs, and arteries) is still possible with improper technique. We recommend that the EJ vein be accessed at the most proximal site available, to avoid iatrogenic injury to the lung or other structures. Venous valves are usually located more distally (at the entrance to the subclavian vein and approximately 4 cm superior to the clavicle) and should be avoided.

When attempting EJ vein cannulation, the patient should be placed in Trendelenburg position (i.e., head down) to engorge the vein, with the neck turned to the opposite side, as depicted in Fig. 3.19. The vessel will be noted to collapse in volume-depleted patients with inspiration but can be engorged with direct pressure to the vein just above the clavicle. Stabilization of the vein can be maintained with direct pressure from the thumb of the non-dominant hand during the cannulation attempt. The vein is usually best accessed at an angle of 10 to 25 degrees, although the angle will be dropped once "flashback" of blood has been noted. Cannulation of the EJ vein is relatively contraindicated when the patient cannot tolerate lying flat, has a ventriculoperitoneal (VP) shunt on the targeted side, or is suspected to have cervical spine trauma.

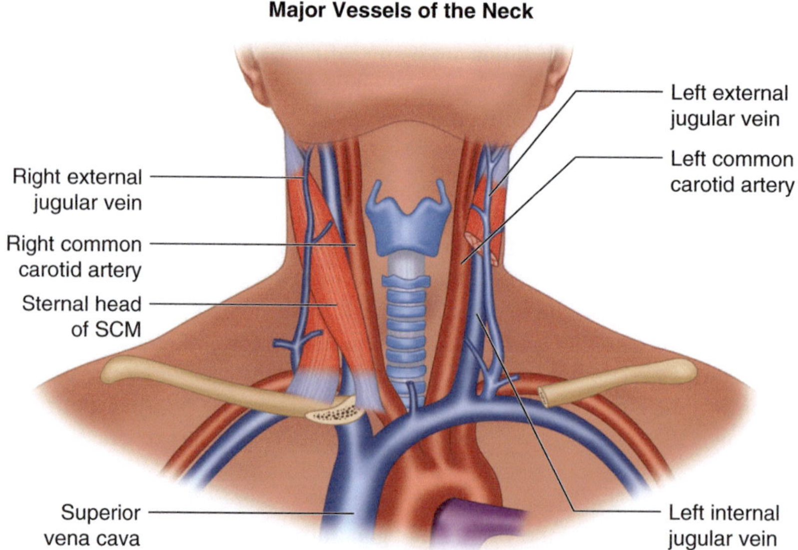

Fig. 3.18 The external jugular (EJ) vein and other great vessels of the neck

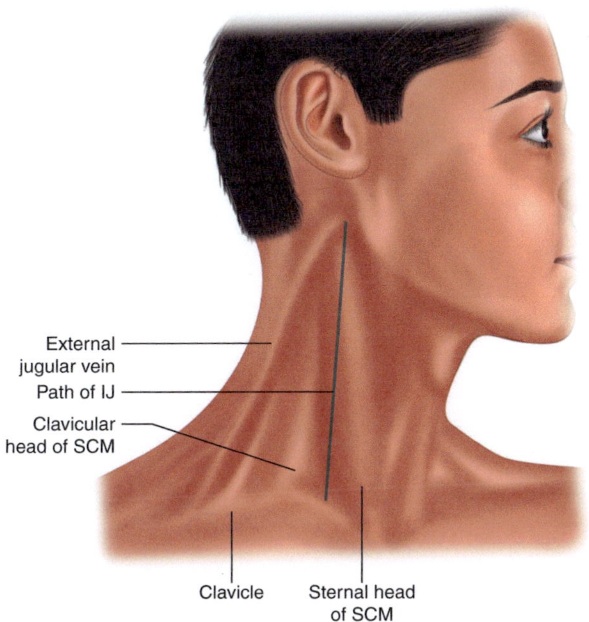

Fig. 3.19 External landmarking for the external jugular (EJ) vein

The Lower Extremity

Veins in the upper torso and legs are usually superficial or tortuous and represent a suboptimal site for PIV insertion. These veins are accessed without a tourniquet, with the catheter inserted at a shallow angle with a smaller-gauge catheter. In general, lower extremity peripheral veins should not be accessed in adults, due to increased risk of complications, but may be appropriate for pediatric patients [9]. The veins of the feet should only be accessed in those patients who do not have known risk factors for complications with vascular access, such as diabetes mellitus, poor wound healing, or known peripheral vascular disease [9]. At most institutions, a physician's order is required to place a pedal PIV, due to the increased risks associated with their use. The most frequently accessed veins of the feet are the *lateral marginal*, *medial marginal*, and *saphenous veins*, which are presented in Fig. 3.20. Due to increased risk of swelling, it is often recommended to elevate the foot for several hours after a failed PIV attempt.

Providers should avoid securing catheters over bony prominences. When selecting a target vein for cannulation, providers should not limit themselves to the most commonly accessed sites if these insertion sites are not available. Rather, the emergency care provider should seek to select the best possible PIV insertion site that may be accessed with the largest possible gauge PIV catheter.

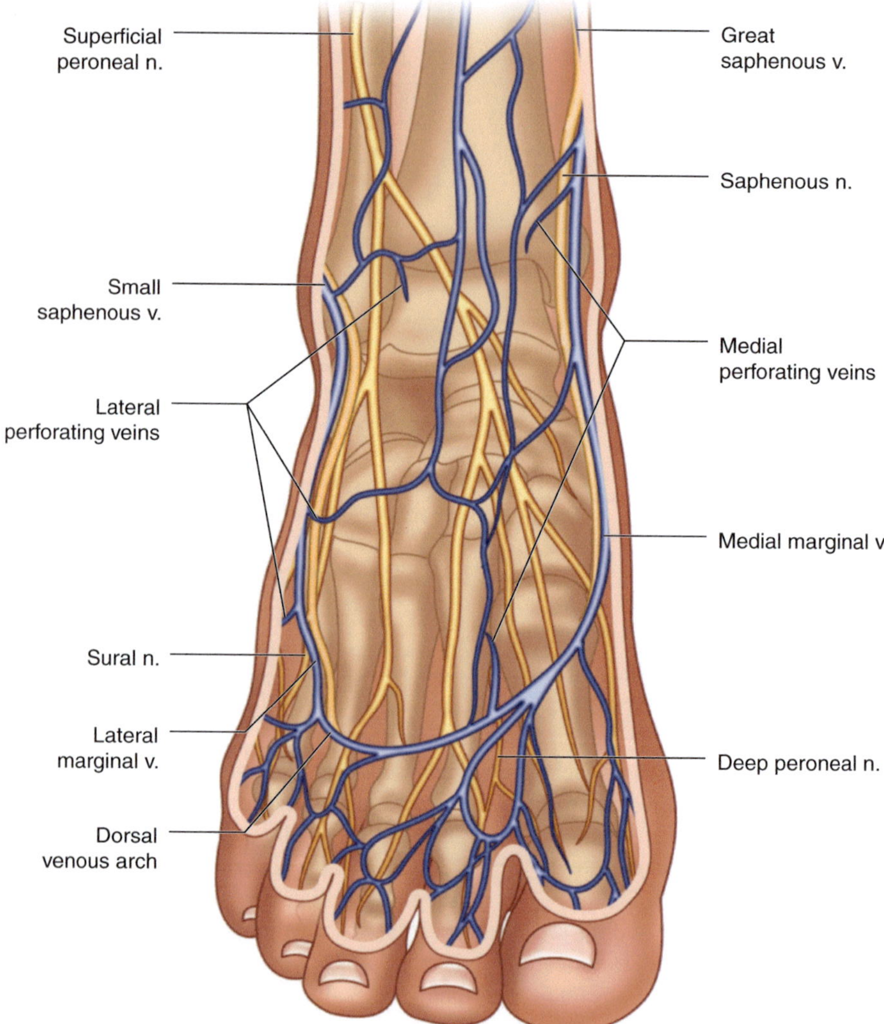

Fig. 3.20 Peripheral veins of the foot

Special Considerations for PIV Insertion

Breast Cancer

Patients with a history of breast cancer should be assessed for a history of mastectomy. If the patient's mastectomy included axillary lymph node removal, the American Cancer Society recommends that the arm on the affected side should not be used for peripheral venous access, due to the likelihood of impaired venous/lymphatic drainage from the extremity [11]. If the patient has had bilateral mastectomies, the arm with the least number of lymph nodes removed or an alternative site should be considered.

Hemodialysis

Patients with end-stage renal disease requiring hemodialysis may have an arteriovenous fistula (AVF) or arteriovenous graft (AVG) [12]. While an AVF anastomoses a native artery and vein, AVGs connect the artery and vein with a synthetic tube or harvested vein. Some patients may have failed AVFs or AVGs at multiple extremities, depending upon the duration of their dependence upon hemodialysis. In the emergent setting, defunct or abandoned AVF/AVG sites should not prevent providers from utilizing the involved extremity, although providers should avoid the AVF or AVG itself, as abandoned AVFs are likely thrombosed and unable to accommodate infusion. However, any extremity containing an AVF/AVG being actively used for dialysis purposes should be avoided. If these active dialysis sites are cannulated, vascular trauma or other complications from the PIV cannulation could cause irreversible damage to the site that may make further dialysis at the site impossible (Fig. 3.21).

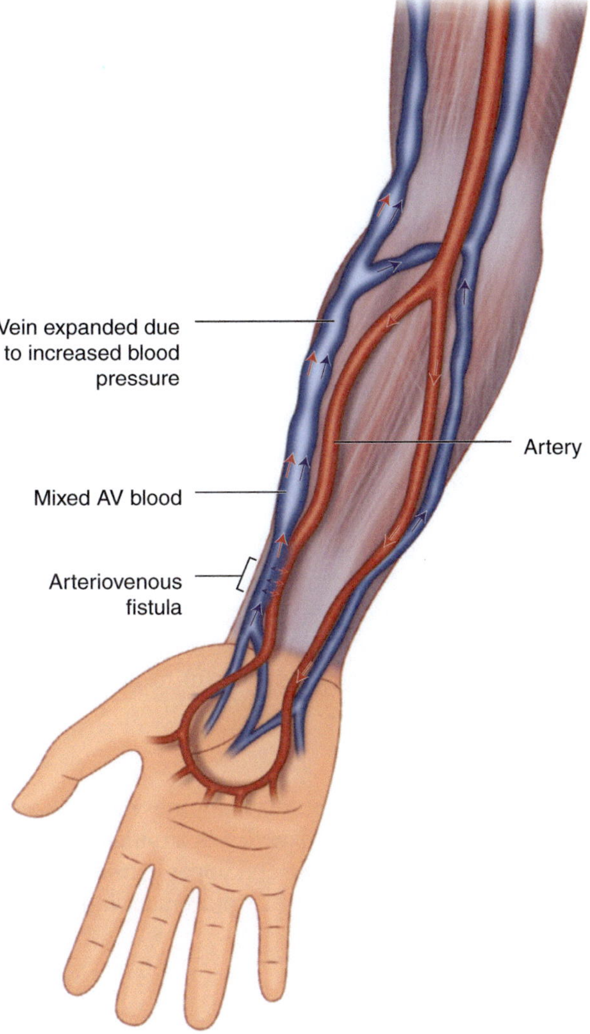

Fig. 3.21 Arteriovenous (AV) fistula

To prevent inadvertent compromise of future dialysis therapy, emergent providers should closely examine the patient for evidence of an AVF or AVG prior to establishing PIV access. The most common site of AVF creation is at the level of the wrist, utilizing the radial artery and cephalic vein [11]. When patients have an inadequate cephalic vein, or have failed distal AVF formation, they may have a more proximal AVF created in the upper extremity, either at the level of the proximal forearm (using the brachial artery and cephalic vein) or the upper arm (brachial artery and basilic vein). In general, more proximal AVFs have a higher rate of complications, so the vascular surgeon will usually attempt a more distal site before resorting to more proximal AVF creation [11].

A viable, functional AVF should have a palpable "thrill" (vibration) and audible "bruit" (rumbling or swooshing sound perceived via stethoscope) at the AVF site. The provider should also observe a bulging of the vessel at the AVF site, which is usually quite visible superficially. However, arteriovenous fistulae can take weeks or months to "mature" to a useable state, so the absence of a bruit or thrill (especially in the presence of a dialysis catheter) does not necessarily suggest that the AVF has been abandoned. The AVF may simply be immature. In general, it is best to avoid cannulating a peripheral vein on an extremity that has evidence of an AVF or AVG. Although most AVFs/AVGs will be in the upper extremities, providers should examine the lower extremities as well, as patients with long-standing dialysis requirements may also have lower extremity AVFs. Consequently, the skilled emergency provider will examine the target extremity fully before attempting vascular access in a patient with end-stage renal disease.

Contractures

Patients with contractures can be a challenge for the emergency provider. Attempting to straighten an extremity that is contracted can damage the underlying structures. The best target veins in "contracted" patients are usually located on the posterior aspect of the forearm, the dorsal aspect of the hand, or the external jugular vein. When placing a PIV in a contracted patient, the provider should seek assistance holding position to avoid unsuccessful IV attempts.

Deep Vein Thrombosis

If a patient presents with unilateral upper extremity edema, consider the possibility for a deep vein thrombosis (DVT). It is not appropriate to place an IV in an extremity that could or does have a blood clot. The risk for dislodgement of the DVT or obstruction of flow could be harmful to the patient. These extremities should be used only as a last resort.

Traumatic Injury

Patients presenting with traumatic injuries require special considerations for peripheral IV placement. If the patient has a unilateral upper extremity injury, place the peripheral IV in the contralateral upper extremity. If the patient has bilateral upper extremity injuries, consider PIV placement in the external jugular (preferred) or a lower extremity.

Scar Tissue

Old scar tissue can create difficulties with PIV insertion. Scar tissue is difficult to penetrate and typically requires a larger-gauge catheter (with a thicker cannula) to bypass. The presence of scar tissue should also alert the provider to the likelihood of underlying chronic vascular injury. Scar tissue is also more sensitive to pain than unscarred skin. Certain vessels may develop sclerotic regions related to a history of previous therapeutic cannulations or certain lifestyle choices (e.g., intravenous drug injection). Scarred veins may be readily palpable to the provider but may not be easily accessed. The provider should ensure when palpating the vein that there is a "spongy" texture and not a "tendon-like" feel before selecting the target vein. In general, it is best to avoid PIV insertion in areas of visible scarring. If venous scar tissue is detected in the target area of interest for the line attempt, the provider should start distal to the scarred region rather than proximally. Scarring of the vein may cause a partial obstruction to blood flow, which could (slightly) engorge the more distal contributing veins and collapse more proximal portions of the venous system. The same principle applies to hematomas, which should be avoided and may reduce venous flow at the site of the hematoma and more proximally.

Soft Tissue Edema

Although it is generally preferred to avoid PIV insertion in an area already edematous, this may be necessary in some patients who have widespread peripheral tissue edema. Peripheral veins in these patients are often deeper than expected, requiring a somewhat steeper angle of skin puncture to reach the target. Additionally, edema fluid in the soft tissues is likely to enter into the needle as it is advanced, which increases the importance of "wasting" the initial aliquot of blood drawn through the catheter, when blood sampling is required. The use of a tourniquet and gauze to absorb the fluid may be necessary, and the provider may also be able to manually "push" the edematous tissue away from the targeted skin puncture site. However, care should be taken to avoid excessive force on the underlying vein, as this may compress the target vein (reducing the size of the target), damage the vein, or cause hemolysis of the drawn blood.

Phlebotomy and Order of Blood Draw

In general, the process by which *phlebotomy* (drawing blood) is performed mirrors that of PIV insertion. Whether the goal is simply to obtain venous blood specimens, or to establish peripheral venous access, the provider will utilize a similar technique to cannulate the patient's vein.

Venipuncture for the sole purpose of phlebotomy often involves either a straight needle (typically 21- or 23-gauge) (Fig. 3.22) or a so-called butterfly needle (typically 21-, 23-, or 25-gauge) (Fig. 3.23) to access the target vein. These needles are not intended to be left in place after the phlebotomy has been performed and are not used for venous infusion. Butterfly needles are typically composed of a narrow (21-, 23-, or 25-gauge) needle with "wings," attached to a short length of tubing which

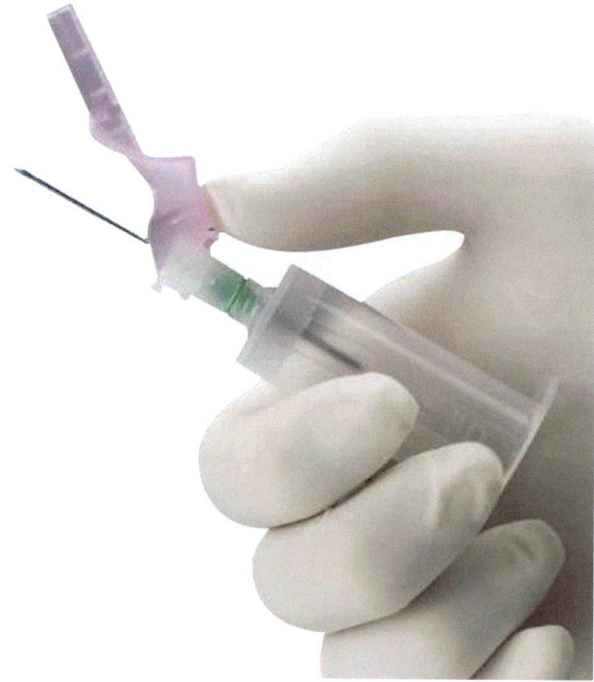

Fig. 3.22 21-gauge straight needle with Vacutainer® tube. (*Image courtesy of Becton, Dickinson and Company Inc. © 2020 Becton, Dickinson and Company Inc. All rights reserved*)

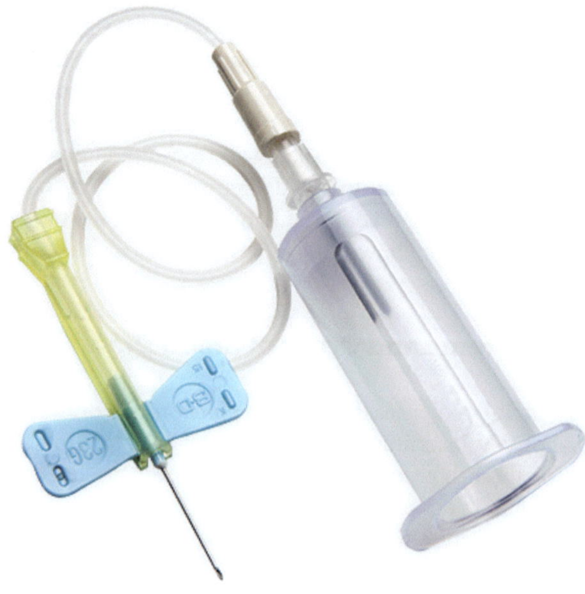

Fig. 3.23 23-gauge butterfly needle with Vacutainer® Safety-Lok® blood collection set. (*Image courtesy of Becton, Dickinson and Company Inc. © 2020 Becton, Dickinson and Company Inc. All rights reserved*)

terminates in a Luer connector. This connector can be attached to a Vacutainer® tube (Becton, Dickinson & Company) or syringe for vacuum-assisted blood extraction.

However, many patients who require emergent vascular access also require blood tests for their care. Thus, it is very common for providers to draw blood directly

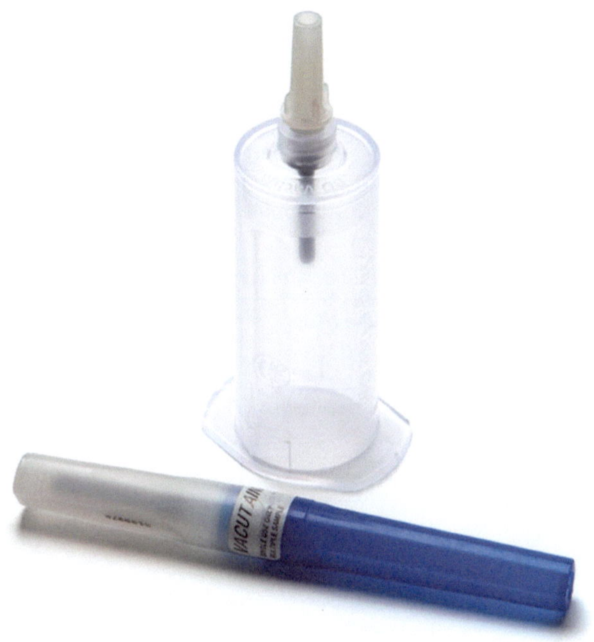

Fig. 3.24 Vacutainer® system multiple sample device with Luer adapter. (*Image courtesy of Becton, Dickinson and Company Inc. © 2020 Becton, Dickinson and Company Inc. All rights reserved*)

from the PIV (or CVC) catheter immediately after the line has been placed, but before the infusion tubing is attached. This may be accomplished with use of a Vacutainer® tube (Becton, Dickinson & Company) system or by direct connection of a syringe to the catheter (Fig. 3.24).

Hemolysis is a common problem with phlebotomy. When it occurs, multiple false laboratory derangements will be resulted, including pseudohyperkalemia. Unfortunately, hemolysis is estimated to occur in up to 8% of all blood draws performed in the emergency department [13]. Hemolysis occurs when red blood cells (RBCs) are fragmented, which may be attributed to a variety of factors. The use of needles that are too large compared to the diameter of the target vein can cause hemolysis, as will excessive vacuum suction force. For this reason, providers should use small (e.g., 5- or 10-mL syringes) to draw blood from PIV starts and should draw the blood as slowly as possible. Larger-capacity (e.g., 20-mL) syringes will generate much larger vacuum force than smaller syringes. The need to reduce vacuum force is especially important with small-diameter PIV catheters, as the blood flows more turbulently and is exposed to greater mechanical friction. The use of smaller volume (e.g., 5-mL) Vacutainer® tubes may also reduce this risk [14, 15]. Fist-pumping, placement of the tourniquet too close to the puncture site, and failure to immediately invert the collection tube after drawing also increase the risk of specimen hemolysis.

Blood sample clotting is another common problem, especially with coagulation studies. Blood begins clotting the moment it first enters the needle, and prolonged blood draws can risk clotting of the blood before the specimen ever enters the collection tube. Drawn blood should be immediately injected into the collection tube, and the provider should immediately and adequately invert the collection tube. Samples should be sent to the laboratory as soon as possible after collection.

The *order of blood* draw must also be respected, whether the blood is obtained through a venous catheter or simple venipuncture. The correct order of draw is depicted in Table 3.3. Additives specific to each tube will differentiate their properties for laboratory processing. If one additive contaminates another one during the blood draw, the test may be rendered ineffective, and blood samples may need to be redrawn. For example, blue (sodium citrate) tubes are used for PT and PTT – it would not be ideal for this tube/test to be contaminated with either a clotting agent or a heparinizing agent.

Table 3.3 Vacutainer® tubes with corresponding labs, in correct order of draw

Order of Draw	Color Tube / Top	Additives	Common Tests*	Number of Inversions
1	Blood culture	N/A	Blood cultures	Invert gently to mix
2	Light Blue	Sodium citrate anticoagulant	D-dimer Factor assays Fibrinogen INR / PT/ PTT Lupus anticoagulant Special coagulation studies	3-4
3	Red Gold "Tiger top"(red and black speckled)	Clot activator (silicone-coated) Clot activator and gel for serum separation	Alcohol level Amylase / lipase Anticonvulsant levels Vitamin B12 / Folate Biochemistry profiles Cancer markers Cardiac markers Digoxin Hormone studies HCG (i.e., pregnancy test) Hepatic / Hepatitis panel Human Immunodeficiency Virus (HIV) Homocysteine (on ice) Insulin Iron studies Lidocaine level Lipid panel Lithium level Rheumatoid factor Salicylate level Thyroid studies Therapeutic drug levels Vitamin D	5
4	Light Green	Lithium heparin, with gel separator for plasma separation	Ammonia (on ice) Biochemistry profiles (STAT) Blood alcohol level Hepatic panel Ionized calcium Lipid Panels Renal function tests Rheumatoid factor Therapeutic drug levels (except Vancomycin) Toxicology tests Troponin	8-10
5	Dark Green	Lithium heparin, without separator (**not used often in acute settings**)	Similar to Light Green Lactic Acid (NOT on ice)	8-10

Table 3.3 (continued)

6		**Lavender / Purple**	Spray-coated K₂EDTA anticoagulant	Adrenocorticotropic hormone (ACTH) Brain Natriuretic Peptide (BNP) Complete Blood Count (CBC) w/differential CD3 / CD4 counts Cyclosporine Erythrocyte Sedimentation Rate (ESR) Factor V Leiden Hemoglobin & Hematocrit HgbA1C Parathyroid Hormone (PTH) RBC folate Reticulocyte count Thalassemia screening Vancomycin	8-10
7		**Pink**	K₂EDTA anticoagulant	Antibody screens Crossmatch Rhogam workup Type & Rh Type & Screen	8-10
8		**Gray**	Sodium fluorideand Potassium oxalate	Glucose Lactic acid (on ice)	8-10
9		**Royal / Navy Blue**	K₂EDTAanticoagulant	Aluminum Arsenic Cadmium Chromium Lead Manganese Mercury	8-10

Images courtesy of Becton, Dickinson and Company Inc. © 2020 Becton, Dickinson and Company Inc. All rights reserved
ªNote: list is not exhaustive and may vary between laboratories

Conclusions

Landmark-based peripheral IV catheter placement remains the "gold standard" for vascular access and should generally be the first type of vascular access attempted for most patients, including those presenting under emergent conditions. Insertion site selection should be informed by a general understanding of the usual human anatomy but also by the patient's specific clinical condition and therapeutic needs. Providers must balance the patient's anticipated therapeutic needs with the availability of peripheral veins for cannulation. A thorough examination is essential to proper site selection, including identification of certain risk factors for difficult or complicated vascular access. When accessing the peripheral veins for simple phlebotomy or for PIV placement, consider the patient's anticipated needs for care, including which medications or fluids may be needed to stabilize the patient.

Key Concepts

- Peripheral intravenous access is best obtained by "feel," not by sight. The provider can usually judge the location and depth of the vein by rebound following gentle direct pressure.
- The provider should use their heart, not just their head, when placing a peripheral IV catheter. They should have an appropriate level of confidence in their abilities, and not "overthink" the process.
- Providers should always place the tourniquet tightly. Even if it seems tight enough, it probably is not.
- Under emergent conditions, always use the largest gauge catheter that can be placed safely without additional risk of complications to the patient. Critically-ill patients often require large-bore vascular access, and it may be difficult to predict what medications and/or fluids may be needed for an undifferentiated and unstable patient.
- Catheters should be inserted from the proper angle, starting superficially. Providers can always "go deeper" if they did not hit the vessel the first time. It is much harder to salvage a vessel after injuring it by going too deep.
- Providers must take care to never obstruct their access to the insertion point with their own thumb or other objects. This will force the insertion angle to be too steep, and put the provider at increased risk of accidental needlestick injury.
- Providers should not reuse a needle once it has punctured the skin. Peripheral intravenous devices are "one poke only" devices and lose their sharpness after the initial puncture.
- When a patient is overly mobile, scared, or combative, providers should always bring a "buddy" to help secure and stabilize the insertion site. Holding the patient's hand, or gently restraining the patient's extremity, may reduce the risk of placement complications for both patient and provider.
- Providers should always exercise caution to avoid accidental blood exposure or self-injury.
- Prior to selecting the appropriate catheter insertion site, providers should fully examine the patient to identify dialysis fistulas/grafts, scar tissue, traumatic injuries, distortion of anatomic landmarks, and other anatomic features that may ultimately prove to be obstacles to placement success.

References

1. Hui YL, Wu YW. The blood pressure of upper and lower extremities in parturients under spinal anesthesia for caesarian section. Acta Anaesthesiol Sin. 1995;33(2):119–22.
2. Lambert JM, Lee M-S, Taller RA, Solomon DD. Medical grade tubing: criteria for catheter applications. J Vinyl Technol. 1991;13(4):204–7.

3. McKee JM, Shell JA, Warren TA, Campbell VP. Complications of intravenous therapy: a randomized prospective study – Vialon vs. Teflon. J Intraven Nurs. 1989;12(5):288–95.

4. Kus B, Buyukyilmaz F. Effectiveness of Vialon biomaterial versus Teflon catheters for peripheral intravenous placement: a randomized clinical trial. Jpn J Nurs Sci. 2020;17(3):e12328. https://doi.org/10.1111/jjns.12328. Epub 2020 Feb 20.

5. Hall JM, Roberts FL. An investigation into the reduction in flow rate of intravenous fluid by antireflux valves. Anesthesia. 2005;60:797–800.

6. Jayanthi NVG, Dabke HV. The effect of IV cannula length on the rate of infusion. Injury. 2006;37:41–5.

7. Reddick AD, Ronald J, Morrison WG. Intravenous fluid resuscitation: was Poiseuille right? Emerg Med J. 2011;28(3):201–2.

8. Smiths Medical [Internet]. Flow rate comparison for peripheral IV catheters – gravity. Cited 2020 June 9. Available from: https://www.smiths-medical.com/~/media/M/Smiths-medical_com/Files/Import%20Files/SS195393EN_112018.pdf.

9. Gorski LA, Hadaway L, Hagle M, McGoldrick M, Orr M, Doellman D. 2016 Infusion therapy standards of practice. J Infus Nurs. 2016;39(1 Suppl):S1–S159.

10. Nursing Made Incredibly Easy! [Internet] How fast should the drops drip? *Nursing made incredibly easy!* Lippincott Williams and Wilkin. 2004;2(4):60–62. Cited 2020 June 9. Available from: https://oce-ovid-com.proxy.lib.wayne.edu/article/00152258-200407000-00012/HTML.

11. American Cancer Society [Internet]. (2019). For people at risk of lymphedema. Cited 2020 June 9. Available from: https://www.cancer.org/treatment/treatments-and-side-effects/physical-side-effects/lymphedema/for-people-at-risk-of-lymphedema.html.

12. Segal M, Qaja E. Types of arteriovenous fistulas [Internet]. Treasure Island: StatPearls Publishing [Updated Feb 2020; cited 2020 June 9]. Available from: https://www.ncbi.nlm.nih.gov/books/NBK493195/.

13. Lippi G, Cervellin G, Mattiuzzi C. Critical review and meta-analysis of spurious hemolysis in blood samples collected from intravenous catheters. Biochem Med. 2013;23:193–200.

14. Cox SR, Dages JH, Jarjoura D, Hazelett S. Blood samples drawn from IV catheters have less hemolysis when 5-mL (vs 10-mL) collection tubes are used. J Emerg Nurs. 2004;30:529–33.

15. Petit N, Ziegler L, Goux A. Reduction of haemolysis rates using intravenous catheters with reduced capacity tubes. Ann Biol Clin (Paris). 2002;60(4):471–3.

Ultrasound-Guided Peripheral Intravenous Catheters

4

Mark J. Favot, Andrew J. Butki, and Eugene B. Rozen

Introduction

The use of ultrasound (US) technology has revolutionized emergent vascular access. Although the first published use of ultrasound-guided vascular access appeared in 1984, pertaining to cannulation of the internal jugular vein, this approach has become increasingly popular over the last four decades [1]. In the 1990s, multiple studies showed increased success rates and reduced procedural time and complication rates with the use of ultrasound for central venous catheter (CVC) placement [2]. This led to the 2001 endorsement of US-guided CVC placement by the US Department of Health and Human Services (HHS) Agency for Healthcare Research and Quality (AHRQ) as *one of the 11 best evidence-based practices that healthcare providers can use to improve patient care and patient safety* [3]. Since that time, the use of dynamic US guidance has become the standard of care for CVC placement [4–5].

Given the apparent benefits of US guidance for CVC placement, this technology has gained increasing attention as a means of improving peripheral intravenous (PIV) catheter placement success in patients with difficult peripheral venous access. Over the last two decades, numerous studies have shown that ultrasound-guided peripheral intravenous (US-PIV) catheter placement is an invaluable technique in the emergency department (ED) and intensive care unit (ICU) for patients who have failed traditional cannulation attempts or are anticipated to have difficult venous access [6].

Electronic Supplementary Material The online version of this chapter (https://doi.org/10.1007/978-3-030-77177-5_4) contains supplementary material, which is available to authorized users.

M. J. Favot (✉) · E. B. Rozen
Department of Emergency Medicine, Wayne State University School of Medicine, Detroit, MI, USA
e-mail: mfavot@med.wayne.edu; erozen@med.wayne.edu

A. J. Butki
Department of Emergency Medicine, Ascension Michigan St. John Hospital, Detroit, MI, USA

Department of Emergency Medicine, McLaren Oakland Hospital, Pontiac, MI, USA

© Springer Nature Switzerland AG 2021
J. H. Paxton (ed.), *Emergent Vascular Access*,
https://doi.org/10.1007/978-3-030-77177-5_4

Among patients with difficult venous access (DVA), ultrasound guidance has been shown to be superior to "blind" cannulation. In head-to-head comparisons, US-PIV placement is associated with *improved success rates over traditional "blind" insertion*, decreasing the time to successful cannulation and reducing the number of required puncture attempts [7–8]. Patient satisfaction scores also appear to be higher with US-PIV catheter placement than with traditional landmark-based techniques [9].

Patients with DVA pose a special challenge to healthcare providers, although as many as 23% of ED patients meet formal criteria for DVA [10]. Prior to the availability of US guidance for PIV catheter insertion, patients with DVA could routinely expect numerous failed attempts at PIV catheter placement, or even the placement of a CVC merely to establish routine venous access. Considering the additional risks introduced by CVC placement, including iatrogenic pneumothorax and central line-associated bloodstream infection (CLABSI), emergency providers have welcomed US-PIV catheter placement as a means of avoiding unnecessary CVC placement. Over the last decade, several studies have concluded that the need for CVC placement can be obviated in up to 80% of patients with DVA with US-PIV placement techniques [9, 11–13].

The widespread adoption of dynamic ultrasound guidance has been one of the most significant advancements in vascular access so far in the twenty-first century. While not all emergent patients require US-PIV, this technique can be readily learned by novice users and is an essential skill in the armamentarium of any emergency care provider [14].

Indications for US-PIV Insertion

Prompt establishment of adequate vascular access is of paramount importance in the emergent management of unstable or critically ill patients. The use of US-PIV placement is especially advantageous when such timely venous access is not available through traditional landmark-based techniques, either because these techniques have already failed or because they are expected to fail. Patients with known DVA risk factors (e.g., children, hypovolemic patients, diabetics, those with a history of IV drug use and sickle cell disease, etc.) or a personal history of DVA are most likely to benefit from US-PIV catheterization [10, 15]. However, patients with readily available peripheral veins should still have landmark-based PIV catheter insertion attempted prior to the use of US guidance. If a target vein is superficial enough to be palpated, US guidance may decrease the likelihood of successful cannulation [16].

Contraindications and Complications

There are very few valid contraindications for US-PIV catheter insertion, other than the usual contraindications for vascular access device (VAD) deployment at a targeted site, such as infection at the insertion site, trauma, or patient refusal. It is important to note that ultrasound-guided venous access is only recommended for accessing deeper veins, such as the basilic and cephalic veins of the upper extremity. Of course, lack of an available US device may also limit the utility of this technique, and patient agitation or inability to maintain control over the insertion site due to excessive patient movement or lack of cooperation from the patient may also increase the risk/benefit ratio. In all cases, the risks of US-PIV catheterization should be weighed against the potential benefits.

The complications of US-PIV catheterization include those risks common to all VAD placement, but certain risks are more prominent with US-PIV placement than with landmark-based approaches. Most of these additional risks relate to the fact that US-PIV is typically used to cannulate veins *deep to the skin surface*. Although venous injury and extravasation may be seen with any PIV catheter insertion, catheter dislodgement may not be as quickly apparent when the deep veins are involved. Delayed identification of extravasation may allow medication, intravenous fluids, or contrast agents to extravasate to a larger degree before the extravasation is noted by the provider [17]. This may increase the risk of complications due to extravasation. Furthermore, ultrasound allows visualization and access to deep vessels that may be adjacent to vulnerable structures, such as the *brachial vein* which runs adjacent to the *brachial artery* and *median nerve*. Attempts at cannulation of these deep veins may be more likely to cause inadvertent iatrogenic arterial puncture or nerve injury [7].

The *risk of infection* may also be theoretically greater with US-PIV catheter insertion than with superficial venous cannulation, as bacterial contamination could be introduced by the ultrasound probe or other components of the US system. It is speculated that pathogens may be harbored on the probe in the interface between the plastic transducer cover and the rubber acoustic window, as this junction cannot be terminally cleaned without specialized equipment. This risk remains theoretical, however, as there has not been any communicable disease transmission attributed to the use of an ultrasound probe to date.

Although peripheral venipuncture is considered a "clean" procedure, and does not require full sterile precautions nor mandatory use of a sterile sheath [7], there are several ways to reduce the potential for disease transmission. We recommend that providers *fully cleanse the probe and cord with a germicidal wipe after each use*. A commercially available probe cover or a disposable film barrier (e.g., Tegaderm™ dressing) should also be placed over the probe (after application of a thin layer of US gel to the probe) prior to venipuncture as an additional level of protection. The use of non-sterile US gel is sufficient for pre-scanning and identifying a suitable target vessel. However, sterile gel (i.e., sterile surgical jelly) should be used during the actual venipuncture procedure itself. The proper application of gel and transparent dressing is illustrated in Fig. 4.1.

The Ideal Vein for US-PIV Cannulation

We suggest that the ideal vein for US-PIV placement is moderately superficial and as large as possible, with a straight path and minimal surrounding or overlying vital structures such as nerves, arteries, or tendons. However, if a vein is superficial enough to be palpated, the use of ultrasound will decrease the likelihood of

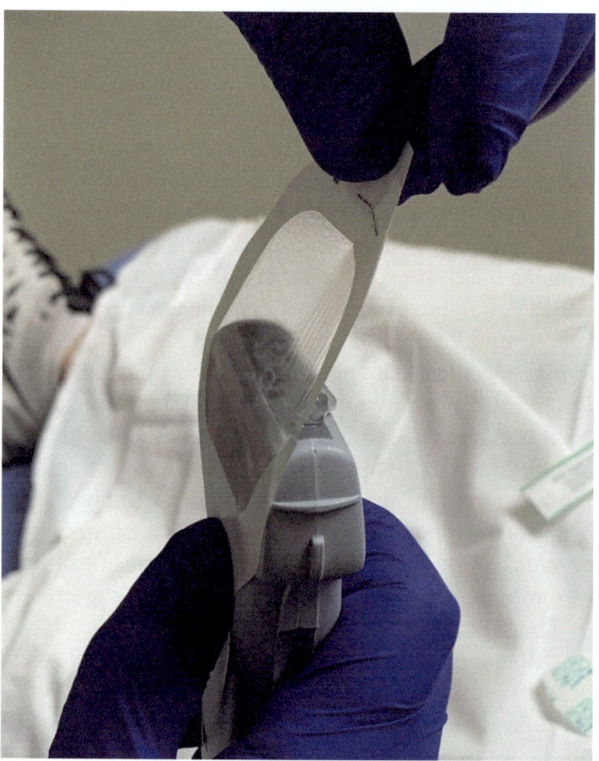

Fig. 4.1 Placement of a transparent film dressing over a linear ultrasound probe

successful cannulation [16]. The course that a vein takes proximally may be unpredictable, so it should be imaged on US prior to attempts at cannulation, to look for branch points, clots, or other anatomical features that may complicate US-PIV catheter placement. These features should be considered when selecting the proper site for targeted insertion.

Common Target Veins for US-PIV Cannulation

The Forearm

The veins of the forearm are abundant and often a good place to begin looking for a vein. Forearm veins tend to be linear, are not located over joints, and are typically superficial. The *cephalic vein* travels along the lateral (radial) side of the wrist, forearm, and arm. It is typically unaccompanied by arteries or nerves. The *radial veins* (*venae comitantes*) are smaller paired veins that usually course through the forearm alongside the radial artery and sometimes adjacent to the radial nerve. The *cubital vein* is often readily palpable for landmark-based insertion but tends to be superficial and may be challenging with US guidance due to the acuity of the angle that the vein makes at the elbow. It may also be more uncomfortable for patients because of its location over the elbow joint. The *basilic vein* is another large vein often unaccompanied by arteries or nerves. Because of its location in the medial forearm, proper positioning of the patient may be a challenge.

The Upper Arm

The veins of the upper arm are essentially continuations of the forearm veins but are typically deeper to the skin surface at this level. As such, they may be more difficult to cannulate and may be more prone to catheter dislodgement [7]. The *cephalic vein*, as in the forearm, is located on the lateral side of the upper arm within the subcutaneous tissue (Fig. 4.2). Although this is an excellent vessel for US-PIV catheterization, it may not be present in all people. This vein continues from the upper arm into the deltopectoral groove and is often used for placement of pacemakers or hemodialysis fistulas. The *brachial vein* and *basilic vein* are usually located on the medial surface of the arm (Fig. 4.3). The median and ulnar nerves are typically found in the same region and should be identified and avoided during the US-PIV cannulation attempt. The brachial vein courses deep to the brachial fascia, and this fascial layer may disguise extravasation from the vein. Caution should be used when selecting this vessel, to reduce the risk of complications.

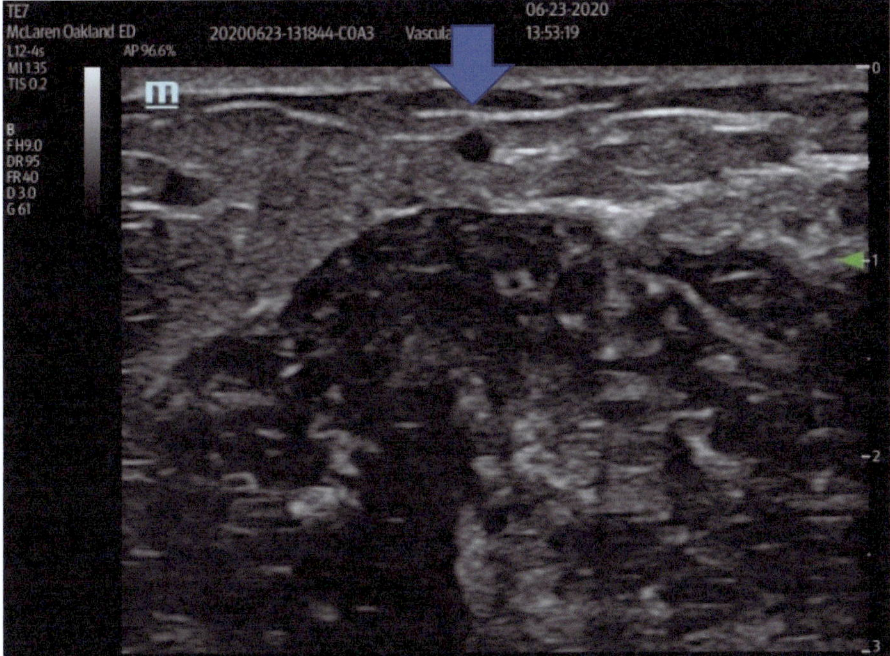

Fig. 4.2 Cephalic vein in superficial tissue lateral to the biceps muscle (blue arrow)

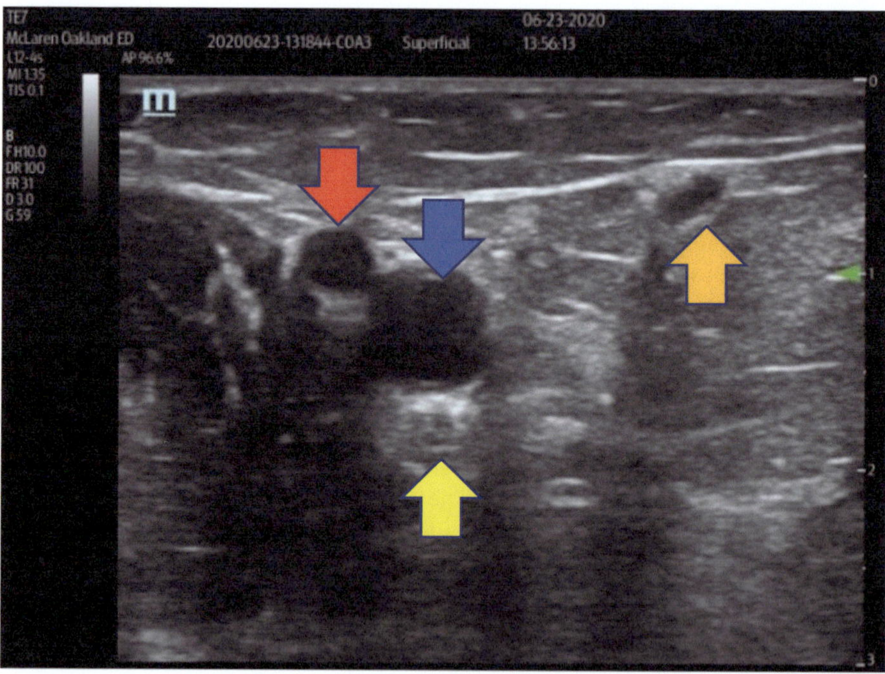

Fig. 4.3 Brachial artery (red arrow), brachial vein (blue arrow), and median nerve (yellow arrow) medial to the biceps muscle. Basilic vein (orange arrow) medial to these in the superficial tissue

The External Jugular Vein

The *external jugular (EJ) vein* is a traditional site for cannulation in patients with otherwise difficult IV access. In patients with obesity, scarring, or thin veins, this may also be a difficult vein to cannulate. It is important to distinguish the EJ vein from the *internal jugular (IJ) vein* during cannulation attempts. The IJ vein is located deep to the *sternocleidomastoid muscle*, while the EJ vein remains superficial to it.

Equipment

In general, the equipment needed for US-PIV placement is no different than that needed for landmark PIV insertion, although a longer (e.g., 48-mm versus standard 30-mm) PIV catheter should be used (Fig. 4.4). Catheters used in ultrasound lines are the same as ordinary PIV catheters but are sometimes referred to as "ultrasound catheters" because of their extended length. Despite this, long catheters do not have any features or any differences that would make them easier to visualize. When using these long catheters for ultrasound-guided PIVs, it is recommended to use

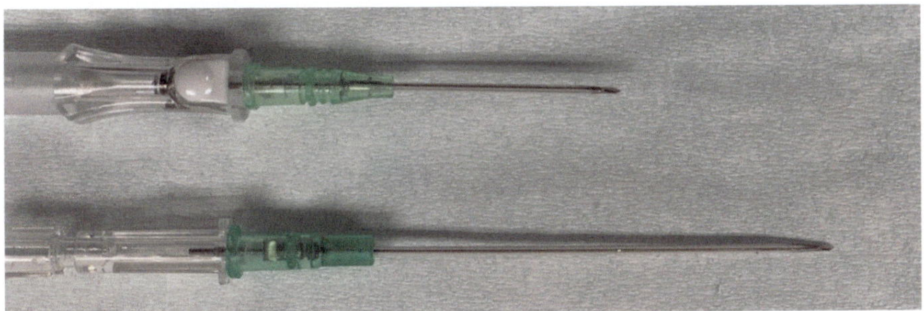

Fig. 4.4 Comparison of 30-mm (short) and 48-mm (long) 18-gauge peripheral intravenous catheters

nothing thinner than an 18-gauge or 20-gauge catheter. The extra catheter length increases the resistance to flow, so larger catheter gauges are preferred [17].

The 30-mm long IV catheters commonly used by nursing for PIVs are typically too short and should rarely be used for US-PIV placement. Deep US-PIV placement usually requires a 48-mm catheter, at a minimum. We recommend that *at least 50% of the length of the catheter should reside inside the lumen of the vein* to secure successful placement of the IV. This is especially true in situations where the contents of the IV are under high pressure, such as during CT angiography or when a pressure bag is used to increase flow rates [18–19]. One recent study on US-PIVs found that 100% of PIVs placed with <30% of the catheter residing in the vein failed within 72 hours, 32% failed when 30–60% of the catheter was in the vein, and no PIV attempts failed when >65% of the catheter was in the vein [18].

Target vessels for US-PIV insertion are often up to 15-mm deep to the skin surface. Even with a steep insertion angle of 45 degrees, the Pythagorean theorem ($c^2 = a^2 + b^2$) suggests that at least 21 mm of catheter will remain subcutaneous en route to a 15-mm deep vessel, with only the terminal 9 mm of the PIV catheter situated within the target vein. If a traditional 30-mm PIV catheter is used, this 9 mm of catheter that is intravascular does not achieve the 50% required to reliably secure the IV. Additionally, the use of ultrasound guidance tends to favor shallower angles of insertion much less than 45 degrees (since ultrasound visibility decreases with steeper angles). This shallower angle will further increase the amount of catheter that remains subcutaneous. Thus, longer catheters are required, and a 48-mm or longer catheter is universally recommended for US-PIV placement, regardless of the depth of vessel. Figure 4.5 compares a standard (30-mm) to a long (48-mm) PIV catheter placement in a hypothetical vein that is 15-mm deep to the skin surface. In this example, $a = b = 15$-mm and $c = 21$-mm.

A *tourniquet should always be used* when placing US-PIV catheters to improve targeting of difficult-to-visualize veins. Sterile technique is not required for peripheral IV placement [7]; however sterile gel (either dedicated ultrasonic coupling gel or sterile surgical lubricant) and a probe barrier are recommended.

There are a few options available when selecting a probe barrier. Dedicated sterile probes and semi-permeable adhesive barriers are made by various

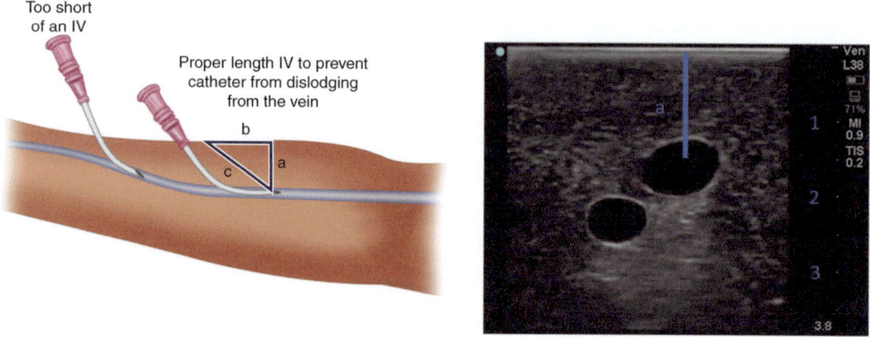

Fig. 4.5 Comparison of standard (30-mm) and long (48-mm) PIV catheter in target vein

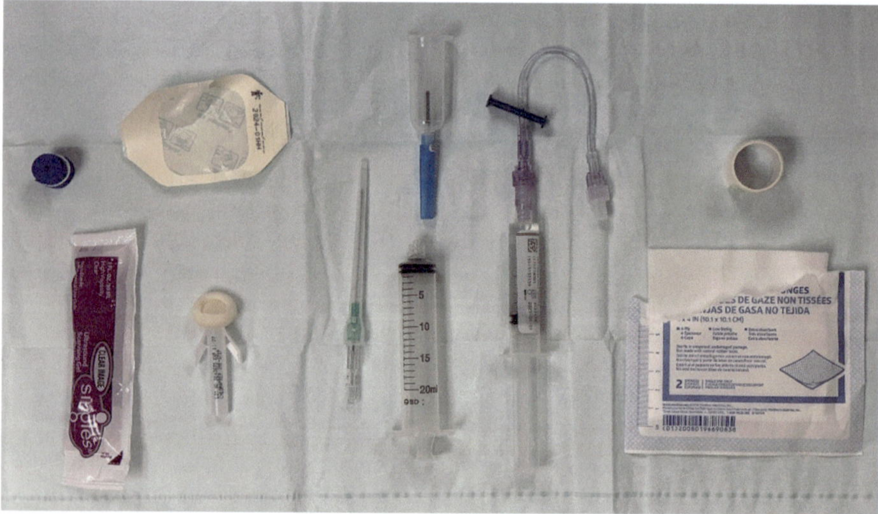

Fig. 4.6 Typical setup for US-PIV, including tourniquet, antiseptic solution, sterile gel, film dressing, gauze, and 48-mm or longer PIV catheter

manufacturers. Little evidence exists on which barrier is best or to what extent they control the spread of infection, but best practice is to use some sort of barrier [7].

The use of gel can make the IV insertion site messy, and it is recommended that this extra gel is removed so that the remaining gel does not interfere with adhesives used to secure the catheter (Fig. 4.6).

Because the US probe will be coursing over an area of skin larger than just the insertion site, a larger area of skin needs to be disinfected prior to beginning the procedure. Following IV placement, the ultrasound probe should be cleansed thoroughly.

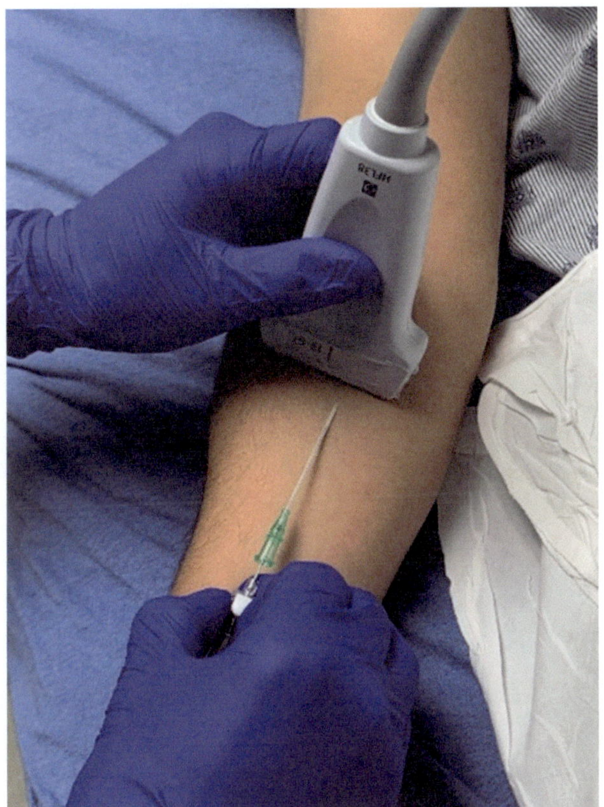

Fig. 4.7 Out-of-plane technique

Technique

A *linear probe* is best used for visualizing both vessels and the needle. A higher frequency setting is preferred to increase spatial resolution of superficial structures. Depth should be set *no deeper than about 3 cm*, as veins deeper than this will have a higher chance of failure. The use of color Doppler US can help identify veins and differentiate them from arteries. It can also help assess for the presence of thrombosis.

The two most common techniques for US-PIV are the *"out-of-plane"* technique (Fig. 4.7) and the *"in-plane"* technique (Fig. 4.10). Consensus has not been established regarding which technique is preferred. The decision to use one or the other of these techniques likely depends upon the provider's previous ultrasound experience and personal preference. With both techniques, the probe is held in the non-dominant hand, and the dominant hand is used for needle insertion. Once the cannula is deployed, the ultrasound probe is set down and the PIV is secured using both hands.

The *out-of-plane (short-axis) approach* involves visualizing a "cross-sectional" slice of vein and needle and making incremental alternating movements of the probe and then the needle until the needle is secure in the vein, at which point the cannula is deployed and the needle is removed. This technique is incredibly powerful, as it

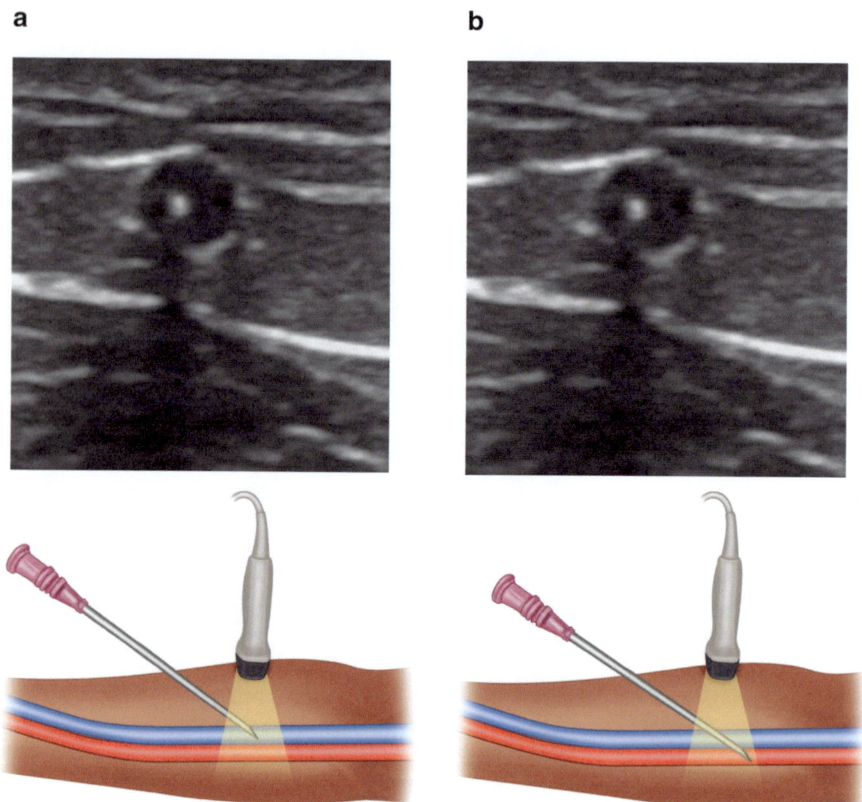

Fig. 4.8 Comparison of different needle cross sections using ultrasound imaging

allows easy visualization of the target vessel and the surrounding anatomy. Identifying the tip of the needle can pose a challenge. However, this can be mitigated by utilizing the following methods which can reliably cannulate even the most challenging of patients with a little practice.

The central concept to consider is that *all parts of the needle look identical in cross section*. This is important to consider because one may visualize the needle and be surprised to learn they are observing the mid-shaft of the needle, and the needle tip is much deeper into potentially dangerous anatomy, as illustrated in Fig. 4.8. Again, all parts of the needle look identical in cross section, so it is key to practice a technique that allows you to identify the *tip* of the needle.

Finding the tip of the needle is facilitated by one simple adjustment to technique: keep the plane of imaging one step ahead of the needle. When utilizing this technique, start by inserting the needle just underneath the skin. Then identify the needle in cross section and follow along down the length of the needle with the ultrasound probe, advancing the imaging plane just until you lose sight of the needle – and then stop. You have identified the tip of the needle and are now just in front of it. Now, advance the *needle* by a tiny amount (about 1-mm) until you visualize the needle in

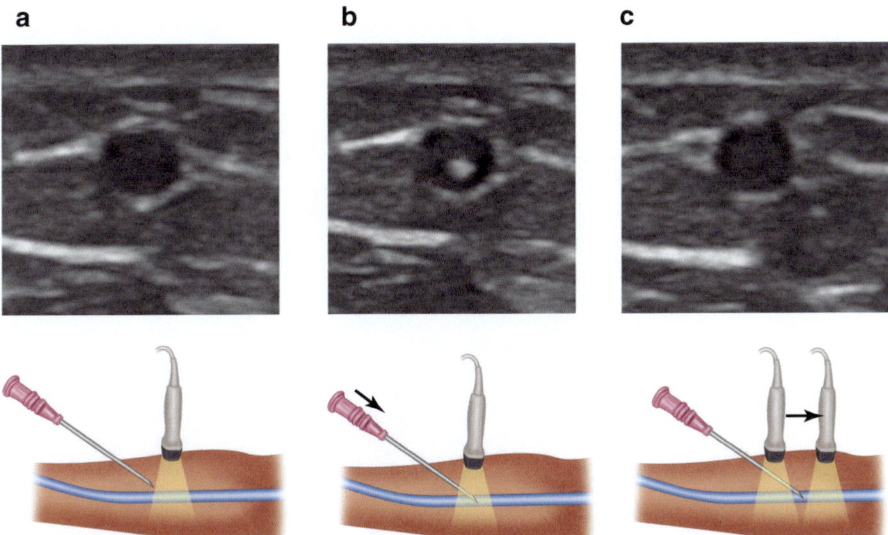

Fig. 4.9 Alternate incremental movements, keeping the imaging plane just in front of the needle, ensure visualization of the needle tip

your imaging plane, and stop. Repeat the process of advancing your imaging plane just until you lose sight of the needle, and then advance the needle until it comes into view again, as depicted in Fig. 4.9 until the needle is centered in the vessel. Once the vein is cannulated, you may flatten your angle of insertion and continue advancing in this alternating fashion up the vessel either until the hub is buried or until you are comfortable sliding the catheter in the remainder of its length. In Fig. 4.9, image "a" shows a needle just above a vein and an ultrasound transducer imaging a cross section of the needle and vein. Image "b" shows the needle advanced slightly, until it encounters the ultrasound plane. Image "c" shows the ultrasound plane advanced slightly until it no longer shows the needle in the ultrasound image. This can be done sequentially until the center of the vessel is successfully cannulated. This is a very useful skill to master. It may seem counterintuitive, at first, to consider that the target image is the area *in front* of the needle path and not focused on the needle itself. This is necessary to ensure that the correct part of the needle (the needle tip) is identified and guided, rather than some other unknown portion of the needle.

The *"in-plane" (long-axis) approach* utilizes a longitudinal section of the vein and offers full visualization of the needle (Fig. 4.10). Aside from minor adjustments to the position of the probe to help visualization, the probe is not moved during this procedure. This method provides improved needle visualization but may present difficulties following tortuous vessels or differentiating veins from arteries.

It is often difficult to keep all three planes (the probe, the needle, and the vein) perfectly co-planar throughout the entire procedure as the needle is advanced. Any amount of stray in one of these results in incomplete visualization. The technique does not require the abovementioned alternating movements to identify the needle

Fig. 4.10 In-plane technique

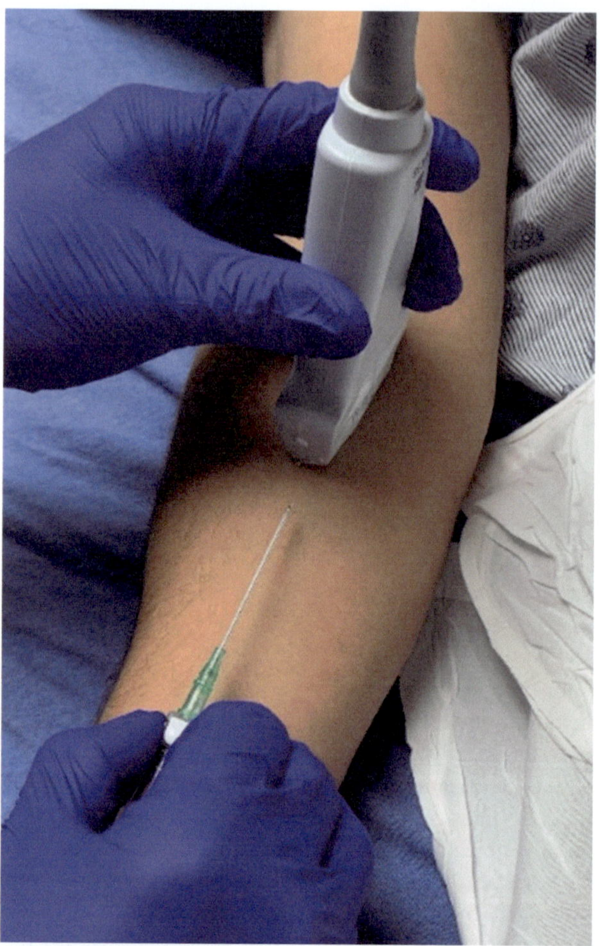

Fig. 4.11 In-plane technique, with the needle (blue arrow) in vessel

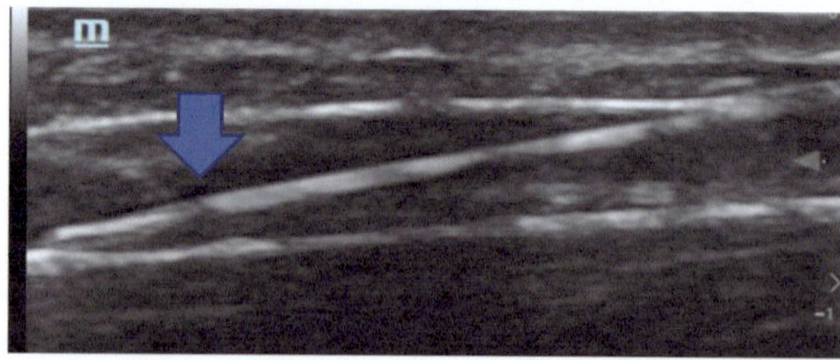

tip, as the entire needle shaft is visualized simultaneously. The in-plane approach can be useful for patients with very straight vessels and no nearby or adjacent arteries or nerves (Fig. 4.11).

Positioning

For operator ease, the best way to prepare for any US-guided procedure, including PIV placement, is to have the procedural field in a straight line between the operator and the US screen, so that the clinician does not have to move their body around during the procedure (Fig. 4.12). This may necessitate the US machine being placed on the opposite side of the patient. The height of the bed and US machine should be placed in such a way that the procedure can be done while sitting or standing comfortably. Any items that will be needed should be placed within reach of the operator's dominant hand.

The patient should also be positioned so that they are comfortable, and this position varies depending on what site is being accessed. For US-PIV access in the forearm, the patient should have their elbow extended and either supinated or pronated. They may be seated, supine, or somewhere in between. If a medial arm vein (e.g., the basilic vein) is being cannulated, the patient should have their upper extremity abducted and externally rotated (Fig. 4.13). Their elbow may be partially flexed for better access to the procedure site. This is easier to achieve if the patient is supine.

Fig. 4.12 Optimal room setup for US-PIV insertion

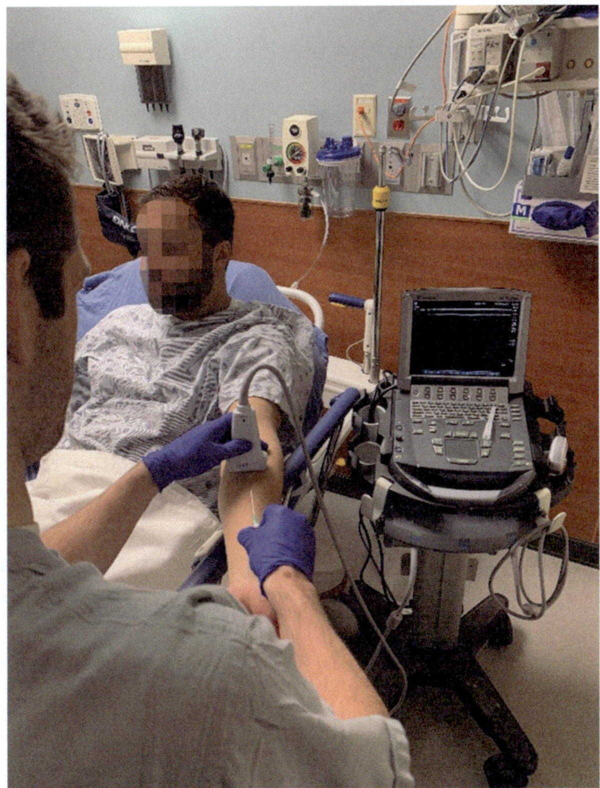

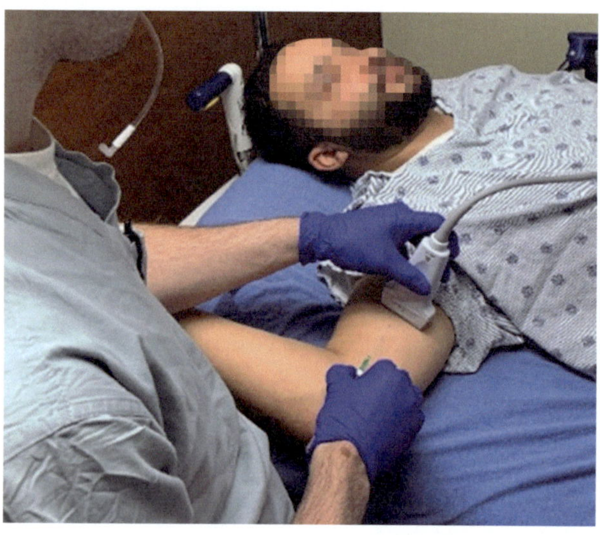

Fig. 4.13 Patient positioning to access the basilic vein

Common Pitfalls

Arterial cannulation is a possible complication of US-PIV placement. Ultrasound can help distinguish arteries from veins in many ways. Pulsatility is the easiest and most readily available of these. *With light pressure, veins will collapse and arteries will pulsate*. Although there may be some ambiguity in peripheral vascular disease or in hypotensive states, this technique should be used in all cases.

As described above, vessel distribution follows a predictable format. One common anatomical formation is that of a central artery flanked by a vein on each side (Fig. 4.14). In this scenario, care should be taken to ensure that the artery is not cannulated. Color flow Doppler can be used to identify the constant low velocity flow in veins or a pulsatile and higher velocity flow in adjacent arteries. Wall thickness also differs between veins and arteries. Arteries often appear double-walled in larger vessels or thicker-walled in smaller ones. *Veins will have thinner walls than nearby arteries.*

Bright red blood color and drawback pulsatility may suggest arterial cannulation. Although these signs may be helpful, they are only detectable after the vessel has been cannulated and can be unreliable depending upon various patient or disease factors. If the artery has been inadvertently cannulated, remove the catheter and hold direct pressure for 15 minutes. Do not attempt venous cannulation in the same area if arterial cannulation is suspected.

In addition to arteries, in the forearm there are three nerves to be avoided: the *radial*, *median*, and *ulnar nerves*. They are all located in the volar half of the forearm and are distributed laterally to medially. These nerves are typically deep to the forearm veins and may not present a problem, but knowledge of their anatomy and typical appearance may help to avoid this complication. In the medial arm, nerves may be located superficial to the target veins and should be carefully investigated.

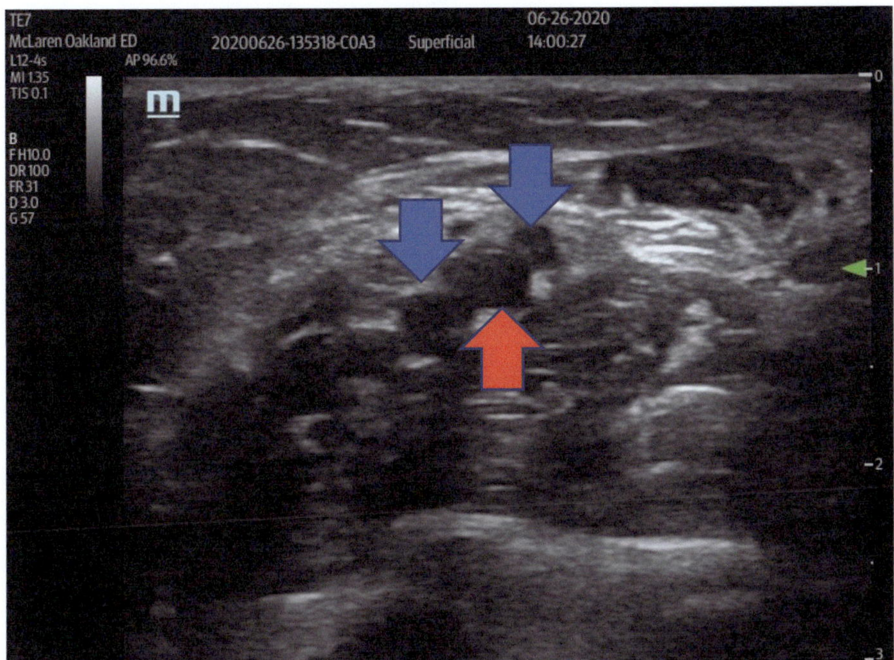

Fig. 4.14   Brachial artery (red arrow) with brachial veins (blue arrows) on both sides

Nerves and tendons display a sonographic feature termed "*anisotropy*," in which they gain or lose echogenicity depending upon their angle to the probe. Tilting the probe back and forth can help to identify these structures, both of which appear hyperechoic (i.e., brighter than the surrounding tissues) when viewed in a plane perpendicular to the plane of the probe.

Both nerves and tendons are discrete hyperechoic structures, so they will appear "brighter" than blood vessels. If such structures are encountered in attempting to locate a vein, they should be avoided (Fig. 4.14). These structures may change position in relation to the vein in a distal or proximal position. The medial arm has many nerves that can overlie veins and should be examined closely before selecting a vein.

Another pitfall is failure to assess or recognize *vein thrombosis*. Thrombosis may be apparent when looking at the vein in B-mode (i.e., regular grayscale), as the venous lumen may appear to have an associated density rather than being anechoic (Fig. 4.15); however, this is not always the case. Figure 4.16 demonstrates a thrombosed basilic vein that appears normal at first glance but does not compress, even with enough pressure to compress the much deeper brachial vein. Thrombosis can be confirmed with lack of compressibility when applying pressure with the probe or by lack of color flow when using Doppler imaging (Fig. 4.13). If using the Doppler method, the probe should be tilted, because flow may not be detectable when the probe is fully perpendicular to the direction of flow (Fig. 4.17).

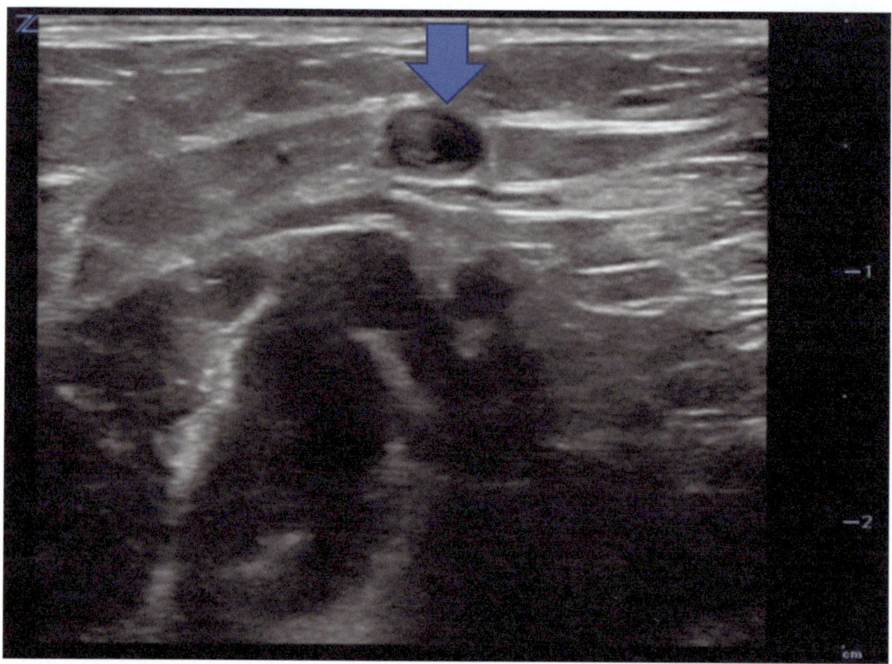

Fig. 4.15 Basilic vein thrombus (blue arrow)

Fig. 4.16 Occult basilic vein thrombus (blue arrow), with deeper brachial vein compression

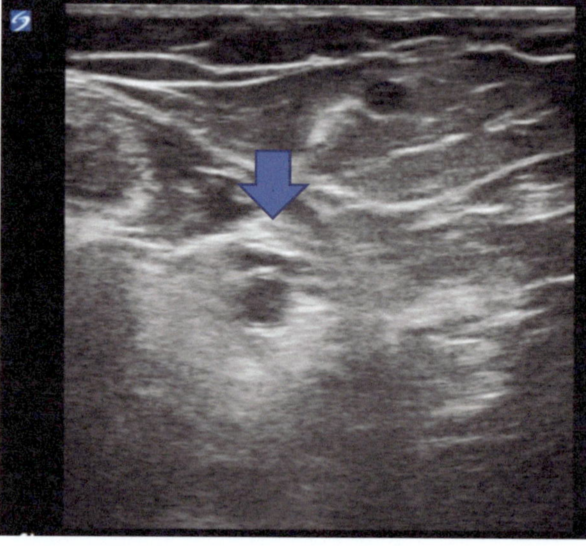

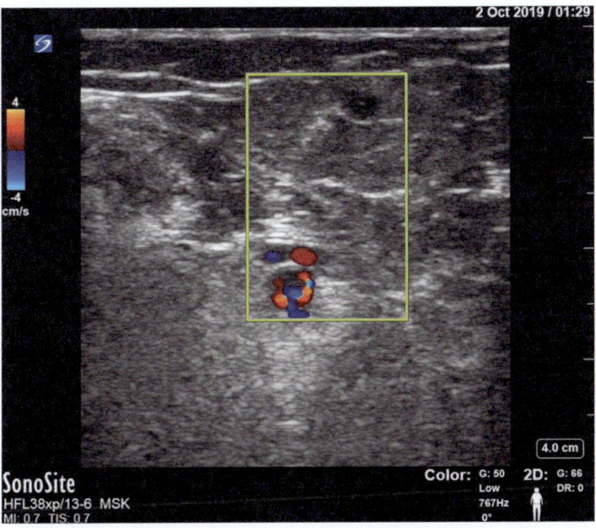

Fig. 4.17 Occult basilic vein thrombus, with Doppler color flow noted in the deeper brachial artery and vein but absent in the basilic vein

There are certain pitfalls that are unique to the veins of the upper arm. The *cephalic vein* is in many ways ideal for US-PIVs when present, but it possesses a high degree of variability in the population. The *basilic vein* is usually reliably identifiable, but it is inconvenient to access as it is on the medial upper arm. The *brachial vein* is more dangerous to cannulate as it lies in approximation to the median nerve and the brachial artery. It also lies underneath an additional fascial layer, so any inadvertent extravasation is less likely to be noticed in a timely fashion.

Conclusions

Ultrasound guidance for peripheral IV insertion is an important technique, which must be familiar to providers of emergent vascular access. Visualization of the deeper veins and nearby vital structures (e.g., arteries, nerves, tendons) allows the provider to avoid iatrogenic complications and more easily identify the target insertion site. However, this technique does have limitations and is not recommended when the vein is superficial enough to palpate. Failure of US-PIV placement is often due to correctable factors, including inadequate catheter length, improper site selection, and lack of adequate training. Before attempting US-PIV access, it is important that the provider consider whether an US-PIV is required and adequately assess the patient's anatomy to identify obstacles to successful cannulation.

Key Points

- US-PIV is associated with improved time to cannulation, higher first-pass success, and increased patient satisfaction over standard landmark techniques in patients with difficult vascular access.
- Catheter dislodgement and extravasation occur more frequently with US-PIV placement than with "blind" PIV insertion, due to the deeper locations of the vessels. This also makes these complications more difficult to identify.
- Ideal target vessel is somewhat superficial (0.5–1 cm deep), straight, and larger in diameter. When such a vessel does not exist, do an adequate pre-scan of both arms to find the most appropriate target.
- Short-axis (out-of-plane) technique is more easily learned than the long-axis (in-plane) technique and is recommended for beginners.
- Diligence is required to ensure you are visualizing the needle tip and not some more proximal point along the needle during the procedure. Advance the needle 1–2 mm at a time, and then advance the probe to the point where the needle disappears on the screen to find the tip.
- Puncture of the posterior wall or failure to advance the catheter into the lumen of the vessel are the most common technical reasons for failure. "Walking" as much of the full length of the catheter into the vessel while continuing to visualize the needle tip will help avoid these scenarios.

References

1. Pandurangadu AV, Tucker J. Ultrasound-guided intravenous catheter survival impacted by the amount of catheter residing in the vein. Emerg Med J. 2018;35:550–5.
2. Legler D, Nugent M. Doppler localization of the internal jugular vein facilitates central venous cannulation. Anesthesiology. 1984;60(5):481–2.
3. Randolph AG, Cook DJ, Gonzales CA, Pribble CG. Ultrasound guidance for placement of central venous catheters: a meta-analysis of the literature. Crit Care Med. 1996;24(12):2053–8.
4. Rothschild JM. Ultrasound guidance of central vein catheterization. On making health care safer: a critical analysis of patient safety practices. Rockville: AHRQ Publications, 2001. Chapter 21, pp. 245–255.
5. Gurney S, Paul R, Price S. Central venous cannulation. Medicine. 2018;46(8):494–5.
6. American Institute of Ultrasound Medicine. AIUM practice parameters for the use of ultrasound to guide vascular access procedures. J Ultrasound Med. 2012;38:E4–E18.
7. Feller-Kopman D. Ultrasound-guided internal jugular access: a proposed standardized approach and implications for training and practice. Chest. 2007;132(1):302–9.
8. Gottlieb M, et al. Ultrasound-guided peripheral intravenous line placement: a narrative review of evidence based best practices. West J Emerg Med. 2017;18(6):1047–54.
9. Bagley WH. Focus on: dynamic ultrasound-guided peripheral intravenous line placement. *ACEP Now* magazine. [Internet] 2009. Cited 20 June 2020. Available from: https://www.acep-now.com/article/dynamic-ultrasound-guided-peripheral-intravenous-line-placement/.

10. Shoenfield E, Shokoohi H, Boniface K. Ultrasound-guided peripheral intravenous access in the emergency department: a patient-centered survey. West J Emerg Med. 2011;12(4):475–7.
11. Fields JM, Piela NE, Au AK. Risk factors associated with difficult venous access in adult ED patients. Am J Emerg Med. 2014;32(10):1179–82.
12. Dargin JM, Rebholz CM, Lowenstein RA. Ultrasonography-guided peripheral intravenous catheter survival in ED patients with difficult access. Am J Emerg Med. 2010;28(1):1–7.
13. Au AK, Rotte MJ, Grzybowski RJ. Decrease in central venous catheter placement due to use of ultrasound guidance for peripheral intravenous catheters. Am J Emerg Med. 2012;30(9):1950–4.
14. Shokoohi H, Boniface K, McCarthy M. Ultrasound-guided peripheral intravenous access program is associated with a marked reduction in central venous catheter use in noncritically ill emergency department patients. Ann Emerg Med. 2013;61(2):198–203.
15. Duran-Gehring P, Bryant L, Reynolds JA. Ultrasound-guided peripheral intravenous catheter training results in physician-level success for emergency department technicians. J Ultrasound Med. 2016;35(11):2343–52.
16. Rose JS, Norbutas CM. A randomized controlled trial comparing one-operator versus two-operator technique in ultrasound-guided basilic vein cannulation. J Emerg Med. 2008;35(4):431–5.
17. Brannam L, Blaivas M, Lyon M. Emergency nurses' utilization of ultrasound guidance for placement of peripheral intravenous lines in difficult-access patients. Acad Emerg Med. 2004;11(12):1361–3.
18. Witting MD, et al. Effects of vein width and depth on ultrasound-guided peripheral intravenous success rates. J Emerg Med. 2010;39(1):70–5.
19. Rupp J, Ferre R, Boyd J, Dearing E. Extravasation risk using ultrasound guided peripheral intravenous catheters for computed tomography contrast administration. Acad Emerg Med. 2016;23(8):918–21.

Landmark-Based Central Venous Catheters

James H. Paxton, James G. Chirackal, and Kinza Ijaz

The History of Central Venous Cannulation

The year 1667 was a very good year in the history of emergent vascular access. In that same year, two major breakthroughs occurred: Major's performance of the first intravenous injection into a live human and Lower's use of the first vascular catheter (composed of silver pipes connected by a quill) to perform a transfer of blood from the carotid artery of a sheep into the external jugular vein of a live human [1].

Aside from these early efforts, the first modern central venous catheterization is believed to have occurred in July 1929, during a bold experiment by Werner Forssmann, a surgical resident at the Augusta Viktoria Hospital, in Eberswalde, Germany. Although he was only 25 years old and had just passed his qualifying medical exams earlier that year, Forssmann devised a plan to prove his theory that medications could be administered directly into the heart through cannulation of the peripheral veins without risk to the patient [2]. His theory had initially been posited on the notion of cannulating the jugular vein of a horse, with the intention of using the catheter to measure intracardiac pressures [3]. In his zeal to advance this theory, he opted instead to perform the high-risk procedure on himself. After locally anesthetizing his own arm, with assistance from an operating room nurse, he inserted a 4-French 65-cm-long urinary catheter into his own left antecubital vein, advancing it into the right auricle of the heart before obtaining fluoroscopic evidence to prove

J. H. Paxton (✉)
Department of Emergency Medicine, Wayne State University School of Medicine, Detroit, MI, USA
e-mail: james.paxton@wayne.edu

J. G. Chirackal
Michigan State University College of Human Medicine, East Lansing, MI, USA
e-mail: chiracka@msu.edu

K. Ijaz
Department of Internal Medicine, Detroit Medical Center, Detroit, MI, USA
e-mail: KIjaz@dmc.org

© Springer Nature Switzerland AG 2021
J. H. Paxton (ed.), *Emergent Vascular Access*,
https://doi.org/10.1007/978-3-030-77177-5_5

the feat [4]. A few years later, Forssmann introduced the notion of cannulating the femoral vein as a means of depositing medications into the inferior vena cava (IVC) for the management of cardiac arrest [3]. Unfortunately, Forssmann retired from the field of vascular access research in the mid-1930s, electing instead to pursue a career in urology [5].

Besides earning him a partial share in the 1956 *Nobel Prize in Medicine or Physiology*, Forssmann's experiment dispelled concerns about the potential risks of arrhythmia and cardiovascular injury previously felt to be unavoidable with central venous access. Subsequent generations of clinical scientists advanced Forssmann's technique, including Andre Counard and Dickinson Richards of Columbia University, who built upon his findings to develop the earliest techniques for diagnostic cardiac catheterization. These scientists ultimately shared in Forssmann's *Nobel Prize* [4]. By the early 1950s, mass-produced polyethylene central venous catheters had become commercially available, and subsequent researchers over the next two decades described methods by which the subclavian and internal jugular veins could be cannulated for therapeutic or diagnostic purposes [6–8].

The greatest deterrent to central venous cannulation prior to 1953 was the significant soft tissue and vascular disruption required to complete the task. Until this time, large metal trocars were used to access target veins, and central venous catheters were inserted through the lumen of the trocars into the target vessel. Because these traditional methods created holes in the target vessel that were larger than the catheters themselves, hemorrhage and other complications were common. Ivar Seldinger, a Swedish radiologist, introduced the notion of a "flexible rounded-end metal leader with increased flexibility of its distal 3-cm" that could be used to guide the angiocatheter into the target vessel in 1953 [9]. While his original technique was described as a means of cannulating arteries, the utility of this method for venous access was quickly grasped, and the Seldinger method became a standard technique for clinicians hoping to establish a central venous access throughout the 1950s and beyond. Although the tip of Seldinger's leader wire was originally constructed as a flexible metal loop, the modern hook-shaped leader wire tip soon replaced it as a less traumatic derivative. Seldinger's technique persists to the modern day as the preferred approach for the placement of both arterial and venous catheters.

The first published report of an ultrasound (US)-based technique for central venous cannulation came in 1982 [9]. In this early study, ultrasound-guided placement was endorsed in the infraclavicular approach to subclavian vein cannulation. The use of ultrasound was expected to ameliorate the high rates of air embolism, pneumothorax, and injury to the subclavian artery and brachial plexus reported in the contemporary literature [9]. Although pioneers of this approach endorsed the use of ultrasound for central venous access in the 1980s, landmark-based methods for CVC placement would continue to dominate the clinical scene for most of the subsequent three decades.

In the modern age, US-guided placement of central venous catheters has become the standard-of-care approach. However, the modern clinician must be well-versed in the landmark-based methods of our clinical predecessors, a fact that becomes readily apparent when ultrasound-based strategies are unavailable or inadequate to provide emergent central venous access. Although US guidance may reduce some of the risks of CVC placement, recent studies have called into question whether the greater cost of US technology is worth this modest reduction in risk [10]. Until reliable US technology is available for all care providers in all clinical settings, value remains in learning the traditional landmark-based methods of our clinical predecessors. Chapter 6 of this book describes the method of US guidance for CVC placement.

This chapter is dedicated to instructing providers in the time-proven external landmark-based techniques allowing central venous access in the absence of a functional ultrasound machine or a trained ultrasonographer. What follows in this chapter is a comprehensive report of the techniques that are known to provide ready access to the most commonly accessed central veins, which may prove to be of special use to the emergency care provider who has neither the time nor the access to ultrasound-based strategies for central venous access.

Anatomy of the Central Veins

As described in the previous chapters, the central veins most commonly used for emergent vascular access are the *internal jugular (IJ), axillary (AX), subclavian (SC),* and *femoral (FEM)* central veins. Because of their superficial location and ready identification on external review of the patient's anatomy, these veins provide convenient access to the central venous circulation without requiring extensive cutdowns or disruption of the overlying soft tissues. What follows in this chapter is a discussion of the techniques by which these central veins are commonly accessed and a description of the relative advantages and disadvantages of each for a variety of clinical circumstances.

As Fig. 5.1 illustrates, the *internal jugular (IJ)* and *subclavian (SC)* veins in the upper thorax coalesce and drain into the *superior vena cava (SVC)*, which, in turn, empties into the right atrium of the heart. These upper thoracic veins are commonly utilized for central venous access due to their superficial location and ease of access through the soft tissues of the neck and superior thorax. Although the IJ and SC vein may seem to be equivalent as sites for venous cannulation, the IJ is often preferred as it is easier to compress in the event of iatrogenic injury, hematoma, associated arterial laceration, or following removal of the catheter. The usual technique for cannulation of the SC vein requires cannulation at a site deep to the clavicle, which prevents compression of the insertion site in the event of hemorrhage. This inability to compress the insertion site becomes especially problematic for patients receiving anticoagulation therapy, as they may be prone to excessive bleeding and hematoma formation. The IJ insertion site is also further from the lung apex, which may reduce the risk of iatrogenic pneumothorax.

The femoral site is generally reserved for those patients for whom IJ or SC cannulation is not possible or has already failed. The femoral vein, located in the lower extremity, is a continuation of the popliteal vein and proceeds until joined by the deep femoral vein to create the common femoral vein. Not only is the FEM

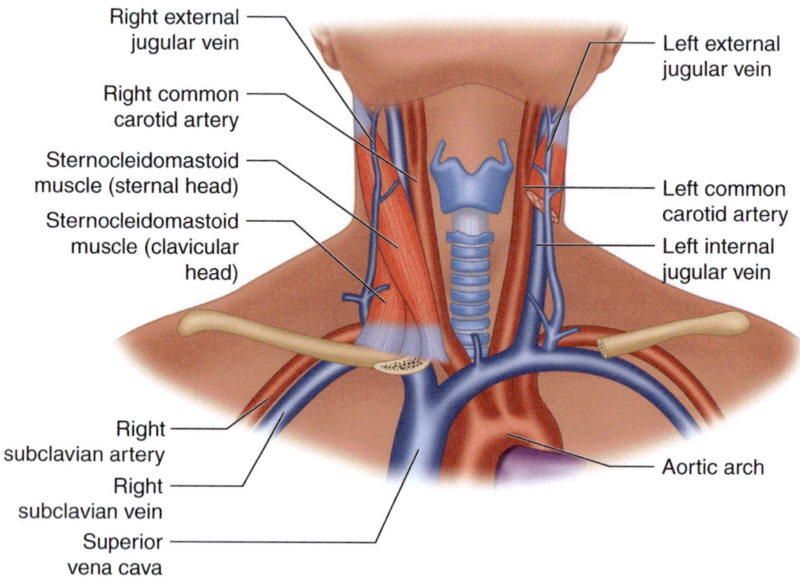

Fig. 5.1 Central vessels of the neck and upper torso

insertion site quite distal to the central circulation, it is also plagued by additional infection risk as compared to the upper thoracic sites [11].

Indications/Contraindications

Indications

Numerous indications for CVC line placement exist, guided primarily by the need for certain medications or fluids that must be infused through a central vein or failure to obtain venous access by any other means when emergent access is truly required. Provider discretion is key to the decision to place a CVC, and providers must weigh the relative risks and benefits of CVC placement when deciding upon the need for central venous cannulation.

Contraindications

There are no absolute contraindications for CVC placement in general, although relative contraindications may exist *according to the insertion site* selected or other patient-specific factors [12]. While we will discuss many of these site-specific factors later, certain relative contraindications may be common to all sites. These universal relative contraindications to CVC placement include the following:

- Medical condition that may be treated adequately with other access routes
- Severe coagulopathy (directs placement to easily compressible sites only)
- Distorted local anatomy (i.e., inability to accurately identify external landmarks)
- Suspected injury, hemorrhage, or disruption of the target vessel or more proximal structures to which that vessel drains (e.g., femoral cannulation in major abdominal trauma)
- Cellulitis or other infection of soft tissues at insertion site
- Thrombus or other structure (e.g., catheter) occluding lumen of target vessel
- Inability to adequately immobilize insertion site (e.g., agitated patients)
- Severe stenosis of target vessel or excessive soft tissue scarring at target site
- Previous failed cannulation of target vessel (especially if failed more proximal attempt)
- Presence of arteriovenous graft (AVG) or fistula (AVF) at target vessel (will influence results of blood gas analyses)

When a relative contraindication exists for a specific insertion site, providers should consider whether other central venous insertion sites may remain viable. Repeated failure to achieve landmark-based CVC insertion should prompt providers to seek other modalities (e.g., ultrasound-based insertion techniques, bridging intraosseous cannulation) to enhance the likelihood of future success.

Types of Central Venous Catheters

Although CV catheters are all designed to cannulate the central veins, a wide variety of basic CVC designs may be found. The primary characteristics that distinguish different central venous catheters include the following:

- Number of lumens (single, dual, triple, quad)
- Length of catheter (e.g., standard, midline, PICC line)
- Implanted (e.g., subcutaneous ports) vs. non-implanted
- Tunneled (e.g., travel subcutaneously before penetrating vein) vs. non-tunneled
- Functionality (e.g., dialysis catheters, introducers)
- Impregnated catheters (e.g., antibiotic, antithrombotic)

The choice of catheter type should be governed by the specific needs of the patient, including the types of medication that are expected to be infused through the catheter and anticipated duration of dwell time.

Infusion rates differ between different CVC types, with multi-access catheter (MAC) flow rates generally higher than those for standard triple-lumen catheter (TLC) lines [13]. Triple-lumen catheters have 18-gauge catheters, allowing a maximum flow rate of 26 ml/min^3. However, a multi-access catheter, MAC, contains a 12-gauge lumen catheter resulting in a flow rate of 155 ml/min^3 [14]. The fluid flow rates through CVC lines depends upon which lumen is utilized, with larger gauge lumens offering a much higher rate of flow than smaller gauge lumens.

Supplies Needed

The supplies needed to place a CVC are listed below and illustrated in Fig. 5.2:

- Sterile drape with fenestration (cover entire patient)
- Chlorhexidine antiseptic with applicators
- Anesthetizing needle (25 gauge, 1 inch or 1.5 inch length)
- Finder needle (18 gauge, 2.5 inch length)
- 5 mL syringe (for anesthetic)
- 10 mL syringe (for finder needle insertion)
- J-tip guidewire with plastic housing and straightener sleeve
- No. 11 scalpel blade
- Skin dilator
- Central venous catheter
- Sterile 4×4 gauze pads
- Suture with curved needle
- Needle driver

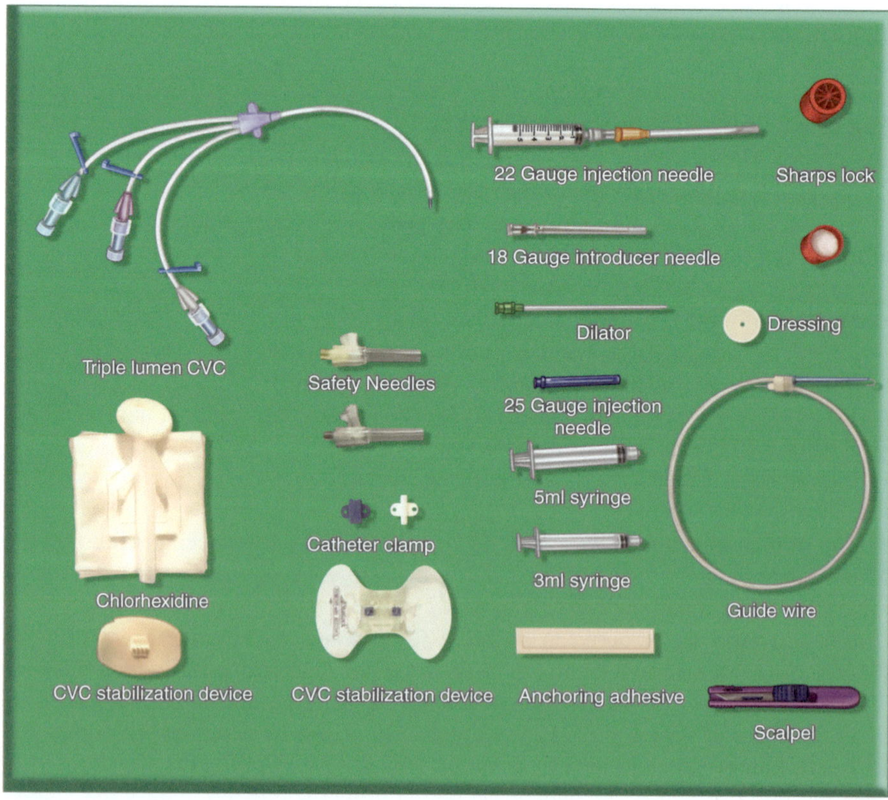

Fig. 5.2 Supplies needed for CVC insertion

- Sterile gloves, gown, cap, and mask with face shield for each provider
- Sterile saline solution for injection/flush
- Sterile Tegaderm dressings
- Local anesthetic (e.g., 1% lidocaine)

The specific components of a central line kit may vary according to the manufacturer, with some kits featuring sterile 10-mL syringes of normal saline (for flushing), transparent film dressings (e.g., Tegaderm™) to cover the insertion site, and suture material for anchoring the catheter clamp to the skin.

After insertion site selection, including preparation of the insertion site and creation of a sterile field, the following steps should be taken:

1. Administer local anesthetic to the skin surrounding the insertion site.
2. Insert needle or angiocatheter into the selected vein.
3. Advance guidewire into the vein through the placed needle or angiocatheter.
4. Remove needle or angiocatheter while holding the guidewire in place.
5. Create incision next to the guidewire to allow room for dilator.
6. Advance dilator over the guidewire followed by CVC over the guidewire.
7. Remove the guidewire through CVC while holding the guidewire in place.
8. Aspirate and flush each of the three lumens for functionality.
9. Anchor CVC in place with suture and/or adhesive [15].

In the sections that immediately follow, we will discuss the most common central veins cannulated in clinical practice, including special considerations for each anatomic site.

Internal Jugular (IJ) Vein Cannulation

The *internal jugular (IJ)* vein collects blood from the brain via the sigmoid sinus, from the superficial face via the facial vein, and from the neck via the lingual, pharyngeal, and thyroid veins. The IJ vein continues down the neck through the carotid sheath into the base of the neck, where it joins the subclavian vein to form the brachiocephalic vein. The right IJ vein is often preferred for cannulation due to its relatively straight pathway to the superior vena cava (as seen in Fig. 5.1), as well as its relatively larger diameter in comparison to the left internal jugular vein [16].

Advantages

- Easily compressible
- Low rate of catheter malposition, providing fast and reliable access [17]
- Low rate of catheter-related infection [18]
- Low risk of pneumothorax, which is especially important for patients presenting with respiratory compromise [19]

Disadvantages

- Requires the head and neck to be held in a fixed position for an extended time; thus, patient compliance can be an issue.
- Challenging in patients with extreme contracture of neck muscles or excessive soft tissue at the neck.
- Complicated by the need for cervical spine immobilization/collar, which is especially important with trauma patients.
- Sterile draping may obstruct access to the chest for chest compressions, thoracostomy, etc.

Patient Positioning

Supine, with neck rotated to the contralateral side. When cannulating the right IJ, the patient's leftward head rotation should be kept to < 45 degree for procedures occurring 2 cm above the clavicle and < 30 degree for procedures occurring 4 cm above the clavicle [20].

Insertion Site Identification

Identifying the Jugular Vein

The preferred insertion site for the IJ vein can be found at the *apex of a triangle formed by the sternal and clavicular heads of the sternocleidomastoid (SCM) muscle*, just lateral to the carotid artery, as illustrated in Fig. 5.3.

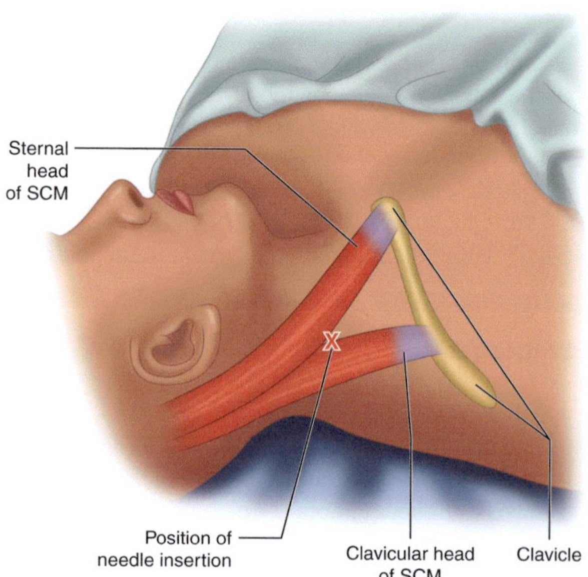

Fig. 5.3 The standard internal jugular (IJ) vein insertion site [21]

At the level of the cricoid cartilage, the IJ vein generally lies anterolateral to the *common carotid artery (CCA)* at the insertion site on the right side. However, in greater than half of cases, the IJ is either completely anterior or anteromedial to the CCA on the left side at this level [22]. When attempting left IJ cannulation, head rotation 30 degrees to the right will usually bring the vessels into a "normal" alignment (i.e., IJ either anterior or anterolateral to the CCA). However, head rotation does not appear to substantially change the relative positioning of the IJ and CCA at this level on the right side [22]. An anterior position of the IJ vein relative to the common carotid artery increases gradually with age, resulting in increasing overlap between the two vessels as they progress inferiorly. Left-sided localization and male sex further increase the probability of an anterior position [23].

Positioning the patient in Trendelenburg (and / or the Valsalva maneuver) can engorge the IJ vein due to increased venous return. Mildly rotating the patient's neck away from the site of insertion will also allow for better visualization of the vein. However, excessive rotation of the neck to the contralateral side causes the SCM muscle to compress the IJ vein, which will present a smaller caliber target for cannulation [24, 25]. Comatose patients who are unable to perform the Valsalva maneuver, or patients displaying respiratory distress with any degree of Trendelenburg positioning, may benefit from slight abdominal compression to engorge the IJ vein during the access attempt [26].

The "Three-Finger Method"

An alternative method of locating the IJ vein is the so-called, "three-finger method" [27]. To achieve access to the right IJ vein, the provider's left ring finger is placed in the patient's sternal notch, with middle and index fingertips at the patient's midline over the trachea. All three fingers are then "rolled over" the trachea and down into the space between the trachea and the sternal (medial) head of the SCM muscle. The pads of all three fingers must stay in contact with the trachea. Utilizing this technique, the left ring finger should be touching the sternoclavicular joint, and the sternal head of the SCM muscle is bunched into a mound lateral to the fingers.

Even if the proper insertion site is assured, anatomic variation may still promote uncertainty regarding whether a provider utilizing the landmark-based method of insertion has cannulated the IJ vein, and not the CCA. In such cases, the following mnemonic may be of use in distinguishing the IJ vein from the CCA:

- *P – Palpation.* The IJ vein is non-palpable and easily collapses with slight manual compression.
- *O– Occlusion.* The IJ vein can be occluded with the index finger compressing the ipsilateral subclavicular area.
- *L – Location.* The IJ vein is located *between* the two heads of the sternocleidomastoid muscle and is usually situated *lateral* to the carotid artery.

- *I – Inspiration.* The IJ venous pressure drops with inspiration, while there is no change in pressure of the carotid artery with inspiration.
- *C – Contour.* The IJ vein has a biphasic waveform, whereas a single pulse is noted in the carotid artery.
- *E – Erect Position.* The IJ venous pulsation drops with an erect body position. Body positioning has little to no effect on the carotid pulse [28].

Cannulation of the carotid artery should be suspected if bright red and pulsatile blood flows out of the catheter. Venous blood is usually darker and under less pressure than arterial blood. If the provider suspects cannulation of the artery, the catheter should be connected to a transducing system (e.g., length of IV tubing). A rising and pulsatile column of blood (especially with pressures > 30 mmHg) in the tubing suggests arterial cannulation. If arterial cannulation occurs, remove the catheter and apply direct, firm pressure to the insertion site for approximately 10 minutes, until no further bleeding from the skin puncture is noted.

The usual insertion site for the IJ cannulation is located approximately *halfway between the mastoid process and the sternal notch*. However, the location of this insertion site may contribute to increased risk of catheter kinkage in the neck as the catheter exits the vein, due to extrinsic pressure on the catheter by the muscles and soft tissues of the neck. This may also be exacerbated by the patient turning their neck. To reduce this effect, a so-called "low" *IJ insertion* may be performed at a puncture site 2 cm superior to the clavicle, between the sternal and clavicular insertions of the sternocleidomastoid muscle. The potential advantage of this approach is that the low neck is more fixed in location; neck movement is therefore less likely to cause catheter kinkage with neck movement.

Needle Direction

The needle should be aimed at the ipsilateral nipple, piercing the skin at a 45 degree angle with insertion.

Site-Specific Risks/Complications

- Puncture or injury of the aorta, carotid, vertebral, or subclavian arteries
- Airway compromise (e.g., tracheal puncture, hematoma compression on trachea)
- Cardiac tamponade
- Pneumothorax
- Hemothorax
- Arrhythmia (due to guidewire contacting cardiac endothelium)
- Injury to the thoracic duct (associated only with left-sided IJ attempts)

A post-procedural one-view chest X-ray is often obtained to confirm intravenous placement of the line and to rule out the presence of complicating pneumothorax [29]. The interpretation of a chest radiograph to confirm appropriate IJ central venous catheter placement requires identification of the carina, which is located at the junction of the left and right main bronchi. Internal jugular vein catheters are generally inserted into the right internal jugular vein, ipsilateral to the superior vena cava (SVC) (Fig. 5.1). In such cases, the catheter may be seen on chest radiograph to descend vertically anterior to the right clavicle, with the tip of the catheter located in the SVC. The optimal anatomic location of the catheter tip in the SVC is above the level of the carina, as depicted in Fig. 5.4 [30].

Electrocardiogram (ECG)-guided line placement has shown some value in ensuring accurate placement, reducing the patient's radiation exposure, and reducing the costs associated with repositioning procedures [31]. When the CVC tip advances from the IJ vein into the SVC, a normal amplitude P-wave is noticed on the ECG monitor. By monitoring the P-wave, the catheter tip is tracked as it travels through the junction of the SVC with the *right atrium (RA)* and into the RA. As the catheter is slowly advanced, while maintaining an eye on the configuration of the P-wave in lead II on the ECG monitor, an abrupt increase in the height of the P-wave is noticed, reflecting the closeness of the intracavitary electrode (the tip) to the sinoatrial node. If the catheter tip is further advanced deep into the right atrium, the P-wave height declines, appears bifid, or even has a negative deflection. In cases of over-insertion, the CVC should be withdrawn at 0.5 cm increments until the P-wave returns to a normal configuration [32].

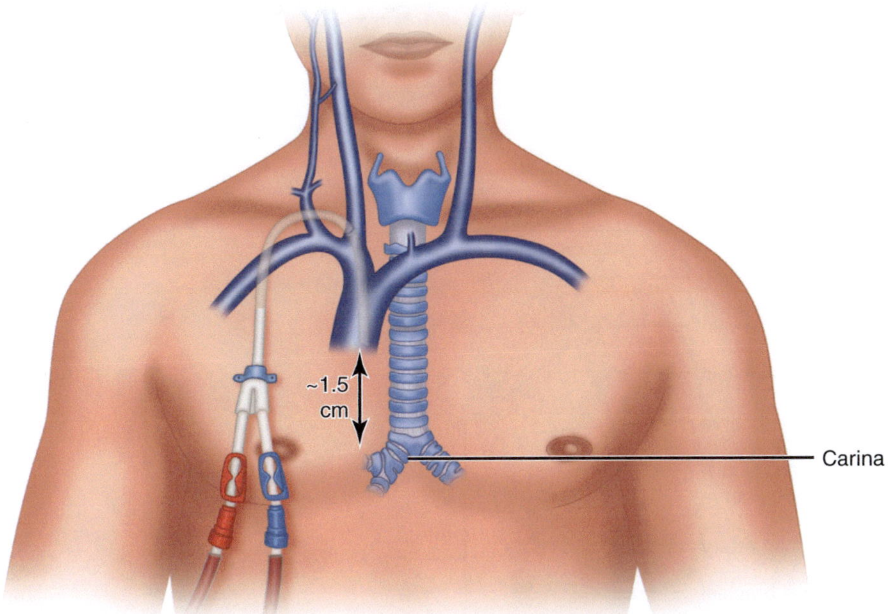

Fig. 5.4 Proper tip position for a right IJ venous catheter

Axillary (AX) Vein Cannulation

The axillary vein is formed when the brachial vein joins the basilic vein in the upper arm [33]. This joining typically occurs at the inferior border of the *teres major muscle* and continues until the lateral border of the first rib, where this vessel continues as the subclavian vein, as depicted in Fig. 5.5. The axillary vein is divided into three parts (i.e., proximal, posterior, distal), according to the vein's location relative to the pectoralis minor muscle. The medial portion of the axillary vein is usually largest, allowing for the easiest cannulation, but its proximity to the pleural space and the axillary artery increases the risk of complications [34].

Landmark-based axillary vein cannulation has largely been superseded in recent years by ultrasound-guided cannulation [34]. Consequently, little published data exist on the reliability of landmark-based cannulation of the axillary vein.

Advantages

- Reduced risk of pneumothorax, when compared to SC site
- Decreased rate of septicemia in tracheostomized patients, as compared to SC site [35]

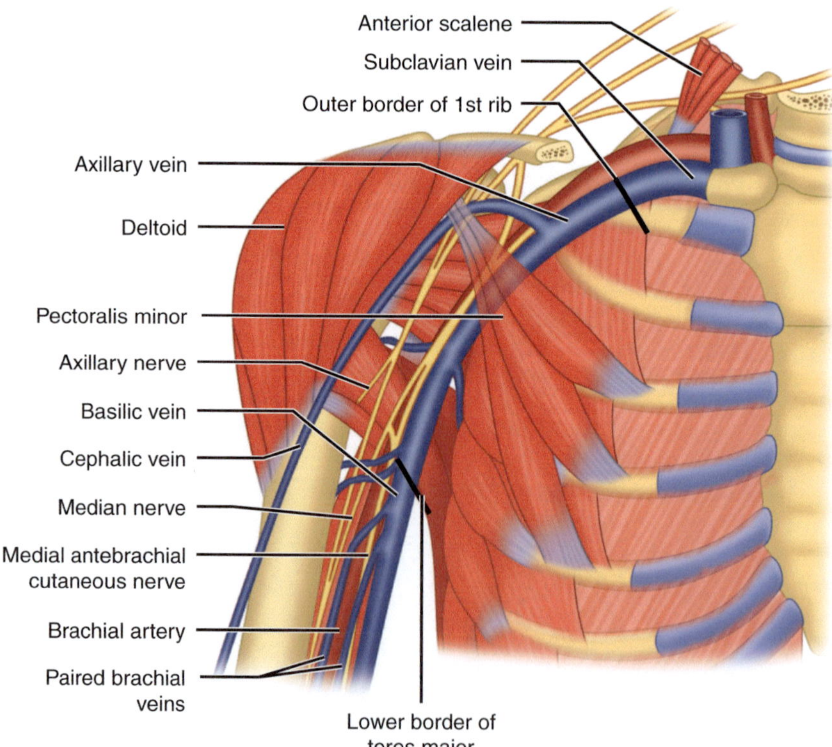

Fig. 5.5 Relevant anatomy for axillary vein cannulation

Disadvantages

- Difficult to cannulate using landmark-based methods.
- Increased length of catheter is needed.
- Risk of iatrogenic injury to adjacent nerves (e.g., axillary nerve, medial antebrachial cutaneous nerve, median nerve) and arteries (e.g., axillary artery).

Patient Positioning

The patient should be in the supine position, with head approximately 15 degrees Trendelenburg. The head should be in a neutral position, with arms placed straight at the patient's side. In the past, it was recommended to abduct the arm to 45 degrees from the trunk, but more recent studies show no significant increase in vein diameter with this technique [34, 36].

Insertion Site Identification

Landmark-based axillary vein cannulation requires an insertion point three fingerbreadths below the coracoid process of the scapula, lateral to the lateral border of the pectoralis minor muscle [34]. At the most lateral aspect of the axillary vein, there are no clinically significant posterior structures that may potentially be damaged during cannulation [37]. An illustration of the proper insertion site and relevant anatomy for axillary vein cannulation is provided in Fig. 5.6.

In the pediatric population, the course of the axillary vein should be determined in relation to the axillary artery, because the axillary vein is often not visible. This vein should be cannulated parallel and inferior to the axillary artery located via palpation [37].

Needle Direction

The needle tip should be elevated 10–15 degrees from the frontal plane, aimed toward the medial quarter end of the clavicle [35–37].

Site-Specific Risks/Complications

- Puncture or iatrogenic injury to axillary artery.
- Iatrogenic injury to adjacent nerves
- Pneumothorax
- Hemothorax
- Upper extremity deep vein thrombosis (DVT), as a delayed complication

Confirmation of axillary central venous line placement can be confirmed with chest radiograph, as shown in Fig. 5.7. Note the catheter emanating from the right

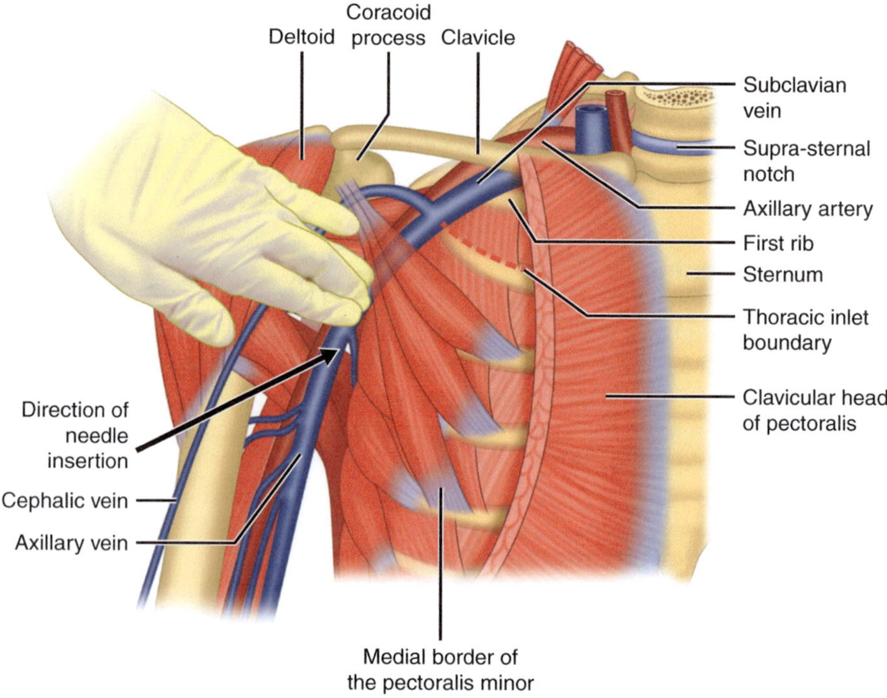

Fig. 5.6 Landmark-based axillary vein cannulation

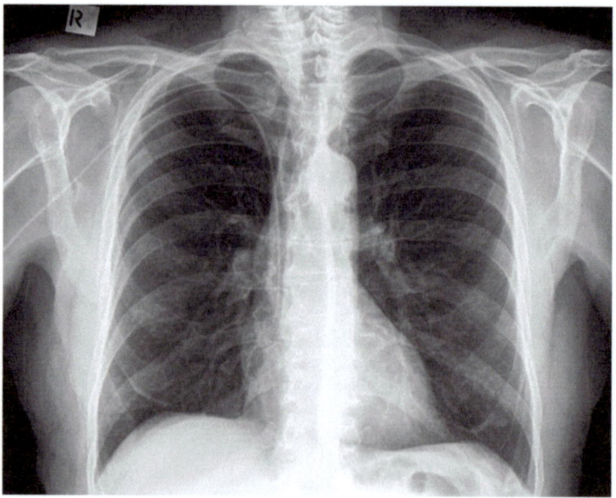

Fig. 5.7 Chest radiograph showing proper right axillary venous catheter placement

upper extremity, then traveling to terminate at the SVC. Optimal placement of the tip of axillary CVCs is the same as other CVC lines.

Subclavian (SC) Vein Cannulation: Supraclavicular Approach

The subclavian vein is a continuation of the axillary vein in the upper extremity. The subclavian vein begins at the outer border of the first rib, terminating at the medial margin of the *scalenus anterior muscle*, by joining with the IJ vein (just behind the sternocostoclavicular joint) to form the innominate vein [38, 39]. Although the subclavian artery lies just deep to the subclavian vein, the two vessels are usually separated by the *scalenus anterior* muscle medially [40]. The right subclavian vein is the preferred insertion site, due to the anatomic location of the left subclavian vein in relation to the thoracic duct and increased projection of the left pleural apex [41].

Advantages

- Large vein, with a diameter measuring up to 2 cm in adults [40].
- Easily landmarked (even in obese patients) due to the superficial location of the clavicle and its position just deep to the clavicle.
- Shorter access time (approximately 1.5 minutes) when compared to the infraclavicular SC approach [41].
- The direction of needle insertion (i.e., anterior to the coronal plane) ensures that the needle tip progressively deviates away from the pleura and the subclavian artery as it is advanced [40].
- Distance between the skin surface and the vein is less than that for the infraclavicular SC approach (0.5 cm to 4 cm vs. 3.8 cm to 6.2 cm) [41, 42].
- Both subclavian approaches are characterized by increased ease of dressing maintenance, improved patient comfort, clearer anatomic landmarks, and lower infection rates than other CVC insertion sites [11].

Disadvantages

- As the venous cannulation site is located posterior to the clavicle, direct pressure to the venous cannulation site is difficult, increasing the risk of clinically significant bleeding and hematoma formation [11].
- Relatively higher risk of iatrogenic pneumothorax can worsen respiratory efforts by patients presenting with respiratory distress.
- Not recommended for patients with clavicular or upper rib fracture, due to the likelihood of associated SC vein injury.
- Risk of subclavian vein stenosis complicating future hemodialysis access attempts via shunt or fistula [43].

Patient Positioning

Supine, with neck turned as far as achievable away from the insertion site.

Insertion Site Identification

According to Yoffa's initial description of this approach (1965), the insertion site is "the junction of the lateral margin of the sternomastoid muscle with the upper border of the clavicle – [at] the 'clavisternomastoid angle'" [38]. In the awake patient, these muscular borders can be more easily visualized by asking the patient to lift their head off the bed. Most (84%) of the time, the subclavian vein lies immediately posterior to the clavicle for 28–38% of the total clavicular length as measured from the sternoclavicular joint [44].

One quick way to locate the insertion point for supraclavicular subclavian vein access is to visually draw a line medially from the anterior most aspect of the shoulder to the intersection with the clavicle. This should approximate one-third of the clavicle length from the sternoclavicular joint.

Needle Direction

The needle should puncture the skin just superior (1–2 cm) to the superior edge of the clavicle, at a position 1 cm lateral to the insertion of the clavicular (lateral) head of the sternocleidomastoid muscle (SCM). The SCM border and the superior edge of the clavicle create a 90 degree angle. The provider should attempt to bisect this angle, forming a 45 degree angle between the needle length and the superior border of the clavicle in the sagittal plane. The needle should then be advanced forward at an angle approximately 15 degrees relative to the coronal plane of the clavicle [38–40]. The needle tip should be kept as anterior as possible, just barely sliding under the clavicle, to reduce the risk of arterial puncture or pneumothorax. The technique for supraclavicular cannulation of the subclavian vein is illustrated in Fig. 5.8.

Site-Specific Risks/Complications

- Puncture or injury to the aorta, carotid, vertebral, or subclavian arteries
- Cardiac tamponade
- Pneumothorax
- Hemothorax
- Cardiac arrhythmia (if guidewire contacts cardiac endothelium)

With both the supraclavicular and infraclavicular SC insertion techniques, providers should plan to "walk down" the clavicle in 1 mm increments. After

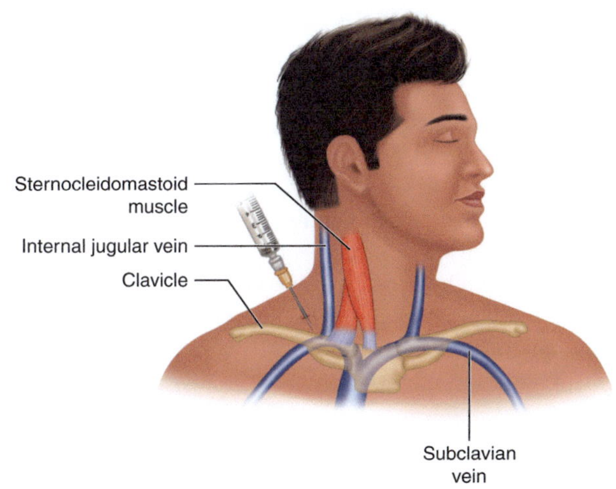

Fig. 5.8 Technique for supraclavicular cannulation of the subclavian vein

careful injection of local anesthetic (e.g., 1% lidocaine) to the periosteum of the clavicle and surrounding soft tissues, the provider will advance the needle until contact with the clavicle is made. The angle of this initial insertion attempt should be intentionally flatter (i.e., lower angle relative to the coronal plane) than what is expected to need to reach the vein. Contact with the clavicle is confirmed when the provider experiences firm resistance to additional advancement of the needle tip. This resistance confirms contact with the clavicle and provides additional information to the provider on the depth of the clavicle relative to the skin puncture site. Once contact with the clavicle is made, the provider then retracts the needle a short amount (e.g., 5 mm) and then readvances the needle at a slightly greater (1–2 degrees) angle relative to the coronal plane until contact is again made with the superior surface of the clavicle. The goal of this exercise is to contact an incrementally (e.g., 1 mm) more posterior point on the superior aspect of the clavicle. This process is repeated until the needle just barely slides under the clavicle. This approach will minimize the risk of iatrogenic injury to the subclavian artery and lung pleura caused by an excessively high angle of insertion relative to the coronal plane.

Subclavian lines are often considered to have the highest rate of catheter malposition among common CVC insertion sites [45]. The most common patterns of malposition include the catheter tip crossing midline to the contralateral subclavian vein, ascending into the internal jugular vein, or advanced laterally into the axillary vein. This risk of malpositioning can be minimized by ensuring that the proper insertion angle is respected and that the "hook" of the J-tip of the guidewire is pointing inferiorly when the guidewire is inserted into the introducer needle [46]. Once the guidewire has been inserted, the provider should be careful to maintain this tip direction by not rotating the guidewire.

Subclavian (SC) Vein Cannulation: Infraclavicular Approach

Since Aubaniac's original (1952) description of this technique, the infraclavicular approach has been extensively modified and further popularized by a variety of authors [6, 42, 47, 48].

Unlike the supraclavicular SC approach, which enjoys a relative lack of soft tissue between the skin puncture site and the target vein, the infraclavicular approach requires penetration of the *pectoralis major muscle* to reach the vein. Due to extensive fascial anchoring to the surrounding structures of the upper torso, this site may be less collapsible than other central venous sites in the setting of hypovolemia, although maneuvers to engorge the vein prior to line placement (e.g., Trendelenburg positioning, leg lift, abdominal compression) are recommended.

Advantages

- Large vein, with diameter measuring up to 2 cm in adults [40].
- Easily landmarked (even in obese patients) due to the superficial location of the clavicle and the vein's position just deep to the clavicle.
- Both subclavian approaches are characterized by increased ease of dressing maintenance, improved patient comfort, clear anatomic landmarks, and lower infection rates than other CVC insertion sites [11].

Disadvantages

- As the venous cannulation site is located posterior to the clavicle, direct pressure to the venous cannulation site is difficult, increasing the risk of clinically significant bleeding and hematoma formation [11].
- Relatively higher risk of iatrogenic pneumothorax can worsen respiratory efforts by patients presenting with respiratory distress.
- Potentially more difficult to place in patients receiving concomitant chest compressions or other thoracic procedures (e.g., thoracostomy).
- This insertion site is not recommended for patients with clavicular or upper rib fracture, due to increased likelihood of associated SC vein injury.
- Presents increased risk of subclavian vein stenosis complicating future hemodialysis access attempts via shunt or fistula [43, 45]. However, multiple studies have concluded that both frequency and duration of catheter placement contribute to the development of central venous stenosis [49].

Patient Positioning

- Positioned with head and neck in neutral position, with bed in 15 degrees Trendelenburg, to maximize venous filling and minimize the risk of air embolism [43, 45]. It is helpful to place a "bump" (e.g., rolled towel or sheet) between the patient's scapulae to open the clavicular angle, thus elevating the clavicle anteriorly and helping the shoulder to "fall away" from the insertion site [50].

Insertion Site Identification

The infraclavicular SC insertion site can be identified using two anatomical landmarks: the "clavicular transition point" (i.e., where the concave lateral two-thirds of the clavicle meets the convex medial one-third of the clavicle) and the sternal notch. The provider's index finger is placed at the sternal notch, with the thumb placed at the transition point as seen in Fig. 5.9. The skin should be punctured 1–2 cm inferior and 1–2 cm lateral to the clavicular transition point [43, 47, 50, 51]. Skin puncture too close to the clavicle will complicate insertion as the subclavicular soft tissues will need to be compressed posteriorly to guide the needle tip under the clavicle. Skin puncture performed too far laterally will lead to excessive soft-tissue "tunneling" required to reach the vein.

The insertion site for the infraclavicular approach is within the "*deltopectoral triangle*," defined inferiorly by the *pectoralis major muscle*, laterally by the medial aspect of the deltoid muscle, and medially by the clavicle [47]. The target space for vein puncture lies between the clavicular origins of the pectoralis major muscle and the deltoid muscle, where the cephalic vein joins the axillary vein. Skilled providers may also identify the insertion site based on palpation of the subclavian artery. The subclavian vein is located anterior and interior to the subclavian artery. After palpation of the subclavian artery below

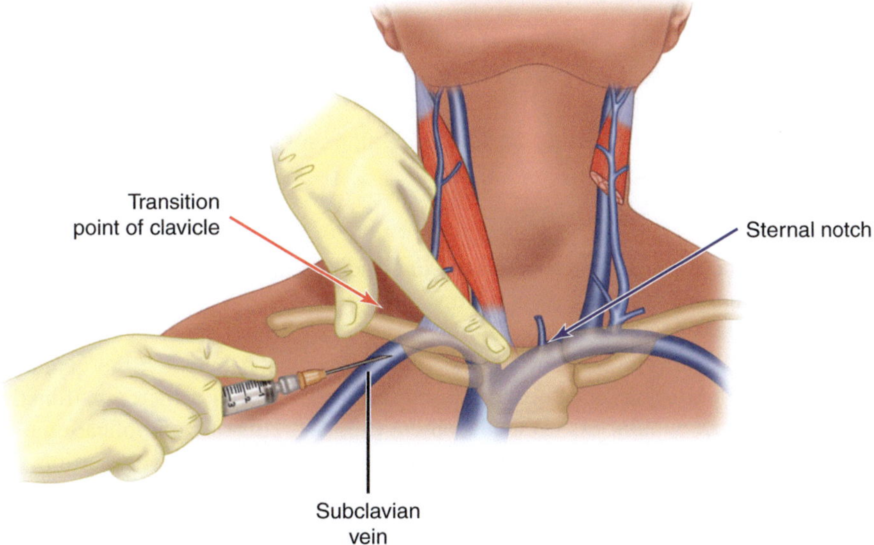

Fig. 5.9 Infraclavicular approach to SC vein cannulation

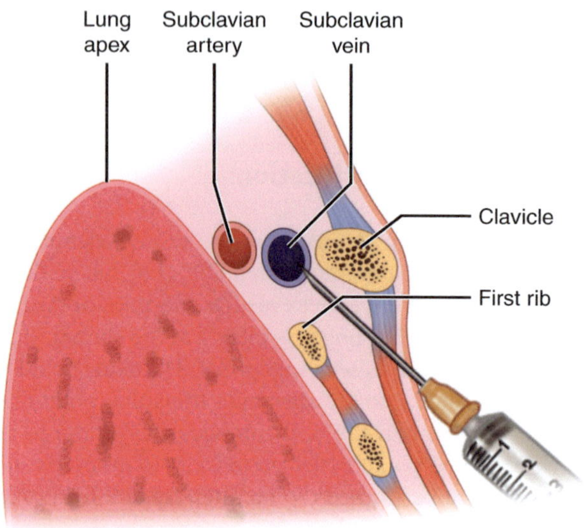

Fig. 5.10 Relative locations of vital subclavian structures (viewed in sagittal plane)

the clavicle, the needle can be introduced 1–2 cm lateral and inferior to the arterial pulsation [52]. The relationship between the subclavian vessels and the clavicle is depicted in Fig. 5.10.

Needle Direction

The needle should be advanced in the coronal plane (i.e., parallel to the stretcher), through the subclavian muscle [51].

Site-Specific Risks/Complications

- Puncture or injury of aorta, carotid, vertebral, or subclavian arteries
- Cardiac tamponade
- Pneumothorax
- Hemothorax
- Arrhythmia (if guidewire contacts cardiac endothelium)
- Injury to nerves of the brachial plexus
- Chylothorax (if left-sided)

"Pinch-off syndrome" (i.e., compression of the catheter between the ipsilateral clavicle and first rib) has been described and may be a cause of catheter malfunction following infraclavicular SC CVC placement [53, 54]. This rare complication most often presents with the patient complaining of pain at the catheter insertion site, along with catheter dysfunction. When this syndrome is suspected, physicians should promptly remove the catheter to prevent more serious complications, including catheter fracture and embolization [54]. The best way to reduce the risk of this

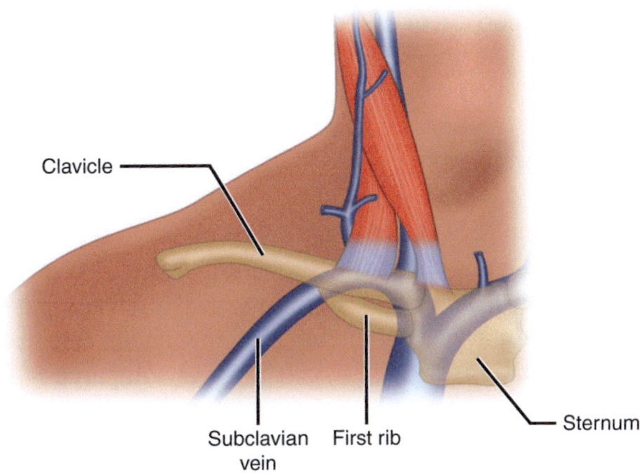

Fig. 5.11 Relevant anatomy of the "pinch-off" site, where the SC catheter can become compressed between the clavicle and the first rib

complication is to ensure that *the catheter insertion site is lateral to the midclavicular line*. Overly medial insertion appears to be a risk factor for this syndrome. The relevant anatomic relationships in pinch-off syndrome are depicted in Fig. 5.11.

Femoral (FEM) Vein Cannulation

The *common femoral vein (CFV)* is formed by the confluence of the superficial femoral vein and the deep femoral vein, and this vein is joined by the saphenous vein just distal to the inguinal ligament to form the external iliac vein, once it has traveled proximal to the inguinal ligament [55]. Since the CFV is of a larger caliber than its tributaries, the optimal site for cannulation of the femoral venous system lies just distal to the inguinal ligament, within the so-called femoral triangle.

Although this site is often readily accessible under emergent conditions, the use of the femoral CVC insertion site remains controversial among providers due to conflicting reports of increased risk of infection, although other studies have shown no increased infection risk when compared to other sites [11, 56–58]. Consequently, FEM cannulation remains less popular than IJ or SC cannulation. Cannulation of the FEM vein offers access to the inferior vena cava (IVC), but not to the SVC. Consequently, this insertion site may not be optimal for introduction of a *pulmonary artery (PA)* catheter. The presence of a FEM catheter may also introduce a higher risk of complicating DVT than the IJ and SC sites [59].

Advantages

- Allows for direct compression of insertion site in cases of coagulopathy or hematoma.
- No risk of pneumothorax or injury to thoracic structures.

- Associated with fewer mechanical complications than the IJ or SC sites [59].
- In comparison to other sites, inadvertent cannulation and dilatation of the femoral artery with a standard catheter do not usually pose significant problems.

Disadvantages

- Contraindicated in the setting of injury to the IVC or its contributing veins
- Does not allow for catheterization of the SVC or PA (e.g., Swan-Ganz catheter)
- May be difficult to achieve in massively obese patients with large pannus
- Suboptimal for ambulatory patients, due to impaired mobility and discomfort
- Potentially increased risk of DVT as compared to IJ or SC site

Patient Positioning

The patient should be positioned supine, with the target leg abducted and externally rotated for ready access to the femoral triangle. It has been proposed that "frog-legging" the target extremity (i.e., flexing the knee with the heel placed on the medial aspect of the contralateral knee) may offer better exposure to the FEM than traditional straight leg positioning, by reducing overlap with the femoral artery and engorging the FEM vein [60]. Reverse Trendelenburg positioning may also help to engorge the vein and facilitate cannulation. Cooperative patients may be asked to hum, cough, or otherwise perform Valsalva maneuvers to increase FEM vein engorgement.

Insertion Site Identification

The FEM vein lies within the femoral triangle, defined superiorly by the *inguinal ligament*, laterally by the *sartorius muscle*, and medially by the *adductor longus muscle*. Contents of the femoral triangle include the femoral nerve, femoral artery, femoral vein, and the femoral canal, including the deep inguinal lymph nodes. An easy method for remembering these contents is the mnemonic *NAVEL* (lateral to medial): **N**erve, **A**rtery, **V**ein, **E**mpty space, **L**ymphatics. This anatomy is illustrated in Fig. 5.12.

Needle Insertion

The proper needle insertion site is located 1 cm medial to the pulsating femoral artery and 2–3 cm inferior to the inguinal ligament (extending from the anterior superior iliac crest of the ilium to the pubic tubercle), as depicted in Fig. 5.13. The needle should be oriented with the bevel up, piercing the skin at a 20 or 30 degree

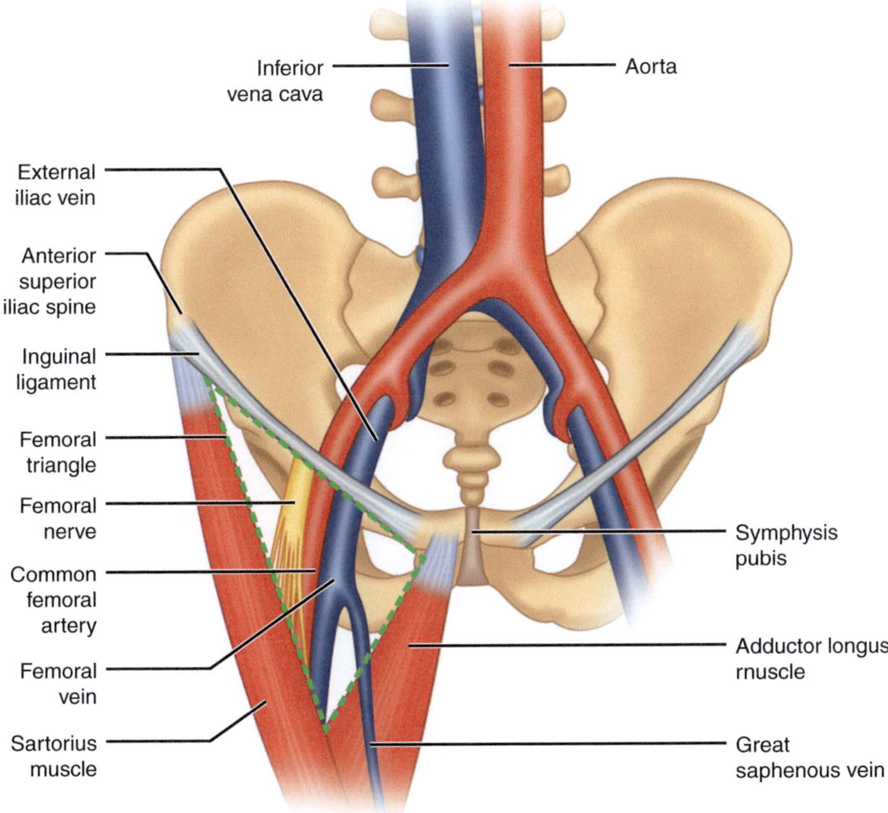

Fig. 5.12 Anatomy of the "femoral triangle" (green)

angle. The vessel is normally reached at a depth of 2 to 4 cm below the skin but may be deeper in obese or edematous patients. When cannulating the right FEM, the provider should keep at least two fingers of the left hand on the artery to maintain a tactile sense of the artery's position while the right hand advances the introducer needle into the vein. This relationship of the hands is reversed when cannulating the left FEM vein. It is recommended that the provider use this technique regardless of the provider's dominant handedness, since the provider will be positioned on the side of the bed lateral to the target site and reversal of this arrangement will force the provider to cross hands during the procedure, which will contort the effort and potentially make cannulation more difficult. In general, right-hand dominant providers may have a preference for right femoral insertions (and *vice-versa*), as the left femoral approach will make proper hand positioning difficult if the patient is not approached from the contralateral side of the stretcher. It is generally easier to insert

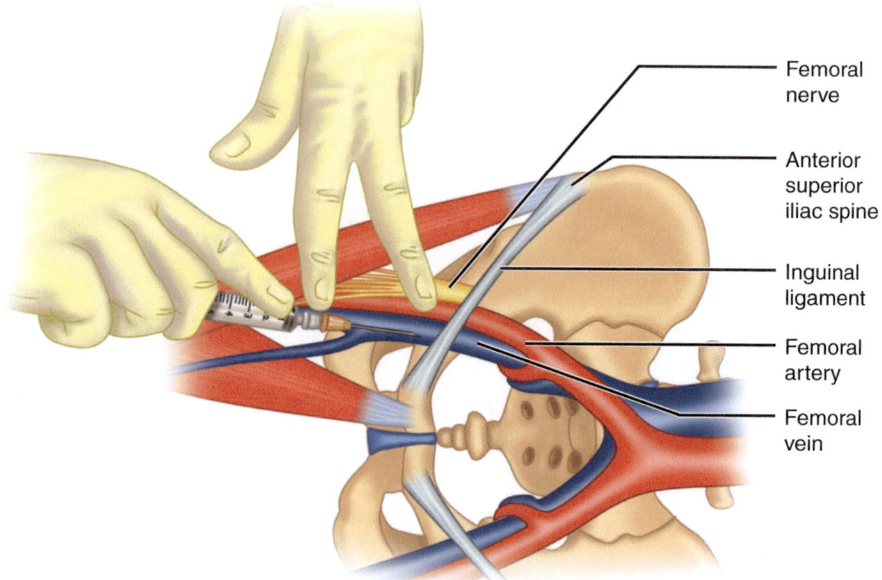

Fig. 5.13 Proper needle insertion technique for FEM vein cannulation

a FEM CVC from the ipsilateral side of the stretcher, rather than leaning over the entire stretcher to reach the insertion site. Providers should consider the importance of provider comfort to procedural success, and try to select an appropriate insertion site that is easily accessed by the provider. Of course, patient-specific factors will limit the availability of specific sites.

Site-Specific Risks/Complications

- Care should be taken when placing FEM lines in patients undergoing cardiopulmonary resuscitation (CPR), as chest compressions can produce femoral vein pulsations that may be misinterpreted by the provider as arterial pulsations. Catheter misplacement at the femoral site occurs in up to 30% of cannulations during cardiopulmonary resuscitation [61].
- Hypercoagulable patients may be at greater risk of DVT at the FEM site than at the IJ and SC sites. It has been suggested that DVTs may form as early as within 24 hours of line placement [62].
- Patients suspected of blunt abdominal trauma, or otherwise at risk for injury to the IVC and associated veins, should be screened carefully for disruption of these veins before FEM vein cannulation is attempted.

Selection of Appropriate CVC Insertion Site

Decisions about which central venous access site to use should always be based on the providers' clinical judgment, considering a variety of factors. Different CVC insertion sites have different complication profiles and offer different advantages for the clinician and the patient. A summary of the preferred insertion sites, according to various clinical circumstances, is provided in Table 5.1.

Complications of Central Venous Cannulation

The major risks of central vein cannulation include both general and site-specific complications and may be grouped according to the time of onset following the procedure:

Immediate Complications (During or Immediately After Procedure)

- Failure to cannulate vein
- Pain
- Bleeding or hematoma formation
- Extravasation of infused substances
- Laceration of the target vein
- Arterial puncture or laceration

Table 5.1 Recommended CVC insertion site, according to specific clinical circumstances [8, 11, 12, 39, 40, 43, 45, 50, 55, 58]

	Subclavicular Subclavian	Supraclavicular Subclavian	Internal jugular	Femoral
Depth	Variable	Superficial	Superficial	Deep
Obesity	Yes	Yes	Yes	Best to avoid
Lower extremity trauma	Yes	Yes	Yes	Best to avoid
Potential C-spine/ head injury	Yes	Best to avoid	Best to avoid	Best to avoid
Bleeding risk	High, due to limited compressibility of the insertion site	High, due to limited compressibility of the insertion site	Low, due to easy compressibility at recommended insertion sites	Variable, depending upon patient body habitus
Recommended during active CPR	No	No	No	Yes
Head and neck trauma	Best to avoid	Best to avoid	Best to avoid	Yes

- Myocardial or great vessel perforation/cardiac tamponade
- Guidewire retention or embolization of guidewire fragments
- Cardiac arrhythmias
- Nerve injury
- Pneumothorax/hemothorax (IJ and SC only)
- Air embolism
- Catheter malposition
- IVC filter entanglement (FEM only)

Early Complications (Days After Procedure)

- Catheter obstruction/blockage
- Chylothorax (IJ and SC only; with injury to thoracic duct (left) > lymphatic duct (right))
- Hydrothorax (IJ and SC only)
- Infection at the insertion site/phlebitis
- Bloodstream infection/sepsis

Delayed Complications (Weeks to Months After Procedure)

- Arteriovenous fistula (when vein and adjacent artery are simultaenously punctured)
- Thrombosis (e.g., DVT)
- Pseudoaneurysm formation (delayed)
- Catheter fracture and embolism
- Vascular erosion
- Vessel stenosis

Some of the most concerning complications and their reported rates, according to insertion site, are provided in Table 5.2.

General Considerations for Central Venous Access

Patient Positioning

Patient positioning is crucial, and the experienced provider will ensure that the patient does not change position during the procedure. In some cases, cannulation may require patient sedation or restraint by colleagues to maintain proper positioning of the patient's head, arm, or leg position throughout the procedure. Assistants should wear gloves and maintain control of the patient's head, neck, or arm beneath the sterile field to prevent inadvertent contamination of the sterile field by the patient. Temporary limb restraints may be required. Trendelenburg (i.e., head-down)

Table 5.2 Site-specific complication rates [8, 11, 12, 39, 40, 43, 45, 50, 55, 58]

	Internal jugular	Subclavian	Femoral
Pneumothorax	+ +	+ + +	–
Hemothorax	–	+ + +	–
Infection	+ +	+	+ + +
Thrombus	+	+ +	+ + +
Arterial puncture	+ +	+	+ + +

Note: Number of "+" represents risk relative to other sites; "–" represents minimal or no risk

positioning >15 degrees is helpful, as this will engorge the central veins and provide the largest possible target for CVC insertion.

Preparation

Providers should ensure that all needed supplies are within reach prior to starting the procedure. Proper preparation prior to the procedure is paramount, and the emergency care provider should ensure that all materials needed for the insertion effort are available before starting the procedure. When possible, it is desirable to have an assistant at the bedside to retrieve items that may become necessary during the procedure. Providers should also seek to optimize the procedural environment, including ensuring adequate lighting, freedom from distractions, and adequate patient counseling or sedation, as needed. The need for documentation of patient consent should be assessed as well. Although "emergent consent" may be implied by certain clinical circumstances, written informed consent for the line insertion (as well as any anticipated complications such as thoracostomy for pneumothorax) should be obtained from alert and oriented patients (or their legally authorized representative) when possible.

Sterility

Sterility is of the utmost importance with CVC insertion, given the relatively higher risk of iatrogenic bloodstream infection as compared to peripheral venous cannulation [63]. Unfortunately, contamination of the provider's gloves or the surgical field may be more common than providers realize [64–66]. Even if providers do not violate the sterile field, field contamination can occur through provider contact with residual bacteria in the deeper layers (e.g., crypts of the hair follicles and sweat glands) of the patient's skin following standard disinfection methods [65, 66]. Chlorhexidine appears to be more effective at achieving sterility of the patient's skin, with bacteria able to be cultured from sterilized skin in only 5.7% of cases, as compared to 32.4% of subjects with povidone-iodine [66]. This has led some authors to suggest routine cleansing of the provider's sterile gloves with antiseptic solution (e.g., 0.5% chlorhexidine plus 70% alcohol) after setting up the field and completing landmark identification, prior to catheter handling. Providers should avoid excessive touching of the patient's prepped skin with the same fingers that will be handling the catheter to reduce the risk of bacteria transfer to the catheter. The placement of "crash" lines (i.e., placement without full sterile precautions) should be avoided unless absolutely required (e.g., cardiac arrest, sudden respiratory collapse), due to the increased risk of iatrogenic infection and injury introduced by lack of proper sterile technique.

Air Embolism

Air embolism is a potential risk with any vascular access attempt but is probably more common with venous cannulation than in arterial cannulation due to the much lower (perhaps even negative) intravascular pressure within the central veins during respiration. Placing the patient in >15 degrees Trendelenburg position should increase central venous return, engorging the IJ and SC veins and providing an easier target while further reducing the risk of air entry through the needle [40]. The frequency of air embolism is largely unknown, but this theoretical risk is easily avoided with proper patient positioning and insertion technique. Saline flush of the catheter lumens prior to insertion may reduce the risk of air embolism, although evidence is limited.

Inability to Advance the Guidewire

Once cannulation of the vein has been achieved, inability to advance the guidewire suggests that the tip of the finder needle may have left the lumen of the vein, or that the veseel lumen is obstructed due to thrombosis or anatomic stricture. If the guidewire cannot be advanced easily, the provider should remove the guidewire, replace the syringe, and attempt to aspirate blood from the finder needle. If no blood is aspirated, it is likely that the needle is no longer within the lumen of the vein. In such cases, the needle should be withdrawn or advanced slowly in 1 mm increments until blood can again be aspirated under syringe suction. Once blood is easily aspirated, the syringe should be removed carefully and guidewire advancement may be again attempted. If the guidewire cannot be passed, it may also be necessary to decrease the angle of the finder needle to be more in plane with the direction of the target vein. If the guidewire can be advanced beyond the tip of the finder needle, it is likely that anatomic obstructions (e.g., bifurcation, thrombus) are preventing further guidewire advancement.

Inability to Remove the Guidewire

When attempting to remove the guidewire from the finder needle, resistance may be encountered. If this occurs, fracture of the guidewire is possible, as the guidewire may be speared on the sharp tip of the finder needle. If retraction of the guidewire is not easily achievable through the internal lumen of the finder needle, it can be helpful to rotate (i.e., clockwise or counterclockwise) the guidewire within the finder needle to determine if this can free-up the guidewire for retraction. If the guidewire cannot be retracted from within the finder needle after rotation, it may be advisable to remove the entire guidewire-finder needle complex from the vein, rather than attempting further guidewire retraction alone, to prevent fracture (i.e., unraveling) of the guidewire. It is generally preferred to remove the entire guidewire/finder needle complex from the vein than to risk guidewire fracture and subsequent embolization of guidewire fragments into the systemic circulation. Unraveling of the guidewire within the vein risks not only damage to the guidewire but also further damage to the target vein during the retraction attempt. If the provider is unable to remove the guidewire with gentle traction, or if embolization of guidewire fragments is suspected, the provider should consult the vascular surgery team for assistance in retrieving the guidewire from the patient.

Confirmation of Proper Line Placement

An anterior-posterior (AP) one-view chest X-ray should be obtained after any CVC insertion in the upper thorax (e.g., IJ, SC), but this is not generally necessary following FEM vein cannulation. The three primary purposes of this chest X-ray are as follows: (1) to confirm that the proper vessel was cannulated (e.g., vein versus artery), (2) to confirm that the catheter was inserted to the proper depth (e.g., terminates at the junction of the SVC and the right atrium), and (3) to rule out the presence of early complications (e.g., hemothorax, pneumothorax). A focused ultrasound (US) examination of the vessel, heart, and ipsilateral lung may also suffice to ensure venous cannulation and rule out pneumothorax, provided that the operator is adequately trained to perform the exam. Transesophageal echocardiography can also accurately identify malpositioned CVCs within the main pulmonary arteries, which is not easily identifiable by CT or ultrasound [67–69]. While *transesophageal* echocardiography may be able to adequately confirm the location of the catheter tip, *transthoracic* echocardiography may not be adequate for this purpose. Direct US visualization of the guidewire within the candidate vessel may also be useful to confirm venous placement prior to dilation [68].

Concern for Arterial Cannulation

The distinction between arterial and venous cannulation is further complicated by the patient's oxygenation status. Dark, nonpulsatile backflow of blood may be seen with arterial puncture in the setting of profound hypoxemia and hypotension [69]. Needle positioning in the vein can be confirmed by the pressure transducer. If there is no access to a pressure transducer, a *venous blood gas (VBG)* can be obtained and compared to an existing *arterial blood gas (ABG)* sample. The differences in various values reported in a blood gas analysis (Table 5.3) can be useful in determining whether the sampled blood is from a venous or an arterial source.

Table 5.3 Comparison of normal ABG and VBG values [70]

	Arterial	Venous
pH	7.35–7.45	7.31–7.41
pCO_2 (kPa)	4.7–6.0	5.5–6.8
pCO_2 (mmHg)	35–45	41–51
HCO_3 (mmol/L)	22–28	23–29
PO_2 (kPa)	10.6–13.3	4.0–5.3
PO_2 (mmHg)	80–100	30–40
SO_2 (%)	>95	75

Securing the Catheter

The suture wing and white rubber clamp/rigid plastic fastener should both be secured to the patient's skin, to reduce the risk of accidental dislodgement or migration of the CVC after line placement. The methods of securing CVC lines include suture and/or adhesive anchoring. Commercial CVC kits include a "bulldog" clamp, which fits over the CVC catheter and is covered by an anchoring device sutured to the skin. Ideally, the anchoring clamp should be placed as close as possible to the insertion site at the skin surface. Transparent film dressing (e.g., Tegaderm®) should be placed so that the dressing is centered on the location at which the catheter penetrates the skin.

Depth of Insertion

Optimal placement of IJ, SC, or AX central lines results in the tip of the catheter being situated in the SVC. *Peres' formula* [71] is a commonly accepted method to determine the optimal depth of CVC insertion needed to achieve this goal and has been shown to be up to 95% accurate [72]. The formula, where "H" is patient height (in cm), is depicted in Fig. 5.14. Some studies have stated that using surface anatomy to determine depth of insertion is superior to formulas, as topographical methods account for anatomical variation [73, 74].

The provider should be sure to document the depth of the catheter insertion from the point at which the catheter penetrates the skin. The "double-hash" marks (Fig. 5.15) represent the full length marked on the manifold ("hub"), while "single-hash" marks are found every 1 cm along the catheter length. The manifold indicates the full length of the catheter as well as the external diameter of the line.

The major veins have differing lengths and diameters, which may influence their availability during conditions of hypovolemia and vascular collapse. The different diameters of the major peripheral and central veins are provided in Table 5.4.

Angle of Bend

Angle of catheter bend influences the rate of flow through the catheter, with more acute angles serving to obstruct flow. Sharp angles or kinking of the external portions of the catheter should be avoided, and the catheter should be secured in such a way that the external portion is kept as straight as possible.

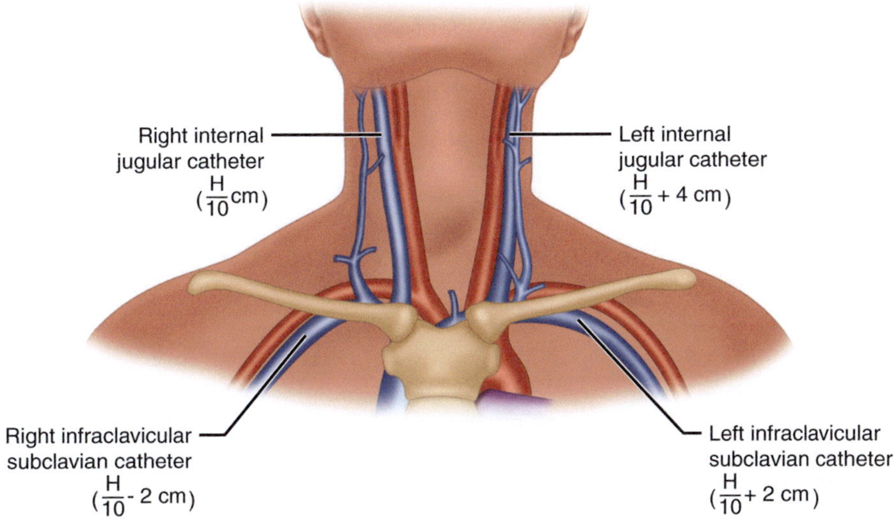

Fig. 5.14 Peres' formula

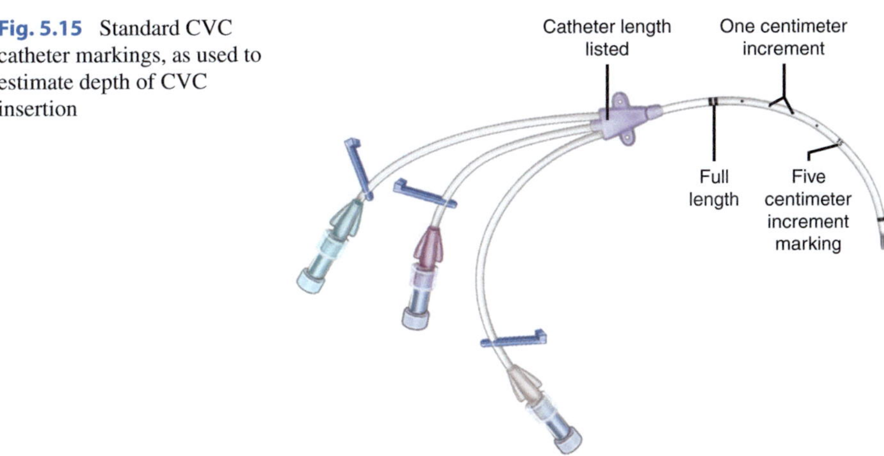

Fig. 5.15 Standard CVC catheter markings, as used to estimate depth of CVC insertion

Conclusion

Landmark-based central venous catheter placement plays a crucial role in the provision of medical care to critically-ill patients under austere conditions. Numerous advantages exist for these techniques, with the main advantage being a quick and reliable method of delivering life-saving medications to provide life-sustaining medications. While each CVC access method has its own unique benefits, it is imperative to remember that each one also poses the risk of complications if not inserted correctly. Knowing which CVC to choose in a specific situation, having sound knowledge of the surrounding anatomy, confirming the correct location of

Table 5.4 Comparative diameter and length of the major veins in adults [75]

Vein	Diameter (mm)	Length (cm)
Cephalic	4–5	35–38
Basilic	8	24
Axillary	16	13
Subclavian	19	6
Right brachiocephalic	19	2.5
Superior vena cava	20	7–9

CVC placement, and detecting complications early on all represent essential skills to reduce the risk of complications.

Key Concepts
- Central venous catheters are often required for critically ill patients, when infusion of non-peripherally compatible infusions or hemodynamic monitoring is required.
- If the provider is unable to cannulate the vein after three attempts, assistance from others should be sought, rather than making additional attempts. Mechanical complications are six times more likely with three or more passes when compared to a single-needle pass.
- Patients should be continuously monitored on telemetry during CVC placement. The presence of arrhythmias suggests that the catheter tip has been advanced too far and may be irritating the right atrial wall.
- Adequate knowledge of vascular anatomy, along with correct patient positioning and physician experience, can allow landmark-based central venous catheter placement within 5 minutes, while ultrasound-guided techniques may require up to 20 minutes to place successfully.

References

1. Geddes LA, Geddes LE. The catheter introducers. Chicago: Mobium Press; 1993.
2. Forssmann W. Die sondierung des rechten herzens. Klin Wochenschr. 1929;8(45):2085–7.
3. Altman LK. Who goes first: the story of self-experimentation in medicine. New York: Random House; 1987.
4. Beheshti MV. A concise history of central venous access. Tech Vasc Interventional Rad. 2011;14:184–5.
5. Agrawal K. The first catheterization. The Hospitalist. 2006; 12. Available at: https://www.the-hospitalist.org/hospitalist/article/123249/first-catheterization. Accessed on 20 July 2020.
6. Aubaniac R. L'injection intraveneuse sous claviculaire. Presse Med. 1952;60:1456.
7. Wilson JN, Grow JB, Demong CV, et al. Central venous pressure in optimal blood volume maintenance. Arch Surg. 1962;85:563.
8. English IC, Frew RM, Piggott JF, et al. Percutaneous cannulation of the internal jugular vein. J Anesth. 1969;24:521–31.
9. Peters JL, Belsham PA, Garrett CP, et al. Doppler ultrasound technique for safer percutaneous catheterization of the infraclavicular subclavian vein. Am J Surg. 1982;143:391–3.

10. Kinsella S, Young N. Ultrasound-guided central line placement as compared with standard landmark technique: some unpleasant arithmetic for the economics of medical innovation. Value Health. 2009;12(1):98–100.
11. Ruesch S, Walder B, Tramèr MR. Complications of central venous catheters: internal jugular versus subclavian access–a systematic review. Crit Care Med. 2002;30(2):454–60.
12. Tse A, Schick MA. Central Line Placement. [Updated 2020 Aug 15]. In: StatPearls [Internet]. Treasure Island: StatPearls Publishing; 2020 Jan-. Available from: https://www.ncbi.nlm.nih.gov/books/NBK470286/. Accessed on 20 July 2020.
13. Teleflex – A Global Provider of Medical Technologies [Internet]. USA: Teleflex Incorporated; 2020. Available from: http://www.teleflex.com/usa/en/index.html. Accessed on 20 July 2020.
14. Thaut L, Weymouth W, Hunsaker B, et al. Evaluation of central venous access with accelerated Seldinger technique versus modified Seldinger technique. J Emerg Med. 2019;56(1):23–8.
15. Rivard AB, Burns B. Anatomy, Head and Neck, Internal Jugular Vein. [Updated 2018 Dec 6]. In: StatPearls [Internet]. Treasure Island: StatPearls Publishing; 2020 Jan-. Available from: https://www.ncbi.nlm.nih.gov/books/NBK513258/. Accessed on 20 July 2020.
16. Giordano CR, Murtagh KR, Mills J, et al. Locating the optimal internal jugular target site for central venous line placement. J Clin Anesth. 2016;33:198–202.
17. Lorente L, Henry C, Martín MM, et al. Central venous catheter-related infection in a prospective and observational study of 2,595 catheters. Crit Care. 2005;9(6):R631.
18. Oner B, Karam AR, Surapaneni P, et al. Pneumothorax following ultrasound-guided jugular vein puncture for central venous access in interventional radiology: 4 years of experience. J Intensive Care Med. 2012;27(6):370.
19. Miki I, Murata S, Nakazawa K, et al. Anatomical relationship between the common carotid artery and the internal jugular vein during head rotation. Ultrasound. 2014;22(2):99–103.
20. Graham AS, Ozment C, Tegtmeyer K, et al. Videos in clinical medicine. Central venous catheterization. N Engl J Med. 2007;356(21):e21.
21. Maecken T, Marcon C, Bornas S, et al. Relationship of the internal jugular vein to the common carotid artery: implications for ultrasound-guided access. Eur J Anaesthesiol. 2011;28(5):351–5.
22. Umaña M, Garcia A, Bustamante L, et al. Variations in the anatomical relationship between the common carotid artery and the internal jugular vein. Colomb Med (Cali). 2015;46(2):54–9.
23. Sulek CA, Blas ML, Lobato EB. A randomized study of left versus right internal jugular vein cannulation in adults. J Clin Anesth. 2000;12(2):142–5.
24. Wang R, Snoey ER, Clements RC, et al. Effect of head rotation on vascular anatomy of the neck: an ultrasound study. J Emerg Med. 2006;31(3):283–6.
25. Beddy P, Geoghegan T, Ramesh N, et al. Valsalva and gravitational variability of the internal jugular vein and common femoral vein: ultrasound assessment. Eur J Radiol. 2006;58(2):307–9.
26. Mendenhall BR, O'Rourke MC. Internal jugular vein central venous access. StatPearls [Internet], Treasure Island (FL), Jan 2019. Available from: https://www.ncbi.nlm.nih.gov/books/NBK436020/. Accessed on 20 July 2020.
27. Abood GJ, Davis KA, Esposito TJ, et al. Comparison of routine chest radiograph versus clinician judgment to determine adequate central line placement in critically ill patients. J Trauma. 2007;63(1):50.
28. Stonelake PA, Bodenham AR. The carina as a radiological landmark for central venous catheter tip position. Br J Anaesth. 2006;96(3):335–40.
29. Gebhard RE, Szmuk P, Pivalizza EG, et al. The accuracy of electrocardiogram-controlled central line placement. Anesth Analg. 2007;104(1):65–70.
30. Krishnan AK, Menon P, Gireesh Kumar KP, et al. Electrocardiogram-guided technique: an alternative method for confirming central venous catheter tip placement. J Emerg Trauma Shock. 2018;11(4):276–81.
31. Felix VB, Dos Santos JAB, Fernandes KJM, et al. Anatomical study of the accessory axillary vein in cadavers: a contribution to the axillary surgical approach. J Vasc Bras. 2016;15(4):275–9.
32. Galloway S, Bodenham A. Ultrasound imaging of the axillary vein – anatomical basis for central venous access. Br J Anaesth. 2003;90:589–95.

33. Gouin F, Martin C, Saux P. Central venous and pulmonary artery catheterizations via the axillary vein. Acta Anaesthesiol Scand. 1985;29:27–9.
34. Nickalls RW. A new percutaneous infraclavicular approach to the axillary vein. Anaesthesia. 1987;42(2):151–4.
35. Khatibi B, Sandhu NP. Real-time ultrasound guided axillary vein cannulation. J Perioper Echocardiogr. 2015;3:42–7.
36. Metz RI, Lucking SE, Chaten FC, et al. Percutaneous catheterization of the axillary vein in infants and children. Pediatrics. 1990;80(4):531–3.
37. Gawda R, Czarnik T, Weron R, Nowotarski J. A new infraclavicular landmark-based approach to the axillary vein as an alternative method of central venous cannulation. J Vasc Access. 2016;17(3):273–8.
38. Yoffa D. Supraclavicular subclavian venepuncture and catheterisation. Lancet. 1965;2:614–7.
39. Deere M, Burns B. Central Venous Access, Subclavian Vein. [Updated 2018 Nov 13]. In: StatPearls [Internet]. Treasure Island: StatPearls Publishing; 2019 Jan-.
40. Bardes J, Lewis M. Central venous catheters. In: Demetriades D, Inaba K, Lumb P, editors. Atlas of critical care procedures. Cham: Springer; 2018.
41. Thakur A, Kaur K, Lamba A, et al. Comparative evaluation of subclavian vein catheterisation using supraclavicular versus infraclavicular approach. Indian J Anaesth. 2014;58(2):160–4.
42. Keéri-Szántó M. The subclavian vein, a constant and convenient intravenous injection site. AMA Arch Surg. 1956;72(1):179–81.
43. Bannon MP, Heller SF, Rivera M. Anatomic considerations for central venous cannulation. Risk Manag Healthc Policy. 2011;4:27–39.
44. Land RE. Anatomic relationships of the right subclavian vein. Arch Surg. 1971;102:178–80.
45. Timsit JF. What is the best site for central venous catheter insertion in critically ill patients? Crit Care. 2003;7(6):397–9.
46. Tripathi M, Dubey PK, Ambesh SP. Direction of the J-tip of the guidewire, in Seldinger technique, is a significant factor in misplacement of subclavian vein catheter: a randomized, controlled study. Anesth Analg. 2005;100(1):21–4.
47. Moran SG, Peoples JB. The deltopectoral triangle as a landmark for percutaneous infraclavicular cannulation of the subclavian vein. Angiology. 1993;44(9):683–6.
48. Bernard RW, Stahl WM. Subclavian vein catheterizations: a prospective study. Ann Surg. 1971;173:184–90.
49. Agarwal AK. Central vein stenosis. Am J Kidney Dis. 2013;61(6):1001–15.
50. James D, Fowler GC. Central venous catheter insertion. Pfenninger & Fowler's Procedures for Primary Care. Elsevier, Philadelphia, PA. USA. 2019;p.1521–28.
51. Sidoti A, Brogi E, Biancofiore G, et al. Ultrasound-versus landmark-guided subclavian vein catheterization: a prospective observational study from a tertiary referral hospital. Sci Rep. 2019;9(1):12248. https://doi.org/10.1038/s41598-019-48766-1.
52. Xu F, Zhang L. Landmark-guided subclavian vein catheterization by palpating the subclavian artery. Am J Emerg Med. 2018;36(4):722–3.
53. Mirza B, Vanek VW, Kupensky DT. Pinch-off syndrome: case report and collective review of the literature. Am Surg. 2004;70(7):635–44.
54. Cho JB, Park IY, Sung KY, et al. Pinch-off syndrome. J Korean Surg Soc. 2013;85(3):139–44.
55. Castro D, Martin Lee LAM, Gossman W. Femoral Vein Central Venous Access. [Updated 2019 Jul 11]. In: StatPearls [Internet]. Treasure Island: StatPearls Publishing; 2019 Jan-. Accessed on 20 July 2020.
56. Palmer ES, Caldwell AK, Newcomb MB, et al. Avoiding the femoral vein in central venous cannulation: an outdated practice. ACP Hospitalist. 2018. https://acphospitalist.org/archives/2018/08/perspectives-avoiding-the-femoral-vein-in-central-venous-cannulation-an-outdated-practice.htm. Accssed on 20 July 2020.
57. Marik PE, Flemmer M, Harrison W. The risk of catheter-related bloodstream infection with femoral venous catheters as compared to subclavian and internal jugular venous catheters: a systematic review of the literature and meta-analysis. Crit Care Med. 2012;40(8):2479.
58. Parienti JJ, Mongardon N, Mégarbane B, et al. Intravascular complications of central venous catheterization by insertion site. N Engl J Med. 2015;373(13):1220–9.

59. Trottier SJ, Veremakis C, O'Brien J, et al. Femoral deep vein thrombosis associated with central venous catheterization: results from a prospective, randomized trial. Crit Care Med. 1995;23(1):52–9.
60. Hopkins JW, Warkentine F, Gracely E, et al. The anatomic relationship between the common femoral artery and common femoral vein in frog leg position versus straight leg position in pediatric patients. Acad Emerg Med. 2009;16:579–84.
61. Emerman CL, Bellon EM, Lukens TW, May TE, Effron D. A prospective study of femoral versus subclavian vein catheterization during cardiac arrest. Ann Emerg Med. 1990;19(1):26–30.
62. Meredith JW, Young JS, O'Neil EA, et al. Femoral catheters and deep venous thrombosis: a prospective evaluation with venous duplex sonography. J Trauma. 1993;35(2):187–90.
63. Ruiz-Giardin J, Ochoa Chamorro I, Velázquez Ríos L, et al. Blood stream infections associated with central and peripheral venous catheters. BMC Infect Dis. 2019;19:841.
64. Kocent H, Corke C, Alajeel A, Graves S. Washing of gloved hands in antiseptic solution prior to central venous line insertion reduces contamination. Anaesth Intensive Care. 2002;30(3):338–40.
65. Levy JH, Nagle DM, Curling PE, et al. Contamination reduction during central venous catheterisation. Crit Care Med. 1988;16:165–7.
66. Sato S, Sakuragi T, Dan K. Human skin flora as a potential source of epidural abscess. Anesthesiology. 1996;85:1276–82.
67. Sawchuk C, Fayad A. Confirmation of internal jugular guide wire position utilizing transesophageal echocardiography. Can J Anaesth. 2001 Jul;48(7):688–90.
68. Gillman LM, Blaivas M, Lord J, et al. Ultrasound confirmation of guidewire position may eliminate accidental arterial dilatation during central venous cannulation. Scand J Trauma Resusc Emerg Med. 2010;18:39.
69. Ezaru CS, Mangione MP, Oravitz TM, et al. Eliminating arterial injury during central venous catheterization using manometry. Anesth Analg. 2009;109(1):130.
70. Higgins C. [Internet] Acute Care Testing.org. Central Venous Blood Gas Analysis, July 2011, acutecaretesting.org/en/articles/central-venous-blood-gas-analysis. Accessed on 20 July 2020.
71. Peres PW. Positioning central venous catheters – a prospective survey. Anaesth Intensive Care. 1990;18(4):536–9.
72. Czepizak CA, O'Callaghan JM, Venus B. Evaluation of formulas for optimal positioning of central venous catheters. Chest. 1995;107:1662–4.
73. Vinay M, Tejesh CA. Depth of insertion of right internal jugular central venous catheter: comparison of topographic and formula methods. Saudi J Anaesth. 2016;10(3):255–8.
74. Jayaraman J, Shah V. Bedside prediction of the central venous catheter insertion depth – comparison of different techniques. J Anaesthesiol Clin Pharmacol. 2019;35(2):197–201.
75. Bullock-Corkhill M. Central venous access devices: access and insertion. In: Alexander M, Corrigan A, Gorski L, Hankins J, Perucca R, editors. Infusion nursing: An evidence-based practice. 3rd ed. Saunders/Elsevier: St. Louis; 2010.

Ultrasound-Guided Central Venous Catheters

6

Lyudmila Khait, Adrienne N. Malik, Michael P. Petrovich, Abdallah A. Ajani, and Mark J. Favot

Introduction

Ultrasound-guided (USG) central venous catheter (CVC) placement is a potentially life-saving technique that must be mastered in order to obtain central venous vascular access quickly with minimal complications. Prior to the routine use of ultrasound, CVC access was performed "blind" via landmark techniques, with failure and complication rates reported to be anywhere from 5% to 19% [1–4]. This chapter discusses the potential advantages and disadvantages of using real-time ultrasound guidance to achieve CVC access, including details relating to the performance of USG CVC placement, confirmation methods, and common pitfalls that may be encountered by clinicians wishing to utilize this technique.

L. Khait · M. J. Favot (✉)
Department of Emergency Medicine, Wayne State University School of Medicine, Detroit, MI, USA
e-mail: lkhai@med.wayne.edu; mfavot@med.wayne.edu

A. N. Malik
Department of Emergency Medicine, Kansas University Medical Center, Kansas City, KS, USA
e-mail: Amalik3@kumc.edu

M. P. Petrovich
Department of Emergency Medicine, Adventist Health, Portland, OR, USA

A. A. Ajani
Department of Emergency Medicine, University of Massachusetts Medical Center, Worchester, MA, USA
e-mail: Abdallah.ajani@umassmemorial.org

© Springer Nature Switzerland AG 2021
J. H. Paxton (ed.), *Emergent Vascular Access*,
https://doi.org/10.1007/978-3-030-77177-5_6

General Considerations

The use of anatomical landmarks alone to guide needle insertion during CVC placement is associated with increased risk of complications. The most common complications of the landmark-guided approach include pneumothorax, arterial cannulation, and hematoma formation. These complications are dependent on the underlying patient pathophysiology, patient anatomy, site of CVC insertion, and clinician experience [1, 2, 5, 6].

The use of ultrasound (US) guidance for CVC placement was first described in relation to the *internal jugular (IJ) vein* by Yonei et al. in 1986 [7], although the same concepts have subsequently been applied to use with the other commonly accessed central veins. In 1993, Denys et al. prospectively compared 302 patients treated with US-guided (USG) IJ vein cannulation to 302 control patients treated with the landmark-guided technique. They found that the use of ultrasound guidance in IJ venous cannulation resulted in a 100% success rate, compared to 88.1% success in the landmark-guided technique. They also demonstrated that US guidance produced fewer cannulation attempts, shorter time to cannulation, lower incidence of carotid artery puncture, lower incidence of hematoma formation, and lower incidence of brachial plexus injury [8]. Since then, additional studies from multiple medical specialties have continued to show similar safety profiles [9, 10]. In 2015, Brass et al. published a Cochrane Review including over 5000 patients that found the procedural safety of IJ venous catheters placed under ultrasound guidance to be superior as compared to landmark placement [11]. That same year, they also published data via Cochrane Review showing superiority in safety of USG catheterization of the subclavian and femoral veins as compared to traditional landmark technique [12].

Previous studies have demonstrated that the use of ultrasound guidance for CVC insertion significantly decreases morbidity and mortality in critically ill patients who require CVC placement [13–15]. Utilizing real-time ultrasound guidance, the clinician can visualize anatomic anomalies, clearly identify and visualize the target central vein, monitor progress of cannulation, and avoid ill-advised attempts to cannulate vessels with intraluminal thrombosis [13–15].

Appropriate patient positioning during IJ venous cannulation (i.e., head turned) inherently increases the risk of *carotid artery (CA)* puncture, as the IJ vein frequently overlaps this structure. In fact, at 90° head rotation away from the midline, the IJ vein overlaps 78% of the carotid artery diameter, vs 29% in a neutral position [16]. In this context, the use of USG for venipuncture is especially helpful to avoid inadvertent CA injury.

Introduction to Ultrasound

Probe/Transducer

The appropriate transducer for any vascular access procedure is a small linear array probe with a high-frequency transducer (5–15mhz) [11]. However, some linear transducers may have a range as high as 20 mhz. This provides an excellent superficial resolution, but image quality may degrade at deeper depths required for direct needle visualization during central venous cannulation [18].

Exam Type

Most commercial ultrasound systems come with preloaded exam types (i.e., vascular, cardiac, RUQ, etc.) It is important to select a "vascular," "small parts," or "needle visualization" exam type to provide you with the spatial resolution required for evaluating the anatomy and for direct needle visualization.

General Tips for Ultrasound Guidance

The reader is encouraged to become familiar with the landmark-based method for CVC insertion detailed in Chap. 5 of this book, including the relevant anatomical considerations, as much of the technique for USG CVC insertion is common with the landmark-based method.

Standard sterile technique should be followed with regard to PPE (personal protective equipment) worn by the practitioner, draping of the patient, and cleansing of the procedural area. A sterile probe cover with sufficient length to cover the probe's cord that will come into contact with the draped area is required. Either a sterile field (e.g., exterior drape or other sterile barrier) to prevent contamination by the US machine or a second person should be employed to operate the US system in case adjustments are needed during the procedure. Sterile lubricant, which usually comes prepackaged with commercially available sterile probe covers, is also needed. Lubricant will need to be applied to the probe itself, as well as on top of the sterile probe cover, to generate optimal US images. Ideal hand, probe, and needle approach positioning are demonstrated in Fig. 6.1. Note that this figure does not include sterile barriers for illustration purposes.

If local anesthesia is to be used, infiltration of 1% lidocaine solution should also be performed in conjunction with US guidance to assure that the location of the skin wheal is in appropriate proximity to the underlying vein of interest.

Cannulation of the vein occurs using either the introducer needle or appropriate angiocatheter. The needle is advanced under direct US visualization using either the out-of-plane (short axis) or in-plane (long axis) (Fig. 6.2) approach toward the target vein.

With the landmark-based approach, negative pressure is typically maintained by pulling back on the plunger of the syringe during insertion until a flash of blood is noted. One important difference with direct US visualization is that negative pressure is not required as the needle is advanced. Although a change in resistance and flash of blood into the syringe may be noted, venous cannulation will be noted via direct US visualization of the needle tip within the lumen of the vessel. Consistent with standard Seldinger technique, the guidewire is then advanced. The introducing

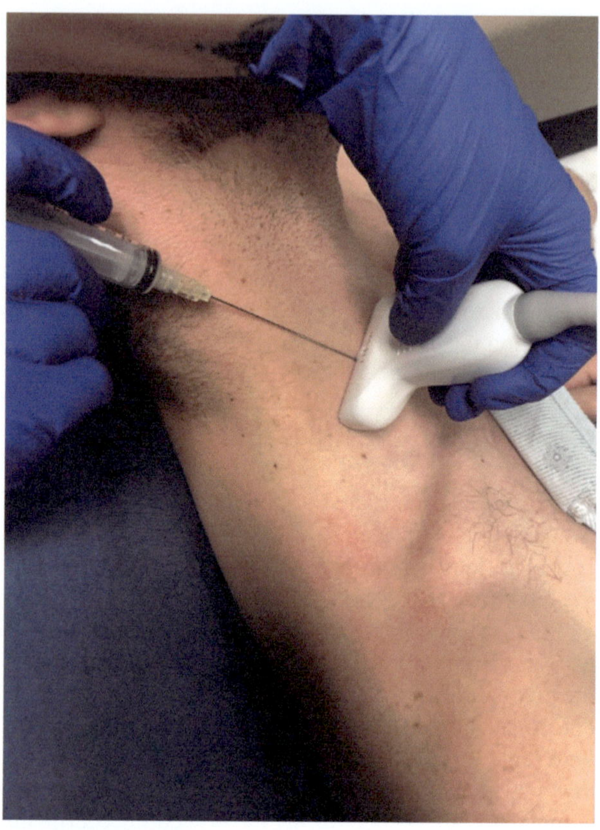

Fig. 6.1 Probe and needle positioning for the IJV out-of-plane (short axis) approach

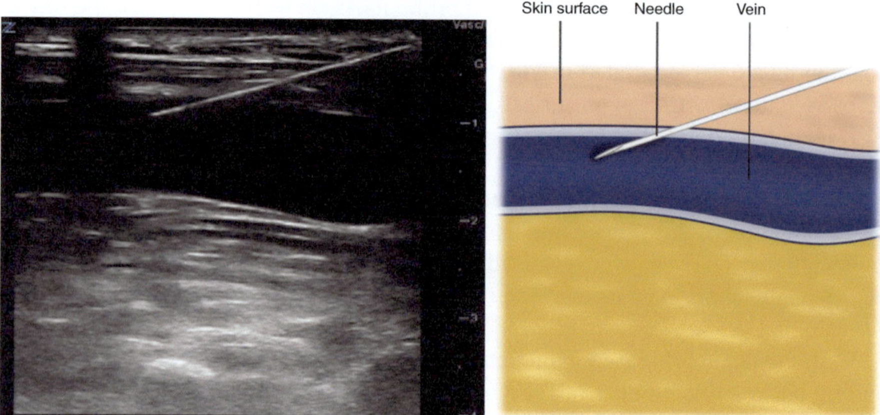

Fig. 6.2 In-plane (long axis) view of USG central venous puncture

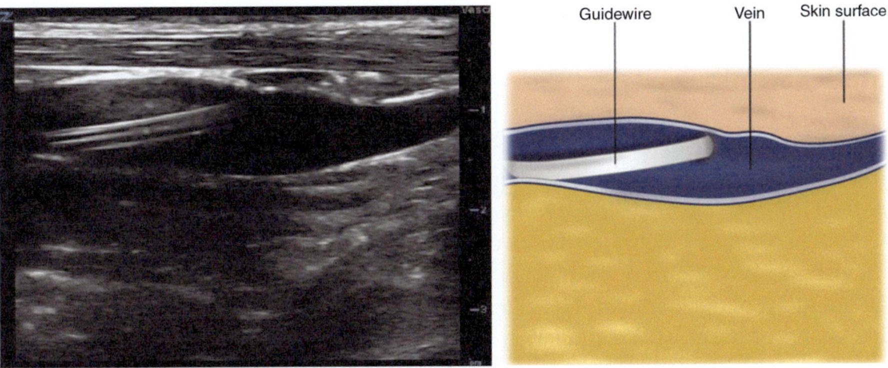

Fig. 6.3 Guidewire visualized with in-plane (long axis) view

Fig. 6.4 Guidewire visualized with out-of-plane (short axis) view

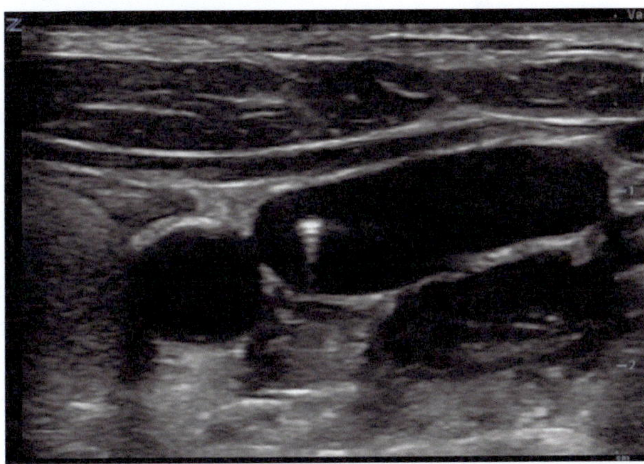

needle or angiocatheter is then removed. As described above, proper placement of the guidewire should be verified by ultrasound prior to soft tissue dilation and catheter cannulation. After cannulation, the positioning of the guidewire should once again be verified with ultrasound (as shown in Figs. 6.3 and 6.4). Note that the guidewire appears as a straight or curved line on the long-axis view, while it appears as a "dot" on the cross-sectional short-axis view. Whichever view is selected, the provider will also see *reverberation artifact lines* below the guidewire, indicating that you are viewing a dense (e.g., metal) structure. Once the guidewire has been confirmed to be in the vein and the catheter has been inserted, all lumens of the catheter should be capped, aspirated, and flushed with sterile saline to minimize the risk of luminal clotting. The catheter should then be sewn into place and secured with an appropriate occlusive dressing. The use of a BioPatch® or other antimicrobial-impregnated dressing at the site of skin insertion is recommended.

Static Versus Dynamic Techniques

Static Technique

Static technique involves using the US to evaluate the patient's anatomy and locate the target vessel but *does not include visualization of the needle as it is inserted into the patient's blood vessel*. Once the relevant anatomy is identified, the US probe is placed out of the field, and the procedure is continued using landmark methods informed by the previously visualized US images. This technique is essentially used to verify the assumptions of the landmark-based approach [12] and has been shown to improve the likelihood of successful cannulation when compared to the purely landmark-based approach [18]. The static technique does not require a sterile probe cover if this vascular survey and target localization is performed prior to sterile field preparation.

Dynamic Technique

Dynamic US guidance not only includes aspects of the static technique but *also involves direct visualization of the needle as it enters the target vein*. Although the static technique may improve the likelihood of successful cannulation, it has not been shown to decrease cost or enhance patient safety [19]. However, dynamic ultrasound guidance has been shown to reduce complication rates and decrease the risk of line-associated infection [19]. Because this additional US-guidance occurs after sterilization of the procedural field, a full-length sterile probe cover must be used for this technique [18]. Dynamic US guidance can be achieved utilizing either the "in-plane" approach or the "out-of-plane" approach.

The "In-Plane" Approach

The "in-plane" (long-axis) approach to the dynamic technique involves orienting both the path of the needle and the US beam in a coplanar path. This allows for continuous real-time visualization of the needle as it is directed toward the vein. However, given the small width of both the US beam and the needle, the margin for error is much greater. *Anchoring the operator's probe hand on the patient is of the utmost importance* to prevent loss of visualization of the needle. If the view of the needle is lost, advancement of the needle should be stalled until visualization of the needle and the needle tip in the vessel are reacquired. The primary benefit of this technique is real-time visualization of the needle in its entirety, decreasing the risk of posterior vein wall puncture [18, 20].

The "Out-of-Plane" Approach

This technique involves a *short-axis approach*, in which the probe is oriented perpendicular to the angle of needle insertion. It allows for visualization of the vein and adjacent structures during the procedure. However, this technique is limited as the needle is only partially visualized. The tip and mid-shaft will appear the same in this orientation, and a stepwise approach of needle advancement is needed to ensure that the needle is not advanced too far, resulting in complications. This technique has been shown to be more easily mastered by emergency physicians [18, 20]. It has also been shown to be associated with an increased first-pass success for operators with varying levels of US expertise [18, 20].

Whether using the static or dynamic technique, identification of the pertinent anatomy is paramount to successful line placement. The vein of interest should be evaluated over a length of several centimeters in the anticipated direction of catheter insertion to identify venous tortuosity or changes in the surrounding anatomic structures. The target vein should be checked for patency. This can be achieved by either compression or by Doppler color flow assessment. Compression of the blood vessel may also help differentiate the vein from the adjacent artery, which must be avoided [18].

Confirming Proper Placement

Proper cannulation of the intended target vein must be confirmed prior to dilation of the tract and venotomy. This can be achieved by using US imaging to verify that the guidewire is in the correct vessel. Verification is often performed using an in-plane (long-axis) view of the guidewire within the vein of choice. (Fig. 6.3). This verification can also be obtained with the out-of-plane (short-axis) view but may be slightly more difficult to visualize (Fig. 6.4). The direct visualization of proper placement should be repeated after the advancement of the catheter to evaluate for possible malposition. This again can be achieved in both the in-plane or out-of-plane technique [21].

Another method of confirming proper venous placement of the CVC is by injecting agitated saline through the newly placed CVC while simultaneously obtaining a transthoracic or subxiphoid view of the heart. The agitated saline is generated using a three-way stopcock and two sterile saline flushes with their contents manually pushed back and forth between syringes to create tiny air bubbles in the sterile fluid. This solution is then injected through the newly placed CVC, while the provider has the phased array probe focused on the right chambers of the patient's heart. The provider monitors the ultrasound screen for a flurry of bubbles to appear in the right heart chambers. If venous placement is achieved, the agitated saline should be visualized in the right atria and ventricle, indicating proper placement and usability of the line. The benefit of this technique is it can prove appropriate line placement, prior to obtaining a confirmatory chest X-ray, and thus has utility when there is a time-sensitive need to start medications through the CVC. However, this technique involves switching between the linear and phased array probe and may be difficult to achieve when a single practitioner is present [21].

Despite the increasing utility of ultrasound imaging, standard of care at most institutions is to obtain a chest X-ray after internal jugular or subclavian central venous catheter placement to evaluate for malposition and possible complications (e.g., pneumothorax).

Needle Versus Angiocatheter

Most commercially available CVC kits contain both an introducer needle and an angiocatheter. Studies have shown that the use of the introducer needle results in fewer complications and increased first-pass success as compared to the angiocatheter [22]. If the angiocatheter is used, however, attempting to refeed the needle into the catheter while inserted into the patient should be avoided. This is due to the thin-walled nature of the angiocatheter and the possibility of the cutting needle damaging the sidewall of the catheter. The dreaded complication is embolization of the sheared tip of the angiocatheter.

Site-Specific Considerations

Internal Jugular (IJ) Vein

The *internal jugular (IJ) vein* is a confluence of the *inferior petrosal sinus* and the *sigmoid dural venous sinus* (Fig. 6.5). This vessel exits the skull through the *jugular foramen* and forms the *jugular bulb*. It descends inferiorly into the neck adjacent to the *internal carotid artery (ICA)* and the *vagus nerve* (cranial nerve X) within the *carotid sheath* before joining with the *subclavian (SC) vein* to form the

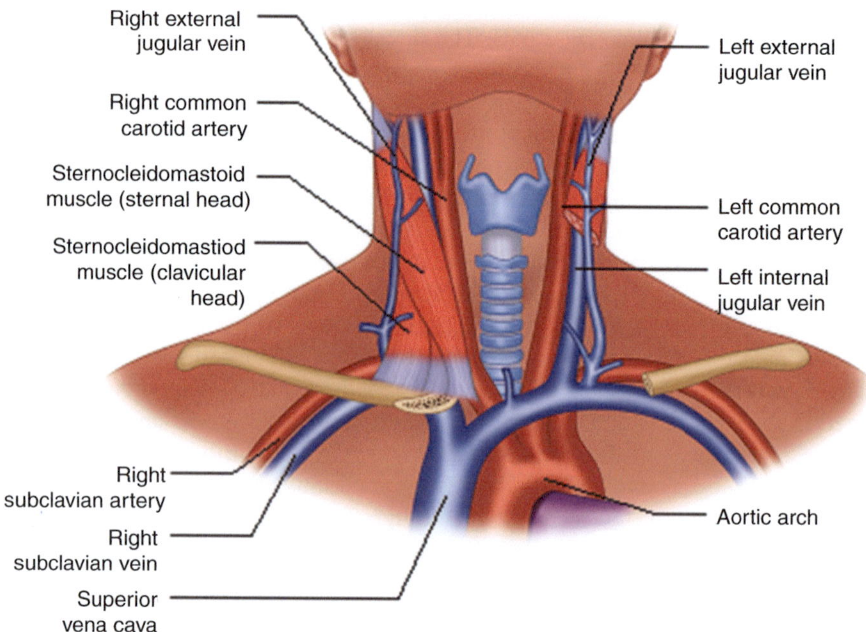

Fig. 6.5 Central vessels of the neck and upper torso

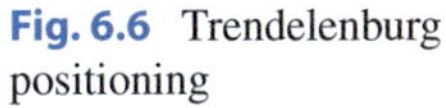

Fig. 6.6 Trendelenburg positioning

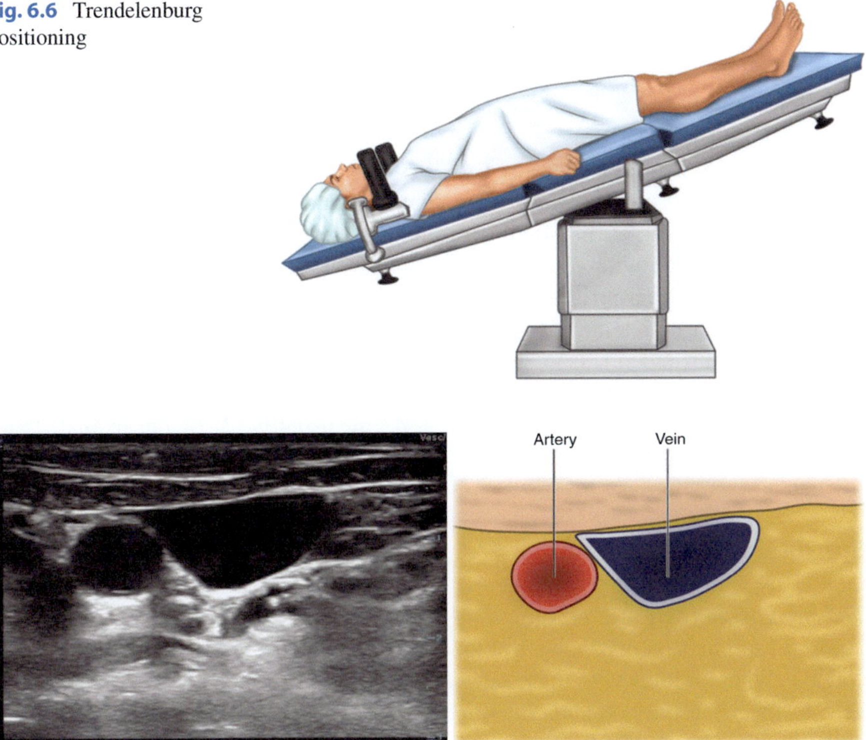

Fig. 6.7 Out-of-plane (short-axis) view of the IJ vein and the carotid artery

brachiocephalic vein. Although the IJ classically lies lateral and anterior to the ICA as it descends, this orientation can be changed with the positioning of the head [18, 23]. The left IJ is classically described as being slightly larger than the right IJ [23].

Proper positioning of the patient will maximize the likelihood of first-attempt success. Place the patient in *Trendelenburg position* (i.e., supine, bed adjusted with feet slightly higher than the head, as in Fig. 6.6) to promote increased venous filling and increase the vein's diameter [20]. This promotes easy identification of the vein and creates a larger target for cannulation. The precise degree to which the head is directed downward will depend upon multiple factors, including the patient's tolerance for this position and the capacity of the patient stretcher.

Turning the patient's head to the contralateral side will bring the IJ into a more superficial position while increasing the depth of the ICA compared to a head-neutral position [20]. This maneuver also affords improved ergonomics with regard to the angle of needle insertion for the practitioner. The IJ vein is typically identified using an out-of-plane approach. As demonstrated in Fig. 6.7, the carotid artery will appear as a thick-walled vessel that is not easily compressible, while the vein appears as a thin-walled vessel that is typically easily compressed with light pressure from the US probe.

Ergonomic positioning of the US provider relative to the patient and US screen is also important. The provider should be at the head of the bed with the US located on the ipsilateral side near the patient's hip. The screen and the point of needle insertion should be in a direct line to minimize any head movement needed by the practitioner [20].

The depth of insertion required for USG CVC insertion at the IJ vein will vary according to the side of insertion, patient gender, and other unique anatomical considerations. Although each patient is different, a good rule of thumb for the length of catheter insertion with *right-sided* IJ CVCs is [patient height in cm]/10. In one study, the average appropriate depth of right-sided IJ catheter insertion was found to be 12–13 cm in males and 11–12 cm in female subjects. The length of catheter required with left-sided IJ CVC placement is greater than that required for the right side. For *left-sided* IJ CVC placement, the required depth of insertion may be estimated by [(patient height in cm) / 10] + 4 cm, usually 13–14 cm in males and 12–13 cm in females [24, 25].

Subclavian (SC) Vein

The subclavian (SC) vein is formed by the *axillary vein* when it crosses the lateral border of the first rib, as shown in Fig. 6.8. It then arches cephalad posterior to the clavicle, where it joins with the *external jugular (EJ) vein*. It is then joined by the IJ vein to form the *brachiocephalic vein*. The SC vein accompanies the *subclavian artery*, which is usually located deep and posterior to the vein. Other structures posterior to the vein include the first rib and the lung pleura. On the left, the *thoracic duct* empties into the beginning of the brachiocephalic vein. The right lymphatic trunk empties into the same position on the contralateral side [27].

Infraclavicular Approach

As with IJ vein cannulation, the patient should be placed in Trendelenburg position (Fig. 6.6) to increase venous filling and provide a more easily identifiable structure and larger target vein [20]. Placing a towel beneath the patient in between the scapulae is also recommended, as this promotes anterior projection of the chest wall with the shoulders drawn back, bringing the SC vein into a more superficial position and reducing obstruction to access by the upper extremities. If the infraclavicular approach is sought, position the patient so that the shoulders are in a "shrugged" position, displacing the clavicle cephalad and opening an acoustic window to facilitate US visualization of the subclavian vein [28]. In neutral position, the clavicle lies over the proximal aspect of the SC vein. Shrugging the shoulder moves the clavicle superiorly, which opens a window that allows the SC vein to be seen on US without obstruction by the clavicle (Fig. 6.9).

The US screen is best placed on the contralateral side of the patient (i.e., opposite the side of the target vessel) for both the supraclavicular and infraclavicular SC approach. The needle insertion site and the US screen should be within a straight line of sight to reduce the amount of movement needed by the practitioner during the procedure [20].

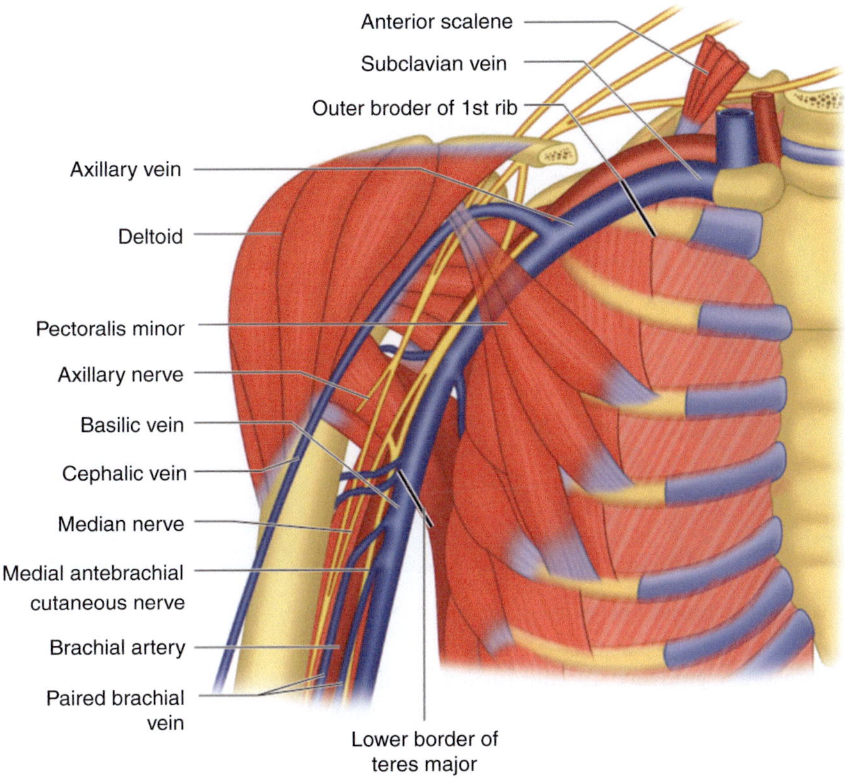

Fig. 6.8 Anatomy of the subclavian and related veins

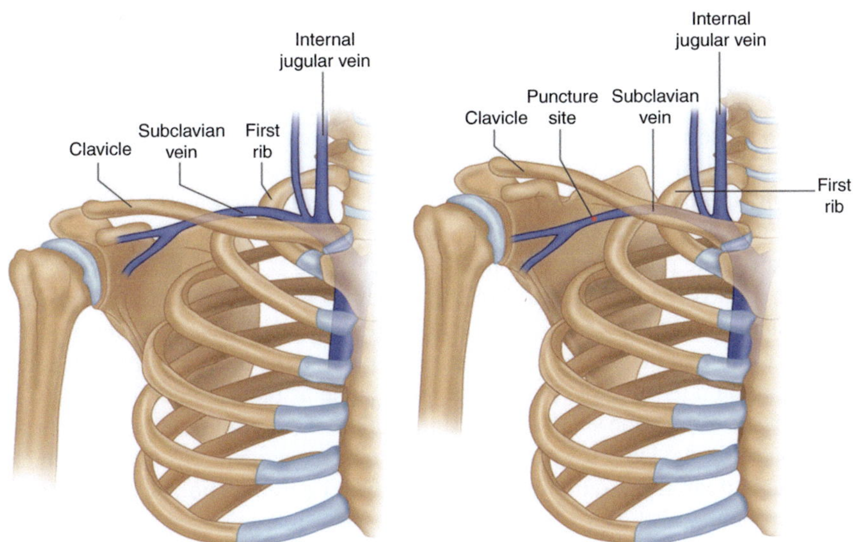

Fig. 6.9 Change in SC vein exposure with shoulder shrug

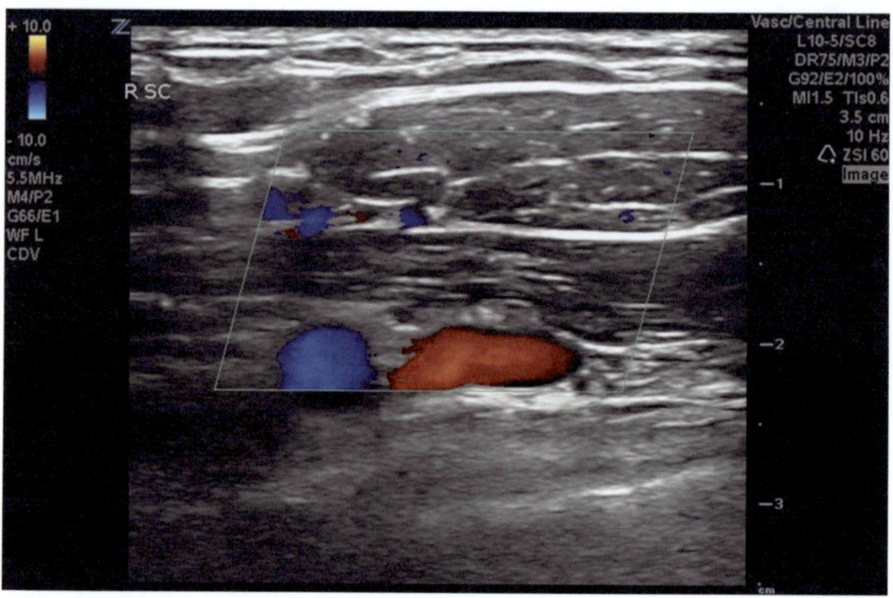

Fig. 6.10 Infraclavicular out-of-plane approach to the SC vein

Ultrasound guidance for the infraclavicular approach can be performed with either the in-plane or out-of-plane technique. Most often, identification of the subclavian vein can be accomplished within the *clavipectoral triangle* (i.e., deltopectoral triangle), which is bounded by the clavicle, the lateral border of the pectoralis major muscle (inferiorly), and the medial border of the deltoid muscle (superiorly). This may be significantly more lateral than the common starting position utilized with the landmark-based approach. The provider should start by positioning the linear probe just inferior to the far lateral aspect of the clavicle in long axis with the probe indicator cephalad and probe placement parallel to the path of the axillary vein. Care should be taken to ensure that the vein is being viewed, not the artery, as their appearance with US may be similar. The vein can be distinguished from the artery in the out-of-plane view (Fig. 6.10) and then the probe rotated 90 degrees to an in-plane approach over the vein (Fig. 6.11). Confirmation can be achieved by assessing for vascular compressibility and a venous hum with pulse wave Doppler. When appropriate positioning is confirmed, the needle is inserted using an in-plane approach (Fig. 6.12) and directed to the center of the axillary vein lumen under direct visualization [29]. The J-loop of the guidewire is fed with the distal J portion of the wire oriented toward the patient's feet to prevent the guidewire tracking cephalad. The remainder of CVC placement is the same as that outlined in the IJ CVC placement section. In one small single-center randomized-controlled trial performed by Fragou et al., the USG long-axis approach to infraclavicular SC CVC placement resulted in increased first-attempt success and fewer complications when compared to landmark methods [30].

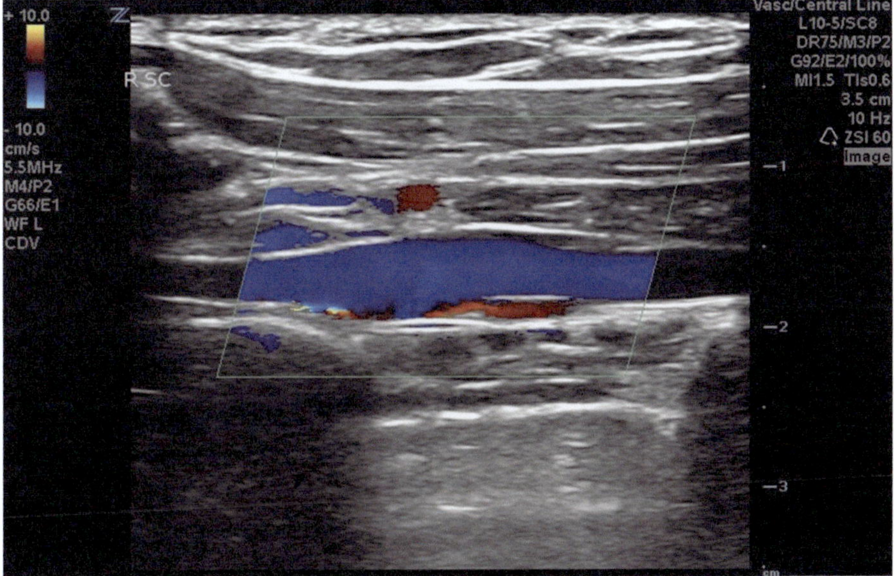

Fig. 6.11 Infraclavicular in-plane approach to the SC vein

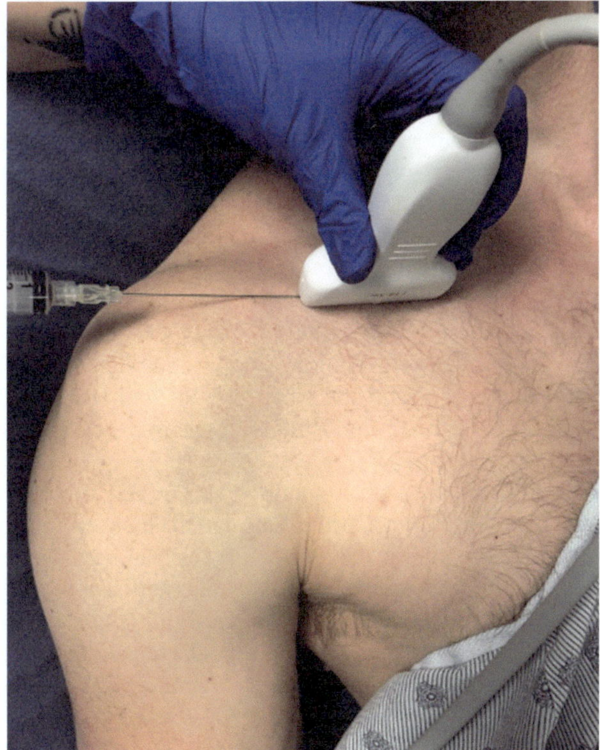

Fig. 6.12 Probe and needle position with the infraclavicular in-plane approach to SC vein cannulation

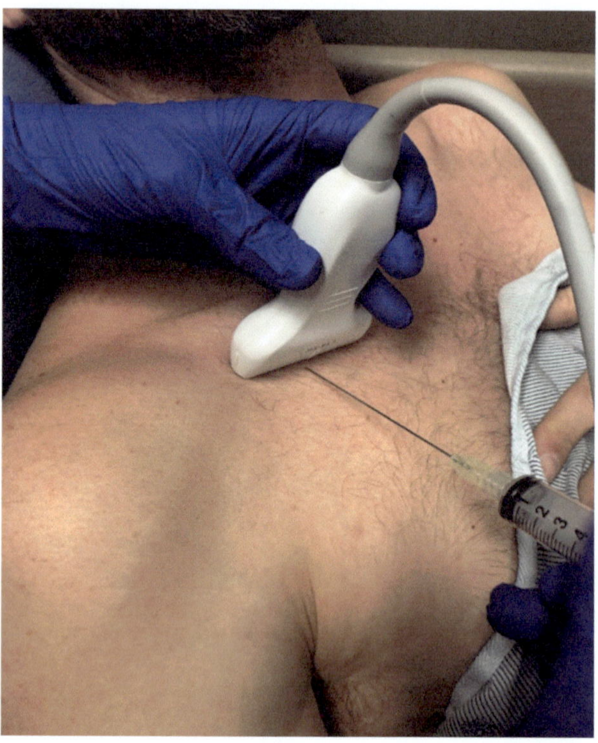

Fig. 6.13 Probe and needle position for the infraclavicular out-of-plane approach to SC vein cannulation

The out-of-plane infraclavicular approach allows for continuous visualization of both the SC artery and vein (Figs. 6.10 and 6.13). However, given the stepwise nature of the out-of-plane technique, there is the possibility of misidentification of the needle tip, leading to the penetration of the needle deep to the vein. However, the out-of-plane technique is easier to master and decreases the likelihood of inadvertent arterial puncture [31].

Supraclavicular Approach

The subclavian vein is more easily identifiable on US using the supraclavicular approach, near to the site where the SC and IJ veins meet to form the brachiocephalic vein. The SC vein is identified above the clavicle, thus negating interference from the clavicle's acoustic shadow, and is also more superficial at this location, allowing for ease of cannulation [18, 29, 32]. However, as the subclavian vein is only visualized for a short distance at this location, dynamic needle guidance can be difficult. The supraclavicular approach has been shown to result in less catheter malposition when compared to the landmark technique. However, limited data exist comparing these two approaches. Depending on the anatomy of the patient and the amount of body surface available in the supraclavicular region, this approach may be optimal compared to an infraclavicular or landmark approach for certain patients [18, 29, 32].

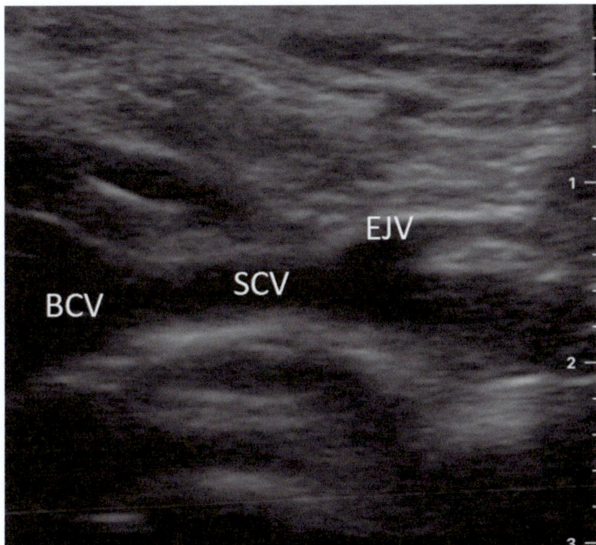

Fig. 6.14 Supraclavicular view of the right subclavian vein

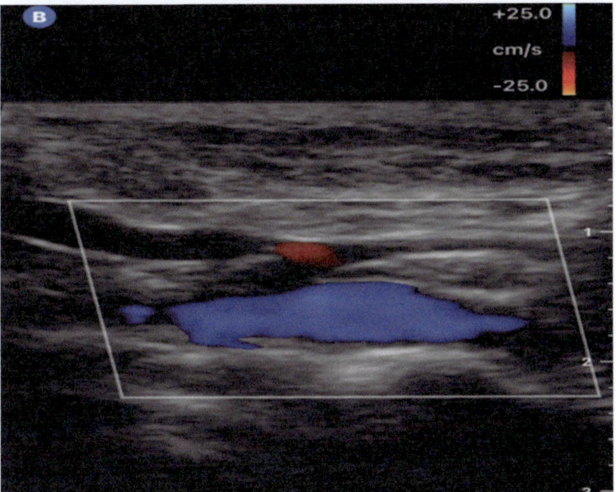

Fig. 6.15 Right supraclavicular view of the SC vein using color Doppler flow imaging

In contrast to infraclavicular SV CVC placement, the supraclavicular USG approach is obtained by first positioning the linear probe on the ipsilateral IJ vein in an out-of-plane fashion. The IJ vein is traced caudally until the probe abuts the patient's clavicle in the supraclavicular fossa, which is approximately the site of the confluence of the IJ vein and the SC vein. The probe is angled toward the patient's chest wall until the SC vein becomes visible in long axis (Figs. 6.14 and 6.15). In Fig. 6.14, note the SC vein (SCV) emanating from the *brachiocephalic (BC) vein* (BCV) on the left side of the image and the *external jugular (EJ) vein* (EJV) arising from the SC vein more superficially. In Fig. 6.15, the blue structure is the subclavian

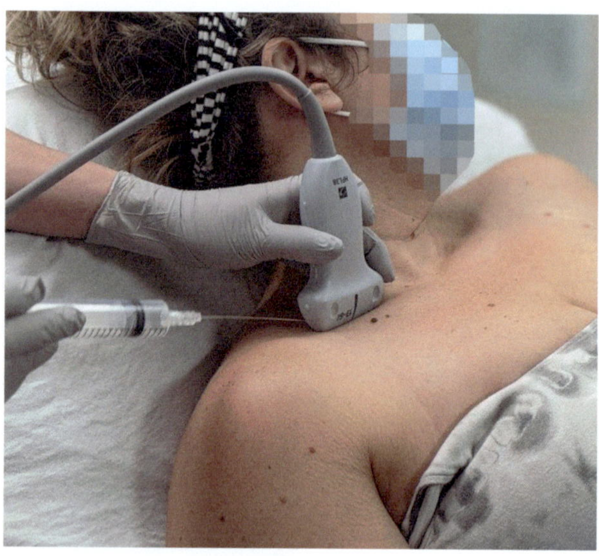

Fig. 6.16 In-plane (long-axis) supraclavicular approach to the SC vein

vein and initial part of the brachiocephalic vein. The red structure is the external jugular vein with flowback toward the subclavian vein.

The *subclavian artery* lies just posterior to the SC vein at this location, and care should be taken to differentiate the SC artery from the vein using Doppler or by fanning the probe prior to any cannulation attempt [18, 32]. The vessel is then cannulated using an in-plane needle approach (Fig. 6.16), followed by CVC line placement, as described above.

Femoral (FEM) Vein

The *femoral triangle* is located inferiorly to the inguinal ligament. Within this anatomic region lies the *common femoral vein*, which is the target vein for femoral CVC placement (Fig. 6.17). The lateral border of the femoral triangle is formed by the medial edge of the sartorius muscle and the medial border formed by the lateral edge of the adductor longus muscle [26]. It is important for providers to distinguish the confluence of the *greater saphenous vein* from the common femoral vein. Inadvertent cannulation of the saphenous vein will result in difficulty advancing the guidewire or malpositioning of the CVC.

When attempting FEM vein cannulation, place the patient in a slight *reverse Trendelenburg* position (i.e., supine, head higher than the feet, as in Fig. 6.18) to increase venous filling in the femoral vein. In cases of cardiopulmonary resuscitation or dramatic volume depletion, this maneuver will allow for a more easily identifiable structure and again a larger diameter target vein.

The appearance of the common femoral vein in out-of-plane probe positioning is demonstrated in Fig. 6.19. If possible, the ipsilateral (i.e., same side) leg of the vein

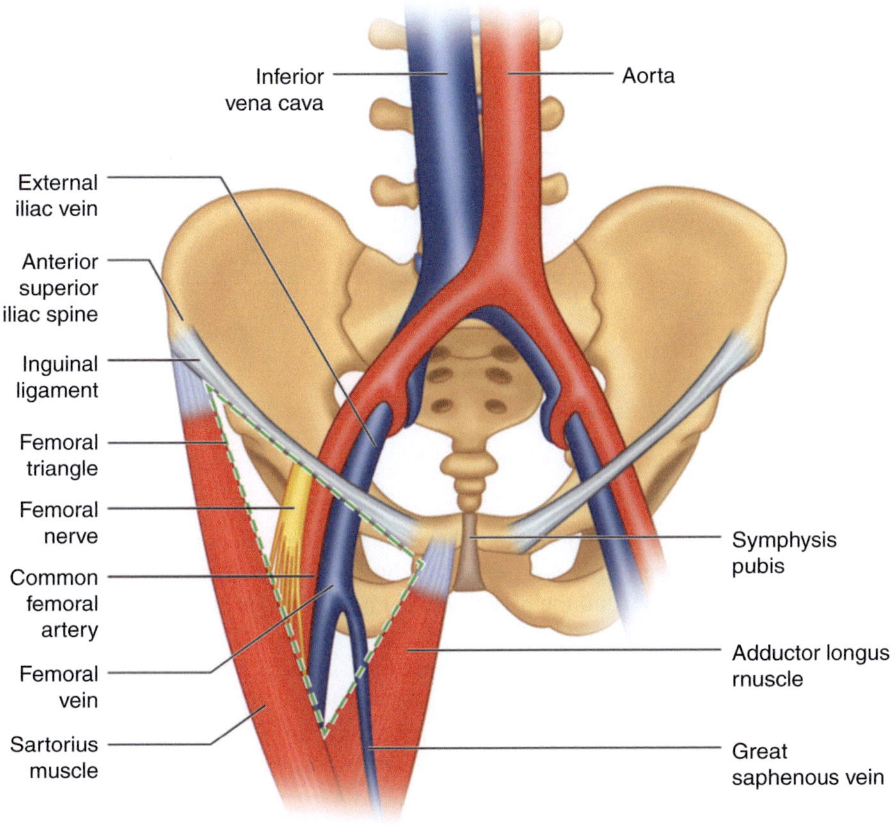

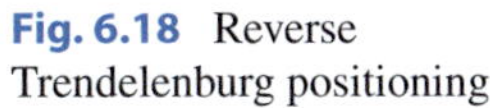

Fig. 6.17 Anatomy of the common femoral vein and related structures

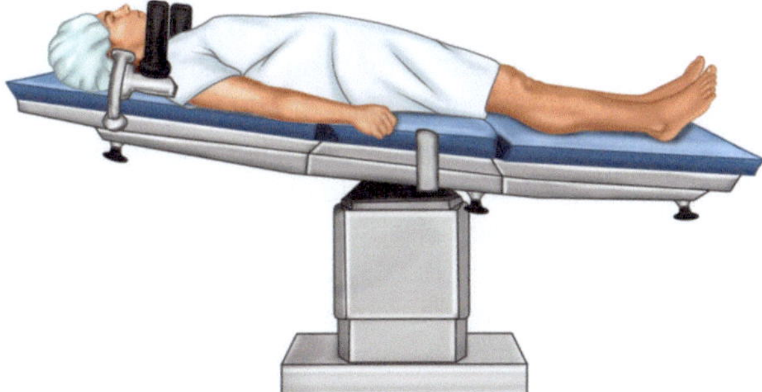

Fig. 6.18 Reverse Trendelenburg positioning

of interest should be externally rotated and flexed to improve the positioning of the common femoral vein, bringing it to a more superficial position [20].

The practitioner should be positioned on the ipsilateral side as the vein targeted for cannulation. The US machine may be positioned on either side of the patient, as

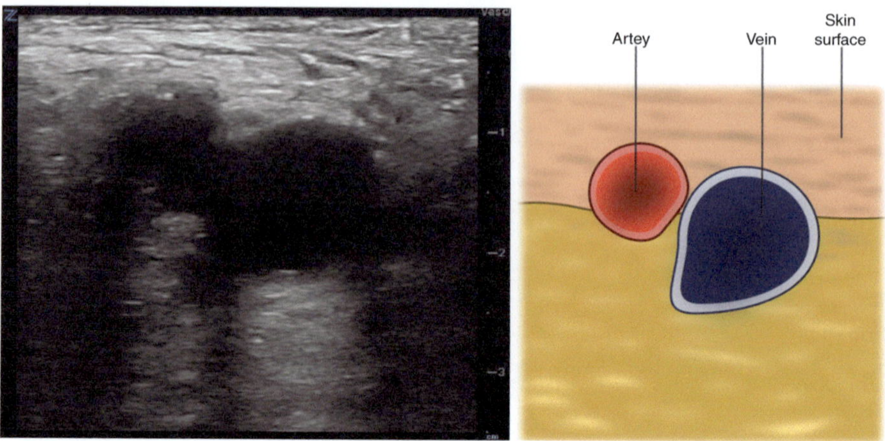

Fig. 6.19 Femoral vein in out-of-plane (short-axis) view

long as the needle insertion point, the US screen, and the patient are within view, so as to minimize the need for head movement by the practitioner during the procedure. Both the US screen and the patient should be at a height that is ergonomically comfortable for the practitioner [20].

Depth of insertion is simpler for FEM vein CVCs than for other CVCs. Femoral CVCs should be fully advanced to their hubs and sutured into position. Unlike CVCs placed in the IJ or SC vein, radiographic imaging is not required to confirm proper placement prior to use. The line is considered usable if each hub of the CVC draws venous nonpulsatile blood.

Pitfalls

Central venous catheter placement is fraught with potential pitfalls, although most of these can be mitigated by proper positioning of the patient, provider, and US machine. As with the placement of any CVC, one common pitfall is the inability to successfully thread the guidewire. This may be alleviated by dropping the angle of insertion of the needle relative to the skin, thus decreasing the initial angle of guidewire insertion into the vessel so that it is less steep and, therefore, less likely to catch on endovascular structures. Dynamic visualization of the needle tip within the central portion of the vessel lumen will also help during advancement of the guidewire [18]. Another common occurrence resulting in the inability to thread the guidewire is that the needle tip becomes inadvertently malpositioned due slight migration either by accidental movement on the part of the practitioner or patient movement due to respiratory variation or inadequate sedation (more common in the IJ and SC veins, as compared to the FEM vein). This occurrence can be addressed by using ultrasound to verify that the needle is within the central portion of the vessel lumen and not in contact with the back wall of the vessel. The needle can be adjusted under

USG intravascularly in long axis so that the tip once again lies in the center of the vessel and guidewire passage may be reattempted [18].

Taking the time to verify the location of the needle tip and to ensure proper dynamic visualization allows for increased first-attempt success rates and decreases the risk of complications. Loss of visualization of the needle tip using either the in-plane or out-of-plane technique can result in arterial puncture or damage to surrounding structures. To help prevent this, advancement of the needle should not proceed until the practitioner can once again identify the needle tip on ultrasound [18].

Complications

There are numerous complications associated with CVC placement. Previous studies have broken them down into several categories, including mechanical, infection, and thrombus formation. The rates of complications are noted to increase secondary to multiple variables including the use of the landmark-based technique for CVC insertion, provider inexperience, individual patient factors, multiple attempts at cannulation, or emergent situations.

Mechanical Complications

As with any procedure, a practitioner must consider the risks, benefits, and alternative therapies available when treating a patient. Numerous mechanical complications of CVC placement have been described, including malplacement, hematoma formation, arterial puncture, pneumothorax, hemothorax, nerve injury, and thoracic duct injury. The incidence of mechanical complications ranges from 6.2% to 19.4% [21, 33]. Arterial puncture is most prevalent in the landmark-based femoral central line placement, but pneumothorax is the most common in the landmark-based subclavian approach. The use of USG to perform CVC placement decreases the risk of all of these complications and thus has become the standard of care [11, 12].

Arterial puncture is the most common of all mechanical complications of CVC placement, although the use of US guidance decreases the risk of this complication by 72% and decreases the rate of hematoma formation by 73% [11]. Ultrasound guidance also allows for quick identification of iatrogenic pneumothorax, by allowing the user to evaluate for lung sliding using the linear probe. The use of US for dynamic guidance has been shown to decrease the number of placement attempts and, in doing so, decreases the rate of all complications [11, 12].

Infectious Complications

Though the overall rate of central line-associated bloodstream infection (CLABSI) is low, infections attributed to CVC placement still represent a significant source of iatrogenic patient morbidity and mortality [17, 34]. The use of aseptic technique for line placement, including the standard PPE, adequate draping of the patient, and an appropriately sized sterile probe cover, is of the utmost importance to prevent infectious complications. The placement of a sterile dressing over a newly placed CVC with either the BioPatch® or other approved form of antimicrobial impregnated dressing is also frequently mandated and may help in decreasing the incidence of infectious complications [34].

Documentation

According to the American College of Emergency Physicians (ACEP), documentation of all USG procedures should include the following data elements: patient demographic data including name, date of birth, medical record number, and gender. Information pertaining to the exam should also be included, such as the date and time of the exam, indication for the exam, the individual performing the exam, and (if applicable) the name of the person reviewing the images for quality assurance. Provider documentation should also contain information on the form of anesthesia used (i.e., local, procedural sedation or other), equipment used, and the technique (i.e., sterile versus emergent). Documentation should also include the anatomic location of the procedure (e.g., right internal jugular vein), compressibility and patency of the target vein, method of guidance (i.e., dynamic or static), the number of attempts, outcome, complications, and method used for confirmation of proper placement [35].

Key Points
- The use of ultrasound guidance for CVC placement increases the rate of successful vessel cannulation and decreases the risk of avoidable complications.
- Placement of USG CVC catheters requires the use of a linear US probe, appropriate US machine exam settings, and aseptic technique including a sterile probe cover.
- Ultrasound can be used to confirm proper CVC placement by guidewire visualization and to detect certain complications associated with this procedure.
- Pitfalls associated with USG CVC placement are similar to those encountered with the landmark technique but may be easier to troubleshoot through direct visualization of the anatomy and/or real-time redirection of the needle tip and guidewire.

References

1. Sznajder JI, Zveibil FR, Bitterman H, Weiner P, Bursztein S. Central vein catheterization. Failure and complication rates by three percutaneous approaches. Arch Intern Med. 1986;146(2):259–61.
2. Mansfield PF, Hohn DC, Fornage BD, Gregurich MA, Ota DM. Complications and failures of subclavian-vein catheterization. N Engl J Med. 1994;331(26):1735–8.
3. Steele R, Irvin CB. Central line mechanical complication rate in emergency medicine patients. Acad Emerg Med. 2001;8(2):204–7.
4. Merrer J, De Jonghe B, Golliot F, Lefrant JY, Raffy B, Barre E, Rigaud JP, Casciani D, Misset B, Bosquet C, Outin H, Brun-Buisson C, Nitenberg G, French Catheter Study Group in Intensive Care. Complications of femoral and subclavian venous catheterization in critically ill patients: a randomized controlled trial. JAMA. 2001;286(6):700–7.
5. McGee DC, Gould MK. Preventing complications of central venous catheterization. N Engl J Med. 2003;348(12):1123–33.
6. Polderman KH, Girbes AJ. Central venous catheter use. Part 1: mechanical complications. Intensive Care Med. 2002;28(1):1–17.
7. Yonei A, Nonoue T, Sari A. Real-time ultrasonic guidance for percutaneous puncture of the internal jugular vein. Anesthesiology. 1986;64(6):830–1.
8. Denys BG, Uretsky BF, Reddy PS. Ultrasound-assisted cannulation of the internal jugular vein. A prospective comparison to the external landmark-guided technique. Circulation. 1993;87(5):1557–62.
9. Hrics P, Wilber S, Blanda MP, Gallo U. Ultrasound-assisted internal jugular vein catheterization in the ED. Am J Emerg Med. 1998;16(4):401–3.
10. Schummer W, Köditz JA, Schelenz C, Reinhart K, Sakka SG. Pre-procedure ultrasound increases the success and safety of central venous catheterization. Br J Anaesth. 2014;113(1):122–9.
11. Brass P, Hellmich M, Kolodziej L, Schick G, Smith AF. Ultrasound guidance versus anatomical landmarks for internal jugular vein catheterization. Cochrane Database Syst Rev. 2015;1(1):CD006962.
12. Brass P, Hellmich M, Kolodziej L, Schick G, Smith AF. Ultrasound guidance versus anatomical landmarks for subclavian or femoral vein catheterization. Cochrane Database Syst Rev. 2015;1(1):CD011447.
13. Gordon AC, Saliken JC, Johns D, Owen R, Gray RR. US-guided puncture of the internal jugular vein: complications and anatomic considerations. J Vasc Interv Radiol. 1998;9(2):333–8.
14. Lichtenstein D, Saïfi R, Augarde R, Prin S, Schmitt JM, Page B, Pipien I, Jardin F. The internal jugular veins are asymmetric. Usefulness of ultrasound before catheterization. Intensive Care Med. 2001;27(1):301–5.
15. Forauer AR, Glockner JF. Importance of US findings in access planning during jugular vein hemodialysis catheter placements. J Vasc Interv Radiol. 2000;11(2 Pt 1):233–8.
16. Wang R, Snoey ER, Clements RC, Hern HG, Price D. Effect of head rotation on vascular anatomy of the neck: an ultrasound study. J Emerg Med. 2006;31(3):283–6.
17. Templeton A, Schlegel M, Fleisch F, Rettenmund G, Schöbi B, Henz S, Eich G. Multilumen central venous catheters increase risk for catheter-related bloodstream infection: prospective surveillance study. Infection. 2008;36(4):322–7.
18. Ma O, Mateer J, Reardon R. Ma and Mateer's emergency ultrasound. 3rd ed. McGraw Hill Professional: New York, NY, USA. 2013;631–44.
19. Peabody CR, Mandavia D. Deep needle procedures: improving safety with ultrasound visualization. J Patient Saf. 2017;13(2):103–8.

20. Saugel B, Scheeren TWL, Teboul J-L. Ultrasound-guided central venous catheter placement: a structured review and recommendations for clinical practice. Crit Care. 2017;21(1):1–11.
21. Smit JM, Raadsen R, Blans MJ, Petjak M, Van de Ven PM, Tuinman PR. Bedside ultrasound to detect central venous catheter misplacement and associated iatrogenic complications: a systematic review and meta-analysis. Crit Care. 2018;22(1):65.
22. Kim E, et al. A prospective randomized trial comparing insertion success rate and incidence of catheterization-related complications for subclavian venous catheterization using a thin-walled introducer needle or a catheter-over-needle technique. Anesthesia. 2016;71:1030–6.
23. Garner DH, Baker S. StatPearls [Internet]. StatPearls Publishing; Treasure Island (FL): Feb 6, 2019. Anatomy, Head and Neck, Carotid Sheath.
24. Czepizak C, O'Callaghan J, Venous B. Evaluation of formulas for optimal positioning of central Venous catheters. Chest. 1995;107(6):1662–4.
25. Kujur R, Roa S, Mrinal M. How correct is the correct length for central venous catheter insertion. Indian J Crit Care Med. 2009;13(3):159–62.
26. Clar DT, Bordoni B. Anatomy, abdomen and pelvis, femoral region. 2020 Sep 18. In: StatPearls [Internet]. Treasure Island: StatPearls Publishing; 2020.
27. Gordon A, Alsayouri K. Anatomy, shoulder and upper limb, axilla. 2020 Aug 15. In: StatPearls [Internet]. Treasure Island: StatPearls Publishing; 2020.
28. Kitagawa N, et al. Proper shoulder position for subclavian venipuncture. Anesthesiology. 2004;101:1306–12.
29. Rezayat T, et al. Ultrasound-guided cannulation: time to bring subclavian central lines Back. West J Emerg Med. 2016;17(2):216–21.
30. Fragou M, Gravvanis A, Dimitriou V, Papalois A, Kouraklis G, Karabinis A, Saranteas T, Poularas J, Papanikolaou J, Davlouros P, Labropoulos N, Karakitsos D. Real-time ultrasound-guided subclavian vein cannulation versus the landmark method in critical care patients: a prospective randomized study. Crit Care Med. 2011;39(7):1607–12.
31. Vezzani A, Manca T, Brusasco C, Santori G, Cantadori L, Ramelli A, Gonzi G, Nicolini F, Gherli T, Corradi F. A randomized clinical trial of ultrasound-guided infra-clavicular cannulation of the subclavian vein in cardiac surgical patients: short-axis versus long-axis approach. Intensive Care Med. 2017;43(11):1594–601.
32. Lieu C, River G, Mantuani D, Nagdev A. Using the supraclavicular approach to ultrasound-guided subclavian vein cannulation – ACEP now. [online] ACEP now. 2020.. Available at: https://www.acepnow.com/article/using-the-supraclavicular-approach-to-ultrasound-guided-subclavian-vein-cannulation. Accessed 12 September 2020.
33. Tsotsolis N, et al. Pneumothorax as a complication of central venous catheter insertion. Ann Transl Med. 2015;3(3):40.
34. The Joint Commission. Preventing Central Line-Associated Bloodstream Infections. Useful Tools, An International Perspective. Nov 20, 2013. Accessed 5/30/19. http://www.jointcommission.org/CLABSIToolkit.
35. EUS-Proc-Guide ACEP, Standard reporting guidelines: ultrasound for procedure guidance, 2015.

Intraosseous Catheters

7

Catalina Kenney and James H. Paxton

History of Intraosseous Access

The earliest investigations into the clinical utility of intraosseous (IO) vascular access occurred more than a century ago. Cecil Kent Drinker (1887–1956), considered by many to be the founder of modern lymphology [1], was only 2 years out of medical school when he first performed a series of experiments that would illuminate the mechanisms by which red blood cells and other bone marrow contents enter the bloodstream. Assisted by his wife, Katherine, he injected a variety of substances, including epinephrine, into the nutrient artery that supplied oxygenated blood to the bone marrow of a live canine tibia [2]. Although Drinker did not inject these substances directly into the intraosseous space, he found that anything that he injected into the nutrient artery found its way back to the general circulation via the intraosseous space [3]. Infusing a hirudinized physiological salt solution at pressures up to 240 mmHg, Drinker was able to increase the rate of blood flow through the dog tibia from the physiological rate of 15 mL/min to as high as 60 mL/min [3]. Although his work was predicated upon the discoveries of many nineteenth-century European anatomists, Drinker's findings represent a pivotal event in our understanding of the potential therapeutic value of IO infusion [4].

In 1922, a medical student at Johns Hopkins University named Charles Austin Doan (1896–1990) independently discovered that venous drainage from the IO space within the radius and ulna was relatively constant, regardless of the systemic blood pressure or the volume of fluid infused [5]. Infusion pressures exceeding the

C. Kenney
Wayne State University School of Medicine, Detroit, MI, USA
e-mail: catalina.kenney@med.wayne.edu

J. H. Paxton (✉)
Department of Emergency Medicine, Wayne State University School of Medicine, Detroit, MI, USA
e-mail: james.paxton@wayne.edu

© Springer Nature Switzerland AG 2021

133

J. H. Paxton (ed.), *Emergent Vascular Access*,
https://doi.org/10.1007/978-3-030-77177-5_7

intrinsic capacity of the drainage system led to capillary rupture and extravasation, but he could not increase outflow beyond this physiological limit. However, he theorized that "functionally dormant" capillaries associated with adjacent pockets of hypoplastic (yellow) marrow might be recruited to enhance outflow in times of physiologic crisis. Doan's work both confirmed and supplemented the work done by Drinker's team.

Over the next two decades, scientist-clinicians began utilizing IO cannulation to infuse a variety of therapeutic substances into the bone marrow space [4]. In an age when hefty metal trocars were routinely inserted into fragile veins with substerile techniques, the IO approach seemed to be a reasonable alternative to peripheral intravenous (PIV) cannulation. However, the availability of convenient "plastic" (polyvinyl chloride) PIV catheters in the 1950s soon led to the abandonment of adult IO cannulation in most developed nations [4, 6]. Sterile Teflon™ and polyurethane PIV catheters would soon supplant IO catheters as the preferred vascular access device for the next four decades.

While IO catheters never really disappeared from use in resource-poor third-world countries, the technique did not regain popularity again in the United States until the 1980s [4]. Pediatrician James Orlowski was among the first Americans to publicly call for a return to the consideration of IO cannulation in 1984. Orlowski had worked in India during a cholera epidemic and witnessed the ability of IO devices to save the lives of pediatric patients firsthand [7]. Realizing the value of IO catheterization for hypovolemic pediatric patients, the American Heart Association (AHA) Pediatric Advanced Life Support (PALS) guidelines soon began endorsing the use of tibial IO cannulation in select pediatric patients as early as 1988 [8].

Unfortunately, the bony cortices of adult patients are much harder than those of pediatric subjects. Early IO devices were exclusively hand-driven into the bone, making IO cannulation much more difficult in adults than in children. As a result, the widespread use of the IO approach would wait for the invention of superior methods of driving the IO cannula into the much-denser bones of adult subjects. These necessary advances began appearing in the late 1990s, with the introduction of the sternal FAST1® (1997), the spring-powered Bone Injection Gun® (1998), and the drill-powered EZ-IO® (2004). By 2005, the AHA had begun recommending the use of the IO route to provide Advanced Cardiac Life Support (ACLS) medications for adult and pediatric patients, but only when IV access was difficult or impossible to achieve [9, 10].

Not much has changed in the landscape of IO cannulation since 2005. Manually driven IO catheters are still commercially available, although they have been greatly replaced (especially in adult subjects) by spring-loaded or drill-driven insertion techniques. At the time of this writing, the AHA still recommends that IO cannulation be considered when PIV access is delayed or impossible, although the medical literature is conflicted with reports of the relative utility of IO access as compared to PIV access for the management of various conditions, most prominently cardiac arrest [11]. In 2010, the AHA ACLS guidelines suggested that, "it is reasonable for providers to establish IO access if IV access is not readily available (Class IIa, LOE C)" for cardiac arrest victims [11]. The AHA chose not to reexamine this recommendation for the use of IO catheterization with its 2015 and 2018 ACLS guideline revisions [12, 13]. Similarly, the 2018 American College of Surgeons (ACS) Advanced Trauma Life Support (ATLS) guidelines recommend that, "if peripheral access cannot be obtained, consider placement of an intraosseous needle for temporary access." [14]. In fact, most major resuscitative organizations currently recommend that IO cannulation be considered for patients requiring emergent vascular access when PIV access cannot be rapidly obtained. Unfortunately, no organization has thus far offered a practical timeframe after which IO cannulation should be considered when other forms of vascular access prove untenable. This leaves the decision of when to declare PIV access "impossible" up to the discretion of the treating clinician. Rescuers must weigh the potential benefits of IO cannulation against the risks of this technique, without substantive guidance from designated authorities on the subject. Consequently, it is especially important that vascular access providers understand the potential risks and benefits of IO cannulation for patients requiring emergent vascular access.

Physiology of Intraosseous Access

Intraosseous access leverages the availability of a non-collapsible route for the introduction of medications and fluids into the central circulation. It is currently theorized that egress from the marrow space may be preserved in shock states, despite collapse of the venous system and impaired forward flow due to shock-related cardiac dysfunction. Consequently, the use of IO cannulation could offer advantages to patients with undifferentiated shock over the use of PIV or central venous catheter (CVC) cannulation.

Traditionally, long bones have been considered the preferred target sites for IO cannulation. Long bones are composed of certain constituent parts: the *epiphyses*, *metaphyses*, and *diaphysis* [15]. The epiphyses are located at the proximal and distal ends of the long bones, bookending the long diaphysis of the bone. The metaphyses are situated between the epiphyses and the diaphysis, in the region formerly occupied by the growth plate in adults [15]. The marrow cavity of long bones is generally located in the diaphysis. The *periosteum* is a fine layer of connective tissue, overlying all external portions of the long bone absent of articular cartilage [15]. The periosteum protects the underlying bony cortex and serves to anchor ancillary blood vessels and nerves servicing the long bone. Because the periosteum is highly innervated, pain perception from the exterior surface of the bone is facilitated by innervation from the periosteum [15]. The anatomy of the intraosseous space is illustrated in Fig. 7.1.

The *medullary cavity* of long bones constitutes the interior of long bones, situated between the bony cortices. This cavity houses both the intraosseous vasculature as well as red and yellow bone marrow [15]. Red bone marrow produces blood elements and is the primary marrow type present in pediatric subjects. However, as humans age, most of the red marrow in long bones is replaced by atrophic yellow (adipose) marrow, which has a higher proportion of fatty tissue and is relatively

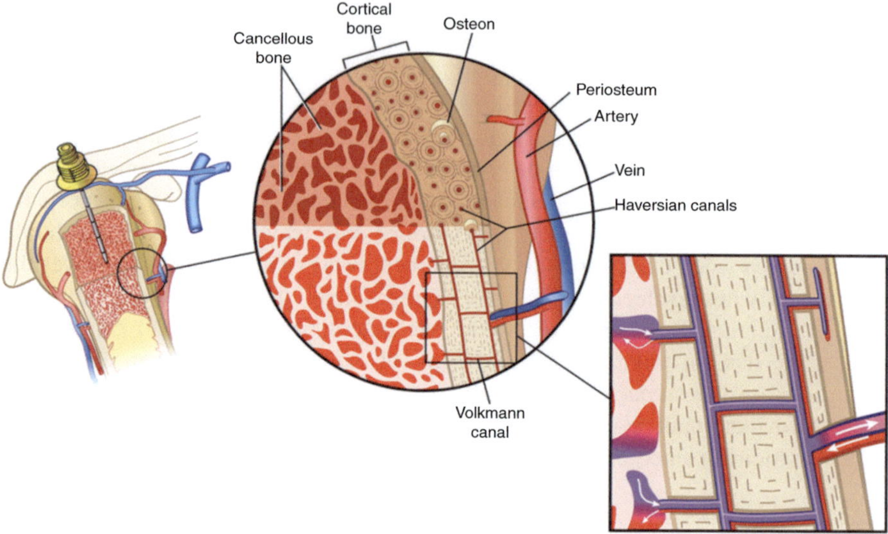

Fig. 7.1 Anatomy of the intraosseous space. (*Image courtesy of Teleflex Inc. © 2020 Teleflex Inc. All rights reserved*)

bereft of hematopoietic cell-producing marrow [16]. Notable exceptions to this are the higher proportions of red marrow seen in adult subjects at the skull, ribs, sternum, and vertebral bodies [15–17]. Nonetheless, adult subjects have a higher proportion of yellow marrow in the medullary cavities of long bones than pediatric subjects [15]. This distinction is important, since red marrow has an enhanced vascular supply, when compared to yellow marrow. This fact led early IO researchers to conclude that IO access could only be successfully achieved in bones that contained red marrow [18]. However, modern data suggest that IO cannulation may be readily and effectively obtained in long bones bereft of red marrow.

In all cases, venous flow from the medullary cavity into the central circulation is achieved via *emissary veins* and *nutrient veins* [15–17]. Interestingly, pediatric subjects enjoy discrete blood supplies for the metaphysis and diaphysis, as native vasculature appears to be unable to cross the cartilaginous growth plate [15]. In both pediatric and adult subjects, substances infused into the medullary space are rapidly picked up by the venous circulation. Much like early resuscitation scientists, modern clinicians typically utilize the superficial portions of the long bones to procure IO access. The proximal tibia and proximal humerus are generally preferred as access routes, though some attention has also been paid to the radius, calcaneus, sternum, and iliac crest as potential sites for IO cannulation [19–22].

Pain is a primary consideration with IO cannulation. The periosteum is highly innervated, and IO catheter insertion leads to the stimulation of periosteal pain fibers, inducing a sharp, highly localized perception of pain at the insertion site. Subsequent infusion of fluid or medication, typically achieved with a high infusion pressure using syringe injection, pressure bag, or infusion pump, leads to additional pain due to the stimulation of pressure sensors within the medullary space. Although local anesthesia of the periosteum and soft tissues at the insertion site is not generally utilized, slow infusion (over 120 seconds, followed by a dwell time of 60 seconds prior to subsequent infusion) of 20–40 mg (1–2 mL) of 2% lidocaine (formulated for IV/IO injection) through the IO catheter is usually recommended immediately after IO placement to anesthetize the intraosseous space in awake subjects to mitigate this pain response prior to pressurized infusion [22–24].

The intrinsic intramedullary pressure inside of long bones is generally believed to be approximately 25% of a patient's systemic systolic blood pressure [25]. Consequently, to achieve forward flow of fluids or medication through the IO device, *infusion pressures must be greater than this intrinsic intramedullary pressure*. So-called "gravity" infusion, achieved without the use of syringe pressure or pressurized infusion devices, is generally not adequate to overcome this intrinsic intramedullary pressure. Consequently, gravity-driven flow rates (i.e., without the use of pressurized infusion) are often inadequate to allow substantial forward fluid flow rates through the IO space. It is also likely that different IO insertion sites (i.e., different target bones) may have different intrinsic intramedullary pressures, depending upon factors such as the volume capacity of the targeted intramedullary space, the cumulative cross-sectional area of the venous drainage system, the type and density of marrow present, proximity to the central circulation, and other patient- or site-dependent factors. Consequently, different infusion pressures may be required at different IO infusion sites.

This chapter addresses the relative indications and contraindications for IO site selection, as well as the known complications of IO access, and those devices currently available for use with this technique.

Indications for Intraosseous Access

In general, IO access is indicated when other forms of vascular access are not readily available for the infusion of fluids and medications. Because the pain associated with IO infusion is not always alleviated with IO lidocaine injection, IO infusion is often reserved for those patients who are unstable or insensate enough for the benefits of immediate venous access to outweigh the risk of infusion pain, especially those patients with severe hemodynamic or respiratory instability. Consequently, most of the existing literature on clinical IO use in the prehospital or in-hospital environment has focused on the use of IO cannulation for cardiac arrest, profound hypovolemia, or imminent respiratory collapse. As analgesic methods improve, the IO route may become more commonly utilized in patients with difficult venous access experiencing less dramatic clinical presentations.

Contraindications for Intraosseous Access

Although no absolute contraindications for the use of IO access exist, relative contraindications have been described in the medical literature, especially pertaining to specific IO insertion sites. Although there is no absolute contraindication for IO placement, relative contraindications do exist, especially at specific bony sites. Intraosseous cannulation is relatively contraindicated under the following conditions:

- *Skin or bony infection at the selected insertion site.* This is due to concerns that the infectious agent (e.g., bacteria) could be transmitted to the medullary space from the dermal surface or that the IO catheter could serve as a nidus for persistent infection.
- *Skin burn at the selected insertion site.* This is due to concerns that the integrity of the skin may be compromised, promoting infection or vascular compromise at the skin surface, leading to increased risk of infection and dermal necrosis.
- *Ipsilateral fracture of the selected extremity.* This is due to concern that fluids or medications infused through the IO device could extravasate into the adjacent soft tissues due to discontinuity in the bony cortex of the selected target bone, or due to disruption of the venous drainage system of the affected limb. This may be more problematic if the fracture is proximal to the IO insertion site, although providers should generally avoid IO cannulation in the presence of any fracture of the ipsilateral extremity, even if the fracture appears to be distal to the potential infusion site.
- *Disorders of bony metabolism.* Conditions such as *osteogenesis imperfecta,* osteopenia, and osteopetrosis have been suggested as relative contraindications to IO cannulation, due to concerns that the force of the IO insertion could lead to bony fracture or allow significant extravasation of infused substances at the insertion site. Substances infused into the medullary cavity will seek out the path of least resistance, which may be retrograde though the gap between the IO catheter and the osteotomy site in cases when bone density is inadequate for the bony cortex to provide a secure grip on the IO catheter.
- *Previous IO attempts at the same target bone.* Preexisting osteotomy (i.e., holes in the bony cortex) produced by recent IO cannulation within 48 hours will provide a low-pressure route for fluid extravasation, as compared to naturally occurring venous drainage tracts from the intramedullary space. This promotes fluid extravasation from the marrow space into the soft tissues adjacent to the previous osteotomy.

While these relative contraindications may prevent utilization of a specific target bone, other bony targets may exist on the same patient. Patients will rarely have contraindications for all potential IO insertion sites.

Common Intraosseous Insertion Sites

Although any intraosseous space can theoretically be targeted for IO infusion, certain insertion sites seem to be preferred for this technique. Each of these sites has its own relative advantages and disadvantages. This section will discuss each of the reported IO insertion sites, including their own unique advantages and disadvantages in the emergent resuscitation of the critically ill patient.

Sternum (Manubrium)

The human sternum has been well-described as a potential IO infusion site. Its position near to the central circulation and the relative absence of overlying soft tissue make it a readily accessible and highly effective route for IO infusion. Comparative studies suggest that the sternum has the greatest potential infusion flow rate of all IO targets [26]. However, the sternum directly overlies the heart and other vital thoracic structures, leading to perpetual concern about the risk of iatrogenic cardiac perforation. Although sternal puncture has been reported with manual IO insertion utilizing manual IO insertions [27], no incidents of cardiac perforation from the clinical use of an FDA-approved IO device have been reported in the modern literature.

Providing external chest compressions for patients experiencing cardiac arrest requires considerable forces to be exerted on the distal sternum, which may interfere with the use of this insertion site. Concerns regarding the risk of inadvertent dislodgement and interference with chest compressions have limited utilization of this site in cardiac arrest. However, it should be noted that the recommended "sternal" IO insertion site is situated on the *manubrium*, and not the sternum itself. Thus, the IO insertion site is far removed from the recommended site of chest compression with cardiopulmonary resuscitation (i.e., distal sternum just superior to the xiphoid process). The recommended sternal IO insertion site is depicted in Fig. 7.2.

Insertion Site 1.5 cm below the sternal notch, inserted at an angle perpendicular to the flat surface of the manubrium.

Available Devices FAST1™ (Pyng Medical) and T.A.L.O.N.™ (Teleflex). Teleflex acquired Pyng Medical in April 2017. No other IO devices are currently recommended by their manufacturers for sternal IO insertion. The FAST1™ device is shown in Fig. 7.3. Note the presence of "stabilizer needles" surrounding the central infusion tube on the FAST1™, which serves to stabilize and hold the device in place during deployment. Substances are only infused through the central infusion tubing. Figure 7.4 shows a cross-sectional view of the infusion tubing seated firmly in the manubrium, with the tip of the infusion tubing emptying directly into the intraosseous space.

Insertion Techniques Downward pressure is applied at the insertion site on the manubrium, utilizing the FAST1™ or similar device. A placement sticker is available from the manufacturer, to guide the provider on identification of the proper insertion site.

Additional Instructions Chest compressions for Advanced Cardiac Life Support (ACLS) can be performed in the setting of a sternal IO device, although some care must be taken to avoid dislodgement of the IO catheter or interference with ACLS efforts. While sternal IO catheters are inserted at the cephalad portion of the manubrium, chest compressions are performed at the distal sternum, which should be adequately removed from the insertion site to avoid accidental dislodgement or

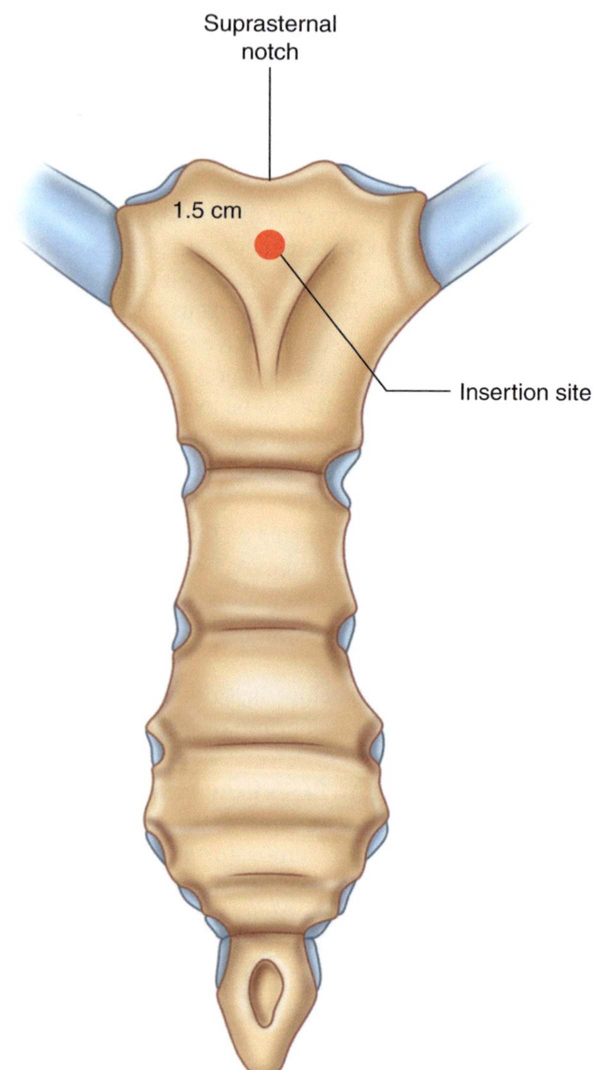

Fig. 7.2 Sternal IO insertion site

compression of the infusion tubing during active chest compression. Sternal IO devices are only recommended currently by the manufacturers for those patients ≥12 years old and >40 kg weight.

Clavicle

The clavicle has been proposed as a potential site of IO cannulation but has not been extensively evaluated in cadaveric or clinical trials. Although it is a long bone with proximity to the central circulation, the intramedullary space of the clavicle is of

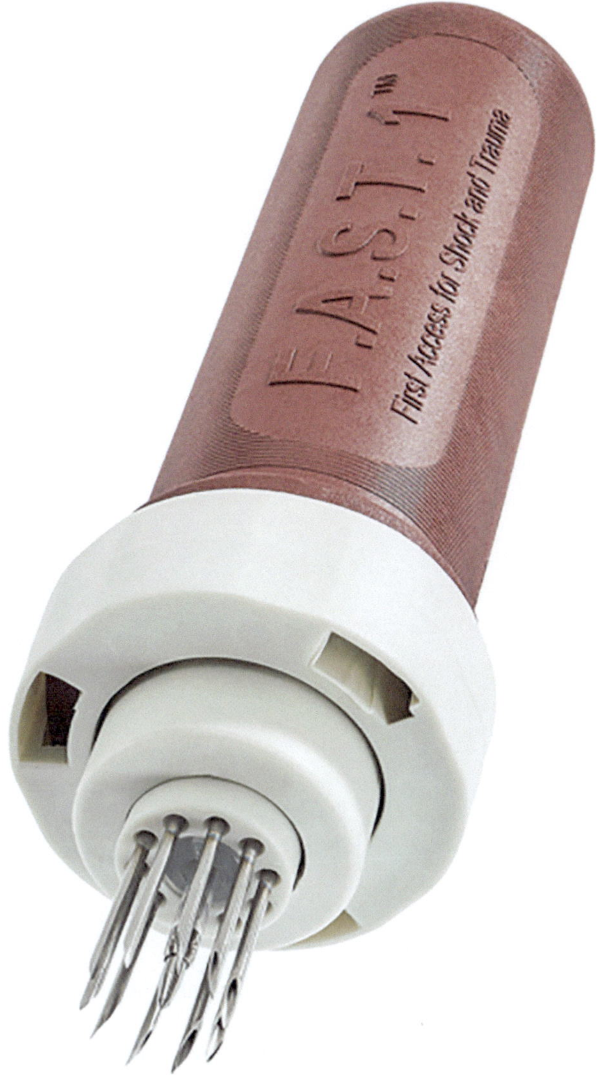

Fig. 7.3 FAST1™ intraosseous infusion device. (*Image courtesy of Teleflex Inc. © 2020 Teleflex Inc. All rights reserved*)

small caliber and may be prone to occult fracture in the setting of major thoracic trauma. Thus, providers should exercise caution in considering its use for patients who may have experienced blunt traumatic injury (e.g., chest trauma, fall). Excessive depth of penetration could also risk injury to the *subclavian vein, subclavian artery*, and other thoracic structures, if the catheter penetrates through the *trans (deep) cortex* of the clavicular bone. Flow from the clavicle into the central circulation appears to occur via the subclavian vein draining into the *superior vena cava* [28]. The IO flow rate from the clavicle appears to be comparable to that achieved with subclavian central venous access, at 11.9 ± 0.68 mL/kg/hr [29]. The insertion site for clavicular IO insertion is shown in Fig. 7.5.

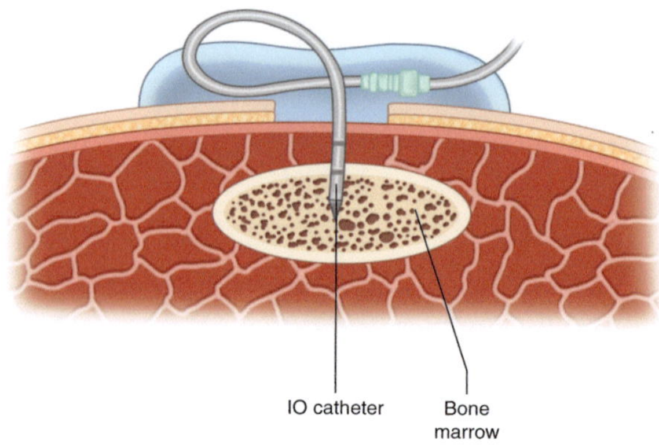

Fig. 7.4 Sternal IO infusion tubing in proper position

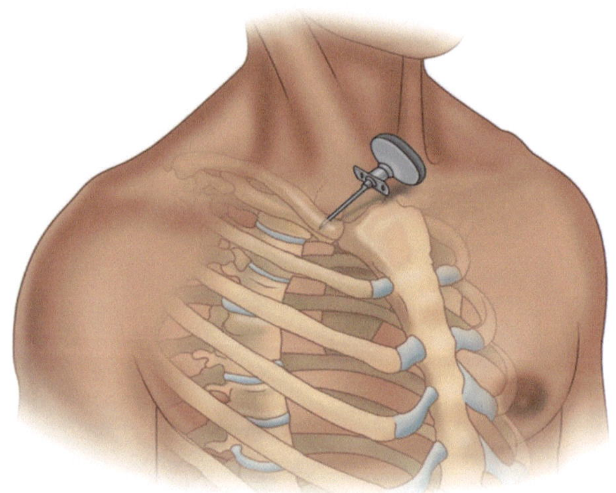

Fig. 7.5 Clavicle IO insertion site

Insertion Site Lateral to the clavicular notch of the manubrium [28].

Available Devices Major manufacturers do not currently endorse the use of their devices at this site.

Insertion Techniques Lateral to the clavicular notch of the manubrium, with insertion angle directed approximately 45 degrees laterally [28].

Proximal Humerus

The proximal humerus offers an optimal combination of anatomic location, accessibility, and venous drainage. Flow rates at the proximal humerus are greater than those seen with more distal insertion sites [22, 30]. This site offers the additional advantage of being sufficiently removed from the site of external chest compressions as to not seem to interfere with the performance of external chest compressions during cardiopulmonary resuscitation. This site has been extensively studied in both trauma and cardiac arrest populations and appears to be easily accessible to providers [22].

Insertion Site 1–2 cm above the surgical neck of the humerus, at the most prominent aspect of the greater tubercle of the humerus.

Available Devices EZ-IO™ (Teleflex), B.I.G.™ (PerSys Medical), NIO™ (PerSys Medical), or various manually-driven IO devices.

Insertion Techniques The recommended insertion technique for the EZ-IO™ (Teleflex) device is illustrated in Fig. 7.6. The patient's hand on the side of interest should be placed over the umbilicus, with the arm adducted (Fig. 7.6a). This arm placement is intended to optimize exposure of the greater tubercle of the humerus and avoid inadvertent placement of the device within the *bicipital groove*. This is exceedingly important for the safety of patients, as the bicipital groove contains the *long tendon of the biceps brachii muscle* (among other tendons) as well as a branch of the *anterior humeral circumflex artery*, both of which are to be avoided with the insertion. The groove is easily palpable on most patients and separates the greater and lesser tubercles of the humerus. When the shoulder is rotated medially, the groove will be felt to move medially.

For right-sided humeral IO insertion, the palm of the provider's right hand should be placed over the proximal humerus anteriorly (hand parallel to the direction of the patient's spine), so that the bulk of the patient's *deltoid muscle* is at the center of the provider's palm and the provider's pinkie finger is at the *anterior axillary crease* (Fig. 7.6b). The fingers of the provider's hand are then extended, and the hand is rotated to rest vertically at the anterior axillary crease (Fig. 7.6c). This is said to look like a "karate chop" of the patient's anterior axillary line. The provider's left hand is then similarly oriented at the *lateral midline of the humerus* (Fig. 7.6d), bisecting the deltoid muscle. Finally, the provider's hands are rotated toward one another, and the point where the provider's thumbs meet represents a site halfway between the anterior axillary line and the midline of the humerus (Fig. 7.6e). This is the approximate location of IO insertion. The recommended insertion site is along a line depicted by the junction of the providers' thumbs. Providers should identify the surgical neck of the humerus, which is the spot where the "golf ball" of the greater tubercle of the proximal humerus meets the "tee" of the surgical neck of the humerus. The insertion site is on the most prominent aspect of the greater tubercle, 1–2 cm above the surgical neck of the humerus (Fig. 7.6f). This surgical neck is commonly described as "where the golf ball [i.e., greater tubercle] meets the tee [i.e., shaft of the humerus]" (Fig. 7.6g). The insertion angle is 45 degrees lateral to the anterior plane, angled posteromedially toward the medial tip of the contralateral scapula (Fig. 7.6h). Figure 7.6i through 7.6n illustrate placement of the stabilizer device and initiation of infusion through the IO catheter.

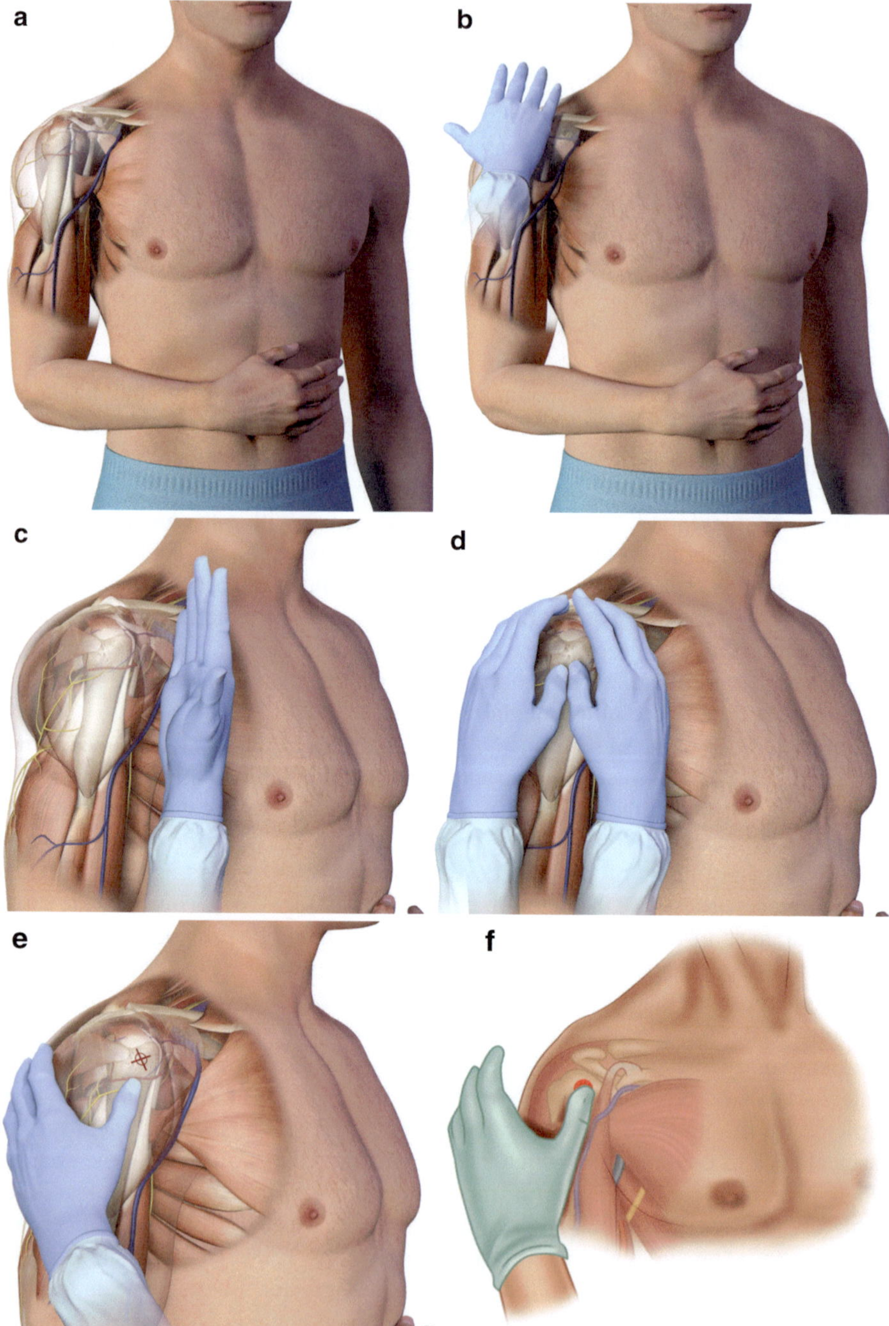

Fig. 7.6 (**a–n**) Recommended insertion technique for EZ-IO™ humeral IO insertion. (*Source images courtesy of Teleflex Inc. © 2020 Teleflex Inc. All rights reserved*)

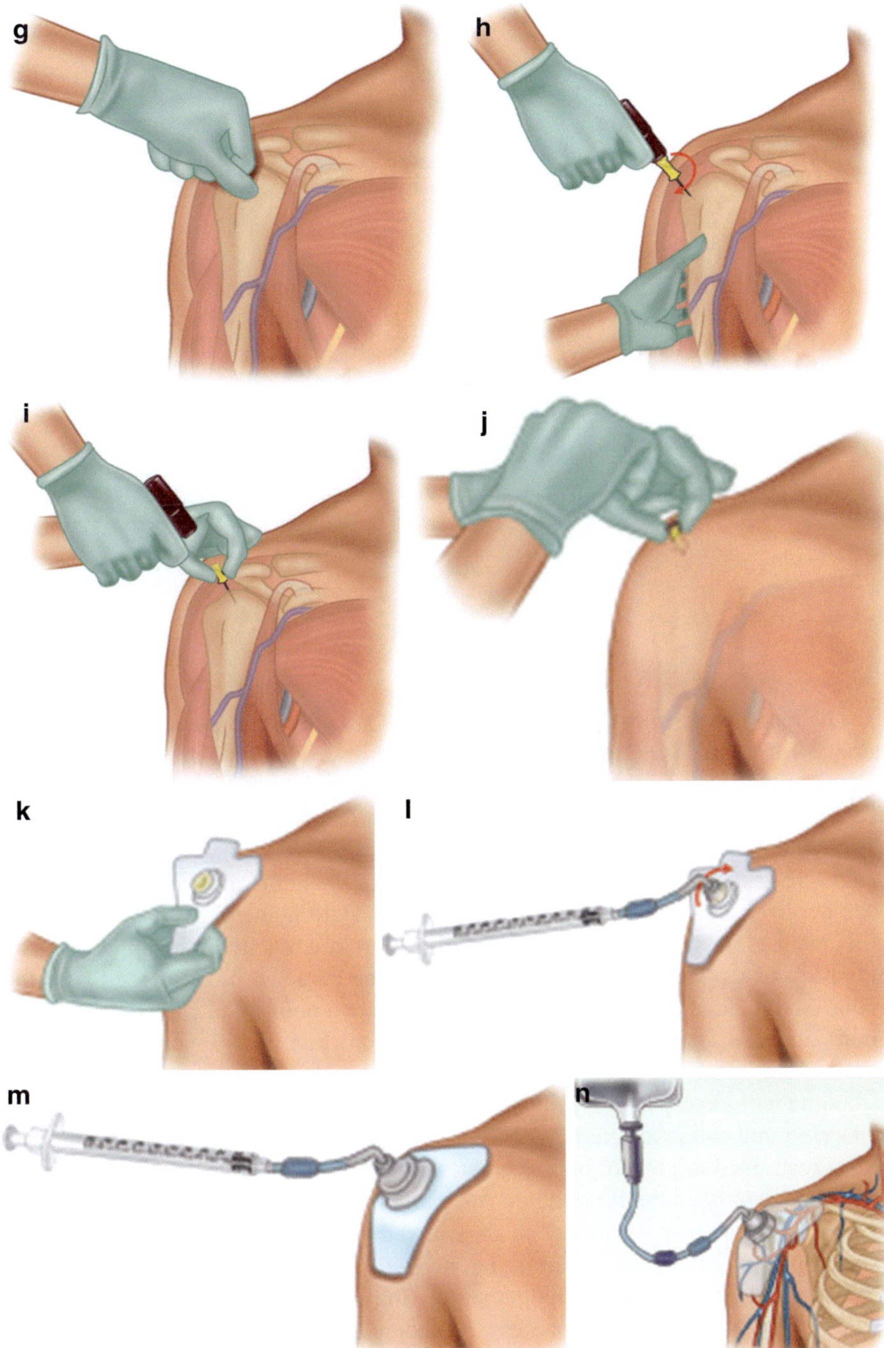

Fig. 7.6 (continued)

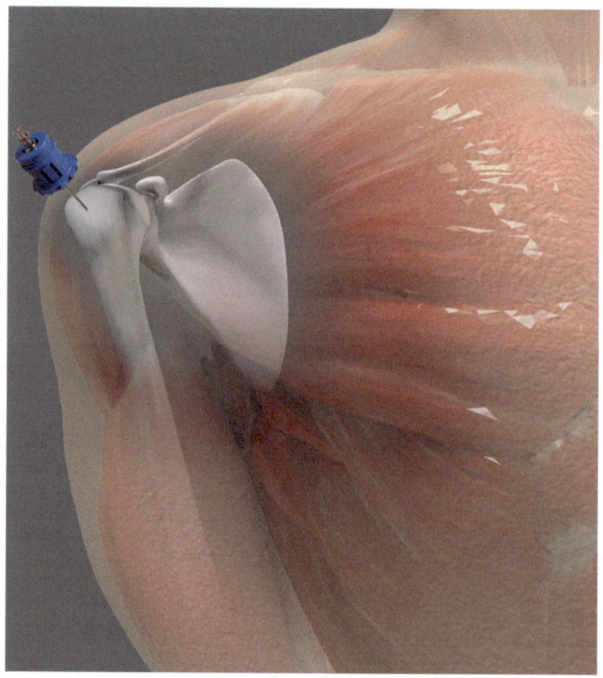

Fig. 7.7 Recommended insertion technique for NIO™ humeral IO insertion. (*Image courtesy of PerSys Medical. © 2020 PerSys Medical. All rights reserved*)

The recommended insertion site for the NIO™ (PerSys Medical) device is the same as for the EZ-IO™, but the recommended insertion angle differs: 45 degrees from the plane of the extremity with the EZ-IO™, and 90 degrees from the surface of the bone for the NIO™ device. The insertion technique for the NIO™ (PerSys Medical) is shown in Fig 7.7.

One alternative method for the identification of the humeral IO insertion site has been described. In this alternative method (for a right humeral IO placement), the provider places their left index fingertip on the patient's acromion process. The thumb tip of the same hand is then placed on the coracoid process, medial to the axilla. An imaginary line is drawn between these two points (the coracoid and acromion), and a spot is identified at the midpoint of this line. The proper insertion location is 2 cm inferior (i.e., toward the elbow) to this midpoint spot. The use of this technique will ideally identify the same IO insertion site as the standard approach.

During and following humeral IO insertion, it is important that the cannulated arm is restrained to prevent inappropriate movement of the upper extremity, which can dislodge or bend the IO catheter. A shoulder sling may be required for immobilization in the poorly compliant or disoriented patient. Elevation of the patient's extremity above the head (as is often done to facilitate thoracic CT imaging) may cause painful bending and dislodgement of the IO catheter, due to torque on the catheter against the acromion process. Providers should provide adequate anticipatory guidance to other members of the care team to avoid inappropriate manipulation of the upper extremity following cannulation. For patients receiving chest compressions, the patient's hand may be placed *behind the patient's back* (i.e., underneath the patient) with the elbow flexed, to expose the relevant anatomy while simultaneously restraining the arm from excessive movement. This provides a similar anatomic arrangement to the placement of the hand over the umbilicus, without the risk of excessive arm movement during chest compressions.

Distal Radius

The distal radius, though far-removed from the central circulation, has been described as a potential site for IO cannulation [31]. Although the radius is a long bone and offers the advantage of being an easily accessible site, it has a smaller intramedullary volume capacity than the proximal humerus and may be at higher risk of occult fracture in polytrauma patients.

Insertion Site At the radial aspect of the base of the styloid process, on the dorsolateral side of the wrist [31].

Available Devices The Bone Injection Gun™ (B.I.G.) is approved in Europe for this site. However, this site is not FDA-approved in the United States. Major manufacturers do not currently endorse their devices at this insertion site.

Insertion Techniques Insertion at the radial aspect of the styloid process, on the dorsal side of the wrist (Fig. 7.8). Great care should be taken to avoid iatrogenic injury to the blood vessels, nerves, joints, and bones of the wrist.

Iliac Crest

The iliac crest has great potential as an IO insertion site, due to its superficial location and access to an extensive intraosseous space, but this site has not been extensively explored in the existing literature. The iliac bone may serve as a large reservoir for fluids and medications, but poor placement technique could theoretically introduce risks of bowel perforation or injury to the deeper pelvic vessels. While existing literature suggests that the iliac crest is an acceptable site for marrow biopsy with IO cannulation, the use of the iliac crest for therapeutic IO access remains speculative [4, 28]. Drainage from the iliac crest appears to be via the inferior vena cava [28], and flow rates appear to be similar to those achieved with clavicular IO infusion and subclavian vein infusion [28, 29].

Insertion Site At the most prominent aspect of the iliac crest, with direction of insertion being perpendicular to the surface of the bone.

Available Devices Manually driven IO devices. No major IO device is currently FDA-approved for clinical use at this insertion site.

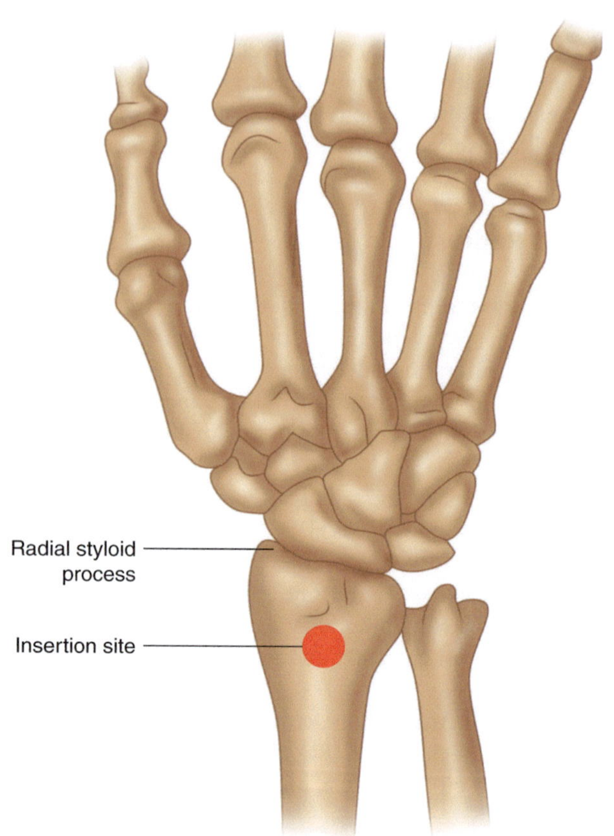

Fig. 7.8 The distal radial IO insertion site

Insertion Techniques Insertion at the most prominent aspect of the iliac crest, directed toward a perpendicular plane from the bony surface. The relevant anatomy for iliac crest IO insertion is illustrated in Fig. 7.9.

Distal Femur

The distal femur IO insertion site appears to be best represented in the pediatric literature, likely owing to the relative lack of muscle and other soft tissue overlying this site in the pediatric population. While the capacity of this bony space has the potential to be superior to tibial sites, flow rates through the femur have never been clinically compared to the humerus or sternum, which appear to be the most similar clinically relevant insertion sites. The utility of the femoral insertion site remains largely unexplored in adults, for whom well-developed quadriceps musculature and excessive adipose may impair its use. This is also a subdiaphragmatic approach, which may suggest poorer performance than the humerus or sternum, due to impaired circulation in low-flow states, such as cardiac arrest. Evidence of the clinical utility of this insertion site in adults remains lacking in the available literature.

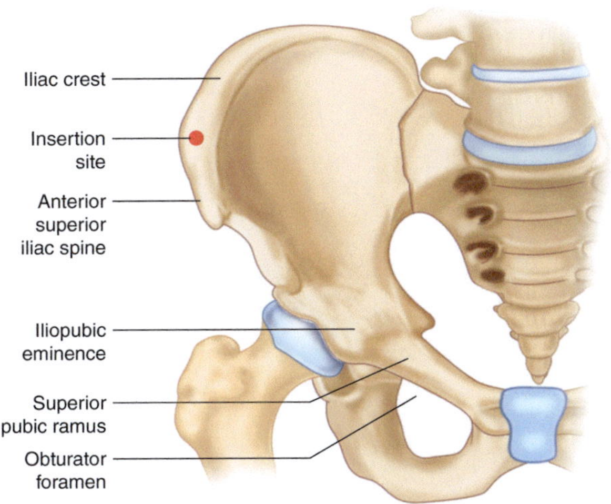

Fig. 7.9 Anatomy of the iliac crest, including IO insertion site

Insertion Site 2–3 centimeters superior to the external condyles of the femur, directly midline along the sagittal plane of this bone [4].

Available Devices EZ-IO™ (Teleflex), or manually driven IO devices.

Insertion Techniques With the patient's leg in full extension, identify the *external (lateral/medial) femoral condyles*. The medial condyle is often larger, and more easily palpated, than the lateral condyle. The needle should be placed 2–3 cm superior to the external condyles, approximately 1–2 cm medial to the midline of the extremity [32]. To minimize risk of injury to the *epiphyseal growth plate*, needle insertion should be angled 10–30 degrees away from the joint in children [4]. Figure 7.10 shows the relevant anatomy for distal femur IO insertion.

Proximal Tibia

The proximal tibia is the most commonly utilized IO insertion site for both pediatric and adult subjects [21, 33]. This preference likely has historical origins, as the canine tibia was one of the earliest sites explored by IO researchers [34]. The tibial site is also far removed from the "action" of external chest compressions during CPR, which has traditionally been perceived as an advantage. Unfortunately, blood flow to subdiaphragmatic sites (including the tibia) is likely compromised in low-flow states such as CPR, which generates only about 20–30% of normal cardiac output [35, 36]. The proximal tibial site also has ready analogues in the canine and porcine models, which have been leveraged by IO researchers to simulate cardiac arrest conditions using these animals. However, tibial IO devices have been shown in many human studies to be inferior to supradiaphragmatic venous access, and the flow rates from proximal tibial cannulation are well-known to be inferior to those realized with supradiaphragmatic sites, such as the humerus and the sternum [37].

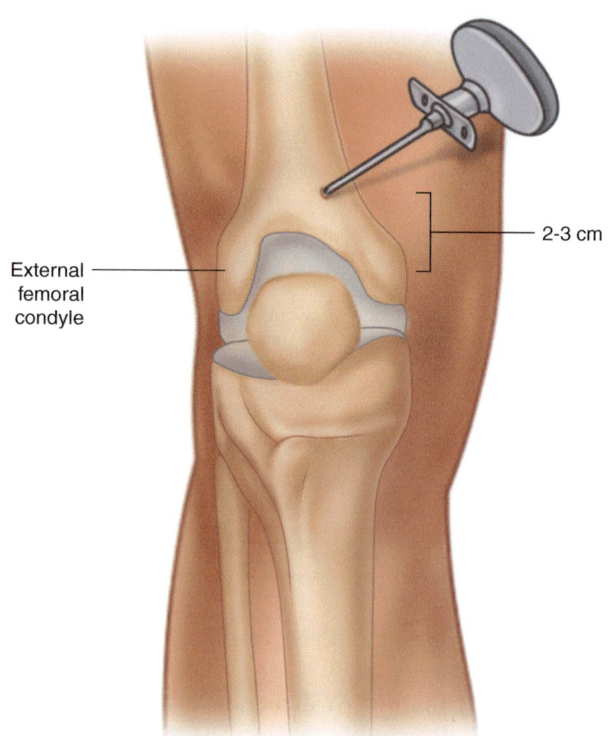

Fig. 7.10 Distal femur IO insertion site

In fact, cadaveric flow from the sternum is 1.6 times greater than in the humerus and 3.1 times greater than at the tibial IO site [37]. In anatomic models, flow from the proximal tibia appears to be via the *popliteal vein* [28].

Insertion Site 2 cm (two finger widths) inferior to the patella bone and then 2 cm medially or 2 cm medial to the tibial tuberosity (in adults) [38].

Available Devices EZ-IO™ (Teleflex), international version of the B.I.G.™ (PerSys Medical) with variable needle length selection, or manually driven IO devices. No devices with single fixed needle length depth of insertion are approved at the distal tibia site.

Insertion Techniques With the knee extended, externally rotate the patient's hip until the flat aspect of the tibia is visualized and parallel to the surface of the patient's bed. With proper positioning, the foot should form an approximately 45 degree angle with the bed. The level of insertion is 2 cm (about two finger widths) distal to the inferior edge of the patella. The insertion site is at this level, but 2 cm medial to the midline of the tibia, at the flat medial surface of the proximal tibia. In pediatric subjects, the insertion angle has been described as 10–30 degrees away from the

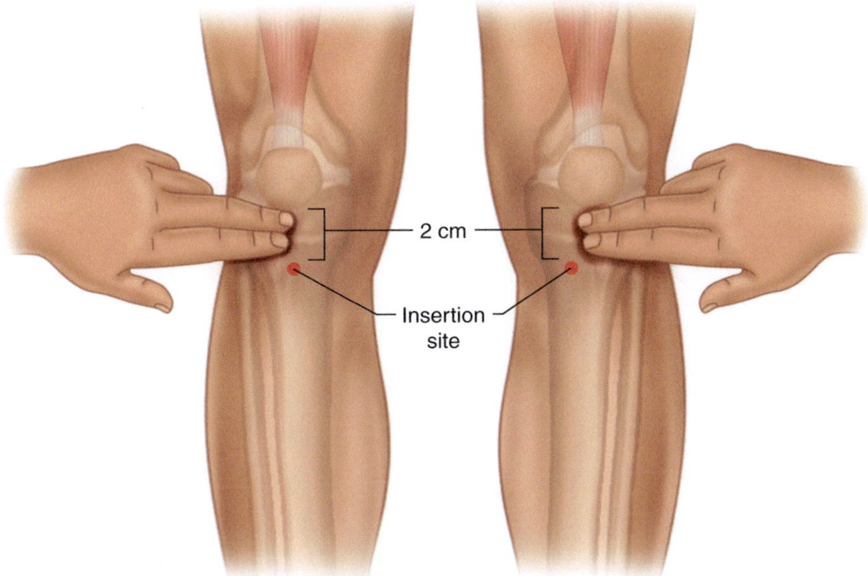

Fig. 7.11 Proximal tibia IO insertion site

knee joint, to prevent theoretical injury to the epiphyseal growth plate [4]. Figure 7.11 shows the site for proximal tibial IO insertion.

Distal Tibia

The distal tibial insertion site suffers the disadvantages of the proximal tibial site, with the added unfortunate distinction that it is even further from the patient's central circulation. Although the use of this site has been described, it should probably be considered a site of last resort. The vasculature emanating from this site is of smaller caliber than that from the proximal tibia. Consequently, both the arterial supply and venous return to this area are highly compromised, in comparison to most other IO insertion sites.

Insertion Site 3 cm superior to the most prominent part of the medial malleolus [4].

Available Devices EZ-IO™ (Teleflex), or manually driven IO devices. The NIO™ and B.I.G.™ (PerSys Medical) are approved for this site in Europe but not FDA-approved in the United States.

Insertion Techniques Insertion site can be located by palpation of the most prominent aspect of the medial malleolus. The provider can locate the anterior and posterior edges of the tibia and place intraosseous device midline to this bone on the flat

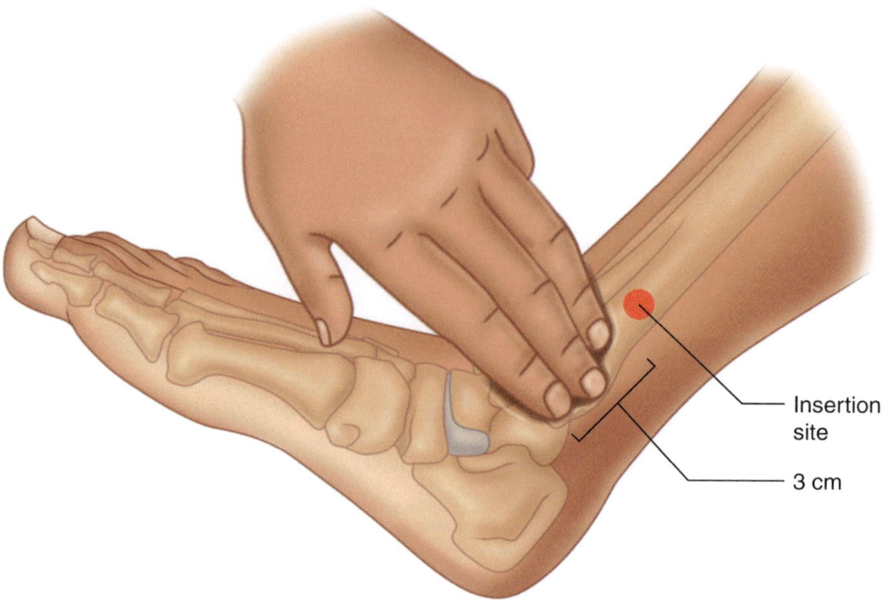

Fig. 7.12 Distal tibia IO insertion site

aspect, approximately 3 cm cephalad. Insertion angle is perpendicular to the bony surface of the tibia, at a depth of approximately 2 cm [4]. Figure 7.12 shows the relevant anatomy for distal tibial IO insertion.

Calcaneus

Insertion of an IO catheter at the calcaneus (i.e., "heel bone") has been described in a cadaveric study [31] and in a single pediatric case report [39], both by the same author. In the case report, 1800 mL of crystalloid fluid was delivered over 6 hrs to a 3-year-old child, without complications [39]. This site does have potential value for IO cannulation, as calcaneal cancellous bone has an open trabecular structure, analogous to the medullary cavity of long bones [31]. However, this site's extremely distal location relative to other IO cannulation sites suggests that the calcaneus should be rarely utilized for IO cannulation in live subjects.

Insertion Site Approximately 2 cm from the calcaneal tuberosity on the ventral portion of the medial process, between the first metatarsal and the calcaneal tuberosity [4]. Alternatively, insertion may be achieved at the anterior portion of the medial tubercle, at the junction of the inferior and medial surfaces of the calcaneus [31]. The medial aspect of the calcaneum has been recommended, "because this can be accessed easily with external rotation/abduction of the ipsilateral hip and slight flexion of the ipsilateral knee and the bone is immediately subcutaneous here" [39].

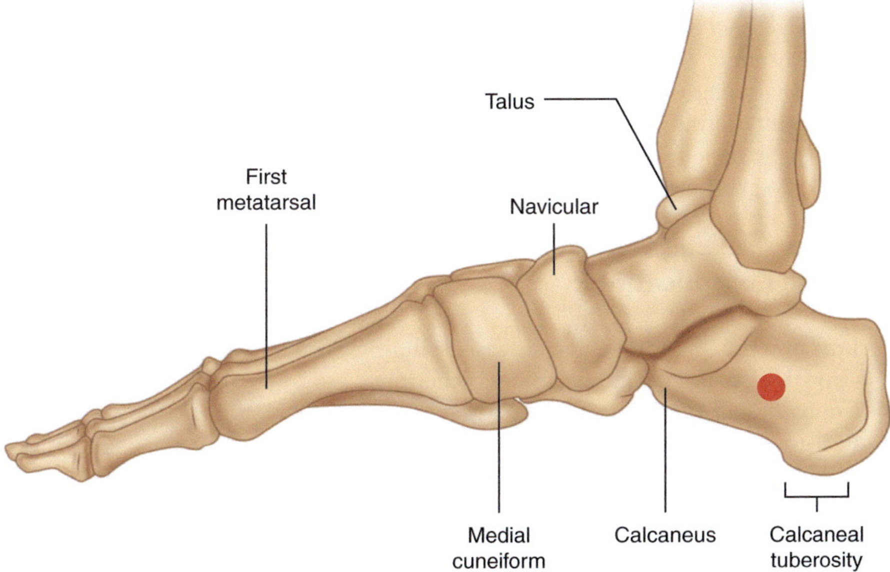

Fig. 7.13 Calcaneal IO insertion site (red dot), including relevant anatomy

Available Devices Major manufacturers do not endorse the use of their devices at this site.

Insertion Techniques According to the described cadaveric technique, the catheter should be inserted at the anterior portion of the medial tubercle, at the junction of the inferior and medial surfaces of the calcaneus [31]. Care should be taken to avoid the epiphyseal plate (posteriorly) and the posterior tibial vessels (anterosuperiorly) as they pass below the medial malleolus. Figure 7.13 shows the relevant anatomy for calcaneal IO insertion.

Complications of Intraosseous Cannulation

Intraosseous catheter placement may be associated with both immediate and delayed complications. *Immediate complications* include those injuries occurring during the insertion process, as well as injuries relating to catheter use that can be clinically identified within minutes or hours of catheter placement. *Delayed complications* are those injuries to the patient that may appear days, weeks, or even months following IO insertion.

Immediate Complications

- Inability to place catheter
- Inability to infuse fluids or medications
- Pain with insertion

- Pain with infusion
- Dislodgement of catheter
- Extravasation
- Pulmonary marrow or air embolism
- Catheter deformity
- Iatrogenic bone fracture
- Injury to great vessels of the chest (only with sternal IO)

Delayed Complications

- Infection (i.e., osteomyelitis, abscess, cellulitis, bacteremia, myonecrosis)
- Growth plate injury (in pediatric subjects)
- Compartment syndrome, with or without limb amputation
- Post-insertion hematoma

Analysis of the existing literature demonstrates a low rate of complications and high success rate overall for clinical IO catheter use. Lewis et al. reported no major complications with 1,014 device deployments over a 5-year period [40]. Santos et al. reported a 1.3% complication rate and 90% success rate with IO insertion [41]. Hallas et al. reported extravasation in 3.7% of cases, and compartment syndrome and osteomyelitis combined occurred in approximately 1% of subjects [42]. Difficulty aspirating bone marrow is encountered in 12.3% of subjects, but failure to aspirate marrow does not necessarily imply malposition of the catheter, as marrow may not be able to be aspirated in all properly placed catheters [42].

The most common complication associated with IO insertion (besides pain) is *extravasation* and fluid infiltration into the surrounding soft tissues, estimated to occur in about 12% of cases [43]. This complication is likely attributable, at least in part, to improper IO catheter insertion technique. Extravasation of infused medication or fluids may be expected when the IO catheter is inserted too deeply or too shallow in relation to the bony cortex. Ideally, the tip of the IO catheter should terminate in the medullary space following a single penetration of the cortex, without significant obstruction from bony spicules, marrow, or debris within the medullary space. Current manufacturers recommend that IO devices be flushed forcefully with at least 10 mL of saline after placement and lidocaine administration, to clear marrow from the potential intramedullary infusion space and facilitate subsequent forward flow. Failure to properly flush the IO catheter before attempted infusion may lead to poor flow, increased intramedullary resistance to infusion, and increased risk of subsequent extravasation.

Extravasation is likely to occur when the imposed volume and pressure upon the IO space exceed its capacitance. Although large volumes of fluid and medication can be safely infused through an IO catheter, providers should monitor the infusion site frequently to identify extravasation early. Once a catheter has begun to extravasate, it will likely continue to extravasate and (depending upon the pressure used for infusion); this can lead to localized soft tissue edema, increased soft tissue compartmental pressures, and even tissue necrosis.

Excessive torque on the IO catheter, which may widen the potential space between the catheter and the corticotomy (i.e., hole in the cortex) could also contribute to extravasation, as this may open a potential space between the catheter and the cortex that could accommodate retrograde passage of infused substances out of the medullary space. Needle length has also been found to contribute to the likelihood of extravasation, as longer needles may be more likely to pass through both the *cis* (superficial, or near) and *trans* (deep, or far) *cortex* of the target bone [4]. This phenomenon underscores the importance of selecting the correct length of catheter according to the selected insertion site. Minimization of over-penetration may be facilitated by ceasing forward penetration of the catheter when a lack of resistance is felt, suggesting that the medullary cavity has been reached after penetrating the bony cortex.

One way to minimize extravasation associated with IO devices is appropriate use of an *engineered stabilization device (ESD)*, which may be sold separately from the IO catheter needle itself or may be bundled into the device packaging. These devices often have a plastic locking hub that interfaces with the IO catheter itself, surrounded by an adhesive film that secures to the patient's skin around the insertion site. These ESDs help to prevent inadvertent pulling and torque on the needle after placement, which can cause loosening between the outer surface of the needle and the surrounding cortex, ultimately leading to catheter migration or dislodgement.

Although needle length is important, needle type does not appear to significantly impact extravasation rates. Insertion of various needle types, including the Sussmane-Raszynski™ needle, nonthreaded needle, Jamshidi™, and Sur-Fast™ catheters, in a randomized animal study demonstrated that extravasation rates under both pressure and gravity were shown to not be significantly different with different needle types. However, the risks of extravasation cannot be overstated, especially when *hypertonic substances* are infused. With certain infusion substrates, extravasation can lead to necrosis of the surrounding soft tissue [44]. Ngo et al. reported that soft tissue necrosis is associated with hypertonic solutions being extravasated into the surrounding tissue [38]. Potentially necrotoxic medications include hypertonic saline, sodium bicarbonate, dopamine, and calcium chloride. Tocantins et al. noted that a minimum of 12 hours in between attempts is necessary for the body to develop a blood clot at the original insertion site [18]. Other studies have shown that as much as 48 hours may be required [4].

Compartment syndrome can occur when excessive extravasation from the IO catheter leads to adequate pressure with the anatomic compartment to critically reduce arterial perfusion [38]. The risk of compartment syndrome is limited by *frequent monitoring* of the extremity and limitation of *one IO access attempt per bony target* [4]. In a recent review, 25% of compartment syndrome cases were attributed to a displaced needle, and at least 30% were associated with iatrogenic fracture or multiple IO attempts [4]. As early as 1945, Tocantins emphasized provider knowledge of IO insertions sites, familiarity with the approach, avoidance of "irritating" substances, and abstinence of IO use in the presence of infection to avoid complications [18]. These principles remain effective at avoiding complications of IO use. Undiagnosed subclinical *fractures at the target bone* have also been shown to contribute to compartment syndrome [45]. The best way to avoid complications of IO use appears to be adequate understanding of the clinical contraindications to IO use at a specific IO insertion site and strict adherence to monitoring of the extremity after cannulation to detect early signs of compartment syndrome and excessive fluid extravasation.

Monitoring distal arterial pressures with a blood pressure cuff distal to the insertion site may also help serve to identify compartment syndrome before adverse clinical effects can develop. Strausbaugh et al. utilized blood pressure cuffs to determine whether an IO needle was placed correctly or not by comparing the flow rate of both correctly placed and incorrectly placed IO needles before and after inflating a blood pressure cuff, both superior and inferior to the site. They discovered that after the blood pressure cuff was inflated, the mean percent flow decreased 48% in correctly placed needles and 95% with improperly placed needles [46]. This is because the intraosseous space will remain patent despite the direct pressure applied at the cuff site, while lymphatic and venous drainage from the surrounding soft tissues is greatly reduced. Small amounts of extravasated fluid and medication are normally picked up by the lymphatic and venous systems, but rapid fluid infusion may overwhelm this drainage system and lead to fluid accumulation adjacent to the insertion site.

Medications

Most medications that can be safely infused through a peripheral intravenous catheter have been infused through an IO catheter in clinical practice. In many ways, the IO route has been "grandfathered" into equivalency with the IV route, although this assumption is largely based upon historical, anecdotal evidence. Very few studies have confirmed the bioavailability of medications infused indirectly via IO catheter as compared to infusion through a direct intravenous line.

Resuscitation efforts with various animal models in the setting of cardiac arrest comparing intraosseous to intravenous access have demonstrated no significant difference in rates of return of spontaneous circulation (ROSC) or central venous concentrations of common resuscitative medications [47–53]. Such studies have led to a consensus opinion that IO and PIV access are bioequivalent when administering common resuscitative medications. Fluid infusion has been similarly assumed to be equivalent, although intramedullary pressures are much greater than the intravenous pressures typically encountered during PIV or CVC cannulation. Additional research is needed to determine whether clinical outcomes following IO infusion are indeed equivalent to those seen with IV infusion of these medications.

The primary considerations with IO infusion relate to the risks of extravasation and subsequent injury to the vascular system and soft tissues. Since medications and fluids injected into the medullary space must be taken up by very small draining veins, *potent vasoconstrictors* could theoretically compromise their own egress from the medullary cavity. The biochemical mediators which regulate drainage from the IO space are poorly understood, and it is likely that certain substances may cause unanticipated damage to the usual mechanisms controlling drainage from the medullary space. It is also likely that certain fat-soluble medications experience a *"depot effect,"* resulting in slower than expected egress from the medullary space in adults due to binding with the adipose tissues within the medullary cavity. This could lead to a slower peak concentration and reduced peak concentrations following IO infusion. Drugs that have already been shown to exhibit a depot effect following IO infusion include ceftriaxone, chloramphenicol, phenytoin, and tobramycin [54].

Flow Rates

The flow rate achievable with an IO catheter depends upon a variety of factors, including the following:
- Gauge and length of catheter
- Anatomic insertion site
- Impediments to flow
- Infusion pressure through the catheter
- Intraosseous medullary pressure
- Venous outflow pressure gradient

While each of these factors should be considered in predicting catheter flow, some of these factors may be outside of the control of the clinical provider. Typical flow rates reported for IO catheters are provided in Table 7.1.

Most modern IO catheters are of a 15-gauge diameter, although length varies according to manufacturer and anticipated use. As stated previously in this book, shorter and wider catheters permit greater fluid flow rates. In addition, the intrinsic resistance to flow is much greater within the bony medullary cavity than within the

Table 7.1 Flow rates associated with various IO insertion sites

Insertion site	Flow rates (gravity)	Flow rates (pressurized)
Sternum	3.4 mL/min [55]	50–100 mL/min with 465–1000 mmHg[a] [37, 56]
Clavicle	11.9 ± 0.68 mL/kg/hr [28]	Unknown
Proximal humerus	81.8–84 mL/min [38, 57]	57.1–153 mL/min [37, 38, 57]
Distal radius	Unknown	Unknown
Iliac crest	32.2 ± 4.48 mL/kg/hr [28], 0.53 ± 0.32 mL/kg/min[a] [58]	1.5 ± 0.60 mL/kg/min[a] [58]
Distal femur	1.03 ± 0.66 mL/kg/min[a] [58], 9.3 mL/min[b] [59]	2.10 ± 0.71 mL/kg/min[a] [58], 29.5 mL/min with 300 mmHg[b] [59]
Proximal tibia	4.96–73 mL/min [38, 57, 60]	7.70–204.6 mL/min [37, 38, 57, 60]
Distal tibia	2.07 mL/min [60]	3.80 mL/min [60]
Calcaneus	5 mL/min [39]	Unknown

Notes: [a]canine study; [b]swine study

venous system. Consequently, a 15-gauge IO catheter should not be expected to realize the same flow rates as a PIV with similar gauge and length, unless additional infusion pressure (e.g., pressure bag) is provided.

Time Required for Placement

Many studies have been performed comparing the insertion speed and first-attempt success rate between currently available intraosseous devices. Jun et al. compared intraosseous insertion speed and success rate among medical students using turkey bones and pork ribs [61]. This study compared students with no training to students who had practiced the insertion technique. In this study, insertion time for the Illinois™ needle was 33 ± 44 seconds, compared to 54 ± 43 seconds for the Sur-Fast™ needle among inexperienced users. However, the speed of placement was essentially the same for experienced users of both devices. The success rate of the Illinois™ needle showed no improvement with practice, although rate of successful placement for the Sur-Fast™ needle improved from 79% to 95% [61].

Other studies have compared manual IO devices to semiautomated IO devices. Brenner et al. compared a manual IO device to the EZ-IO™ system and noted similar insertion times (32 ± 11 seconds for EZ-IO™ placement vs. 33 ± 28 seconds for the manual device) [62]. However, the EZ-IO™ was associated with a higher first-attempt success rate (97.8%) compared to the manual device (79.5%) [62]. Shavit et al. found that 69% (20/29) of students preferred the EZ-IO™ device over a manual device and enjoyed a significantly higher first-attempt success rate with the EZ-IO™ (97%) when compared to the B.I.G.™ (65.5%) [63]. Leidel et al. found no significant difference in placement success rate and overall procedure time between the B.I.G.™ and the EZ-IO™ [64].

Kurowski et al. found that the first-attempt success rate for the B.I.G.™ was roughly 92%, better than the EZ-IO™ (83%) and Jamshidi™ (48%). In this study, the use of the B.I.G.™ was associated with a mean insertion time of 2.0 ± 0.7 minutes, while the EZ-IO™ insertion time was 3.1 ± 0.9 minutes, and the Jamshidi™ required 4.2 ± 1.0 minutes [65]. In another study comparing the EZ-IO™, B.I.G.™, and a manual device, the EZ-IO™ device was associated with a 96% success rate, better than the B.I.G.™ (55%) or manual IO device (50%) [66].

The FAST1™ has been shown to have a 73% rate of successful insertion, with an average procedural time of 67 seconds [67].

The NIO™ device is a semiautomated device, which has also been compared to other available intraosseous devices. In a randomized manikin experiment by Szarpak et al. including 84 paramedics, the first IO attempt success rate of NIO™ was 89.3% for the tibia and 73.8% for the humerus, suggesting that the tibia is associated with an easier and more rapid insertion than the humerus site [68]. Bielski et al. compared the pediatric NIO™ with the Pediatric B.I.G.™, EZ-IO™, and Jamshidi™ in a cohort of 87 paramedics. They found that the NIO™ had roughly a 9-second insertion time, while the B.I.G.™ was associated with a 12-second insertion time, the EZ-IO™ required a 13.5-second insertion time, and the Jamshidi required a 15-second insertion time. This study suggested that the NIO™ device is associated with a much shorter placement time than the EZ-IO™, B.I.G.™, or Jamshidi™. Statistical differences were also seen with the EZ-IO™ and B.I.G.™, when compared to the Jamshidi™ [69].

Banerjee et al. observed 60 pediatric patients with dehydration to determine the average amount of effort required to establish vascular access. In this study, they found that an IO device could be secured within 5 minutes in all patients who had an IO attempted, while PIV access was only successfully achieved in two-thirds of subjects within the first 5 minutes of dedicated effort [70]. Overall, the time taken to adequately administer a PIV was roughly 129 ± 13 seconds, compared to IO cannulation requiring 67 ± 7 seconds. In this study, IO devices required less than half of the time needed to secure a PIV, suggesting that IO may be more rapidly established than PIV in dehydrated pediatric subjects [70].

Manual Intraosseous Devices

Thirty years ago, all intraosseous devices available on the market were manual devices. Despite the recent expansion of the IO market to include mechanically driven devices, manual IO catheters still deserve a place in the provider's *repertoire*. These devices are all characterized by reliance upon the clinician to provide all the force needed for insertion. Consequently, these devices are more challenging to place in hard bones, especially the lower extremities of adult subjects. However, the less calcified bones of infants and children, as well as the upper (i.e., non-weight bearing) extremities of adults, may present less of a challenge for manual IO insertion.

The "traditional" manual IO needles that remain commercially available at the time of this writing include the standard *Cook*™ (Cook Medical), *Dieckmann*™ (Cook Medical), *Sussmane-Raszynski*™ (Cook Medical), *Illinois*™ (Becton, Dickinson, and Company), and *Jamshidi*™ (Becton, Dickinson, and Company) models. These needles all differ regarding the style of their hub, needle length, and shape of the trocar tip and are available in a variety of gauges and catheter lengths. The Dieckmann™ modification of the standard Cook needle (Fig. 7.14) includes a 45 degree angle at the trocar tip and is distinguished from other manual IO models by the presence of laterally opposed side ports positioned near the needle cannula's distal tip to ensure proper flow if the needle tip is obstructed. The Dieckmann™ comes in 3 cm or 4 cm cannula lengths, with 14-, 16-, or 18-G internal diameter.

The Jamshidi™ and Illinois™ devices feature an adjustable depth guard, which can be moved up or down on the needle to theoretically prevent over-penetration. The depth guard can also be removed, allowing for deeper penetration. The Jamshidi™ size used for patients >9 months of age is 15 G with length adjustable from 24 to 48 mm. The manufacturer recommends using the 18-G needle with 14 to 48 mm adjustable length in patients <9 months of age. Although the greater potential length of this needle can be advantageous, this increased length also raises the center of gravity for the device and may increase difficulty of placement [71]. As

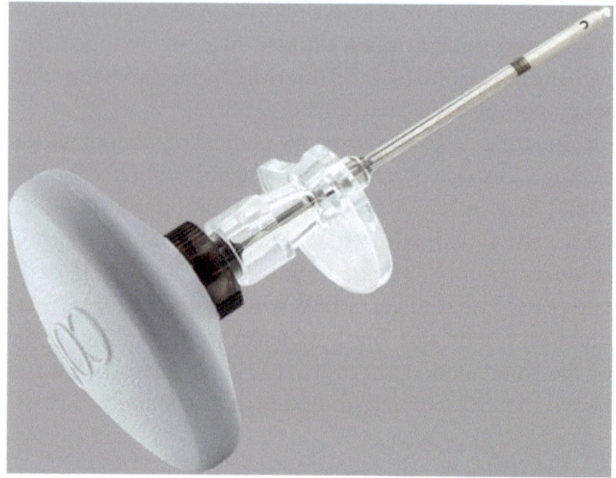

Fig. 7.14 Dieckmann™ manual intraosseous needle. (*Image courtesy of Cook Medical Inc. © 2020 Cook Medical Inc. All rights reserved*)

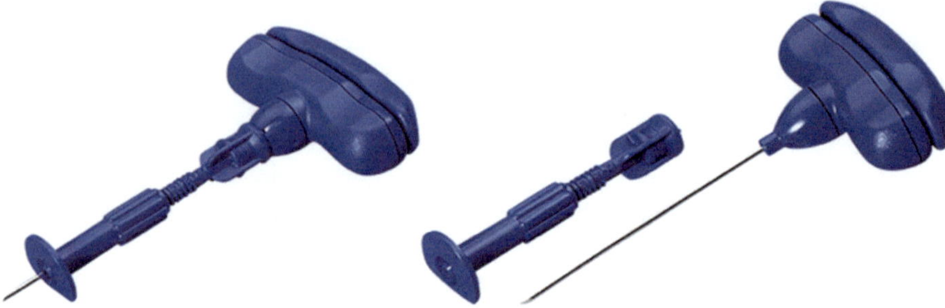

Fig. 7.15 Illinois™ manual intraosseous needle. (*Images courtesy of Becton, Dickinson and Company Inc. © 2020 Becton, Dickinson and Company Inc. All rights reserved*)

illustrated in Figs. 7.15 and 7.16, the Illinois™ needle has a wider handle than the Jamshidi™ needle, and both devices protrude from the patient approximately 2 inches after deployment, which may predispose to accidental dislodgement of the catheter. By contrast, the Cook™ catheters have a detachable handle, lowering the catheter's profile after deployment (Fig. 7.17). However, the depth guard may still be elevated above skin level. Consequently, a silicone Molnar disc and pull tie are recommended to help stabilize the Cook™ catheter at skin level. The original Jamshidi needle was designed circa 1971 and tapers distally toward a non-serrated cutting end [72], intended to minimize crushing of the tissue with placement and reduce the risk of subsequent catheter occlusion [73].

The Sussmane-Raszynski™ and Sur-Fast™ (Cook Medical) manual IO catheters featured a "threaded" external cannula that was "screwed" into the bone. The Sussmane-Raszynski™ uses a fine-screw needle cannula and was available in 3 cm length with 16-G needle and a 45 degree trocar. The Sur-Fast™ cannula featured a coarser thread to secure the catheter in the bone. The insertion kit for the Sur-Fast™ also included a small scalpel used to cut through the overlying skin prior to

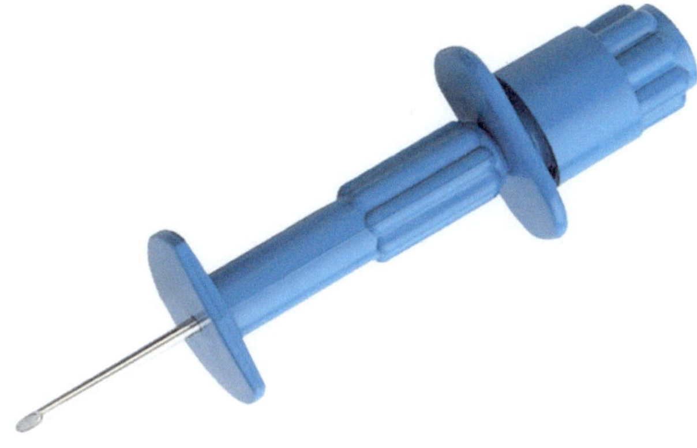

Fig. 7.16 Jamshidi™ manual intraosseous needle. (*Image courtesy of Becton, Dickinson and Company Inc. © 2020 Becton, Dickinson and Company Inc. All rights reserved*)

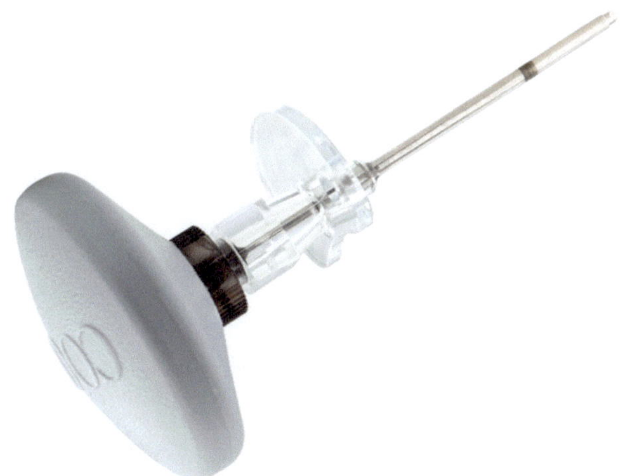

Fig. 7.17 Standard Cook™ manual intraosseous needle. (*Image courtesy of Cook Medical Incorporated. © 2020 Cook Medical Incorporated. All rights reserved*)

insertion. These threaded catheters are shown in Fig. 7.18. Many other eponymous intraosseous catheter designs have been developed and abandoned over the last century, including various modifications. Those with an interest in the history of intraosseous cannulation and manual IO catheter design are directed to a literature review by Parapia [74].

The *T.A.L.O. N.*™ (Tactically Advanced Lifesaving Intraosseous Needle) intraosseous device (Teleflex, Inc.) is the first and only manual IO device currently FDA-cleared for insertion at all seven primary IO insertion sites (i.e., sternum, bilateral proximal humerus, bilateral proximal tibia, and bilateral distal tibia) [75]. As with the other Teleflex IO devices, it is a 15-gauge catheter made from grade 304 stainless steel. The T.A.L.O. N.™ comes in a standard 38.5 mm length and includes a "sternal stabilizer" to help secure the device and prevent overpenetration. The T.A.L.O.N. device is shown in Fig. 7.19, along with the stabilizer device and infusion tubing attachment.

The *SAM Medical*™ IO needle driver is a lightweight (75 grams) manually operated device, powered by repeated trigger compression while guiding the needle

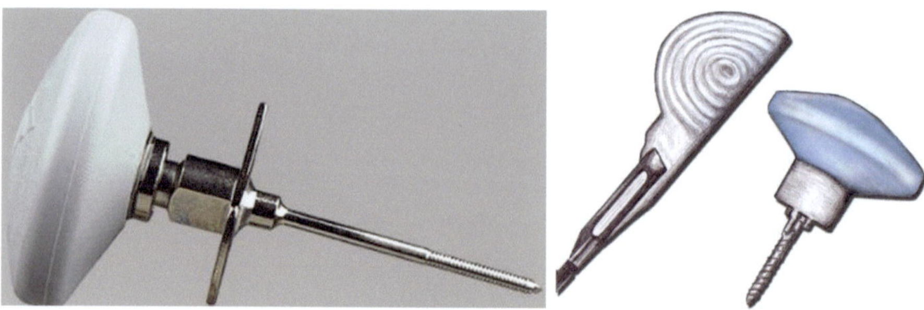

Fig. 7.18 Sussmane-Raszynski™ (left) and Sur-Fast™ (right) IO catheters. (*Image courtesy of Cook Medical Inc. © 2020 Cook Medical Inc. All rights reserved*)

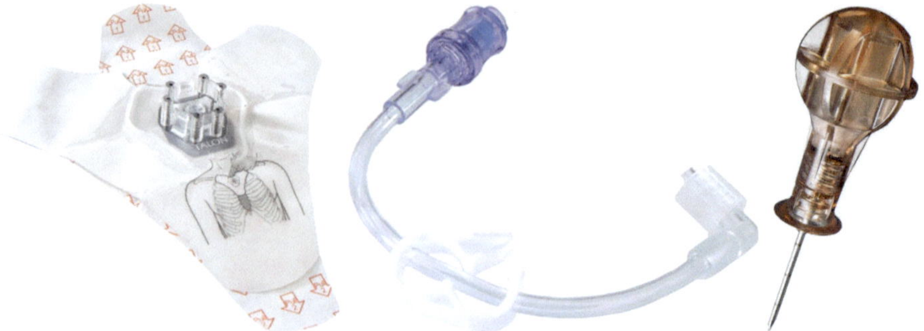

Fig. 7.19 The T.A.L.O. N.™ intraosseous system, including sternal stabilizer and EZ-Connect® extension set. (*Image courtesy of Teleflex Inc. © 2020 Teleflex Inc. All rights reserved*)

assembly into position [76]. The rotational spin of the needle (actuated by the trigger compression), along with forward pressure provided by the user, facilitates a finely controlled insertion when compared to conventional manual IO devices. The driver is made of a polycarbonate material and is reported by the manufacturer to last 10,000 actuations. The standard 15-gauge catheter comes in three lengths (15, 25, and 45 mm), which can be used for both pediatric and adult subjects. The SAM IO Needle Adapter™ allows the SAM IO Driver to accommodate "alternative" IO needles (e.g., EZ-IO™) [76]. The SAM IO manual driver and needle are shown in Fig. 7.20.

The *FAST1*™ was the first IO device approved for sternal placement, receiving FDA approval for use in adults in 1997, and pediatric subjects >12 years old in 2008 [77]. This single-use device is employed exclusively at the sternum. It is a "muscle-powered" device that is designed to project into the sternal medullary cavity of adults through direct application of approximately 45 lbs force by the provider and does not use a spring or other mechanical augmentation of force to facilitate insertion. The user must first place a target patch on the patient's manubrium, focus the introducer on the desired area of insertion, and push firmly on the introducer to

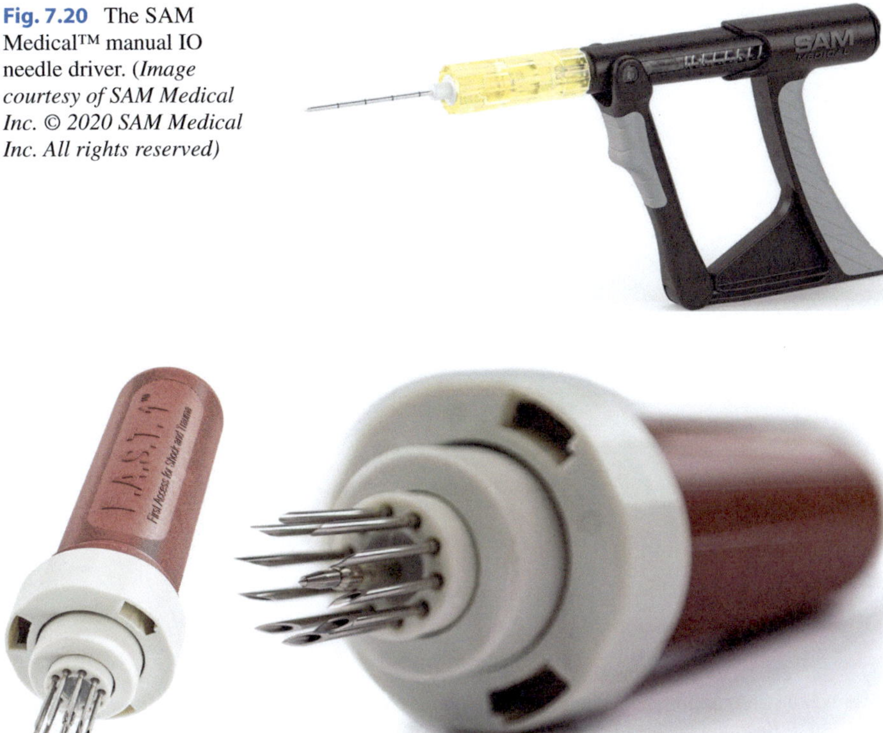

Fig. 7.20 The SAM Medical™ manual IO needle driver. (*Image courtesy of SAM Medical Inc. © 2020 SAM Medical Inc. All rights reserved*)

Fig. 7.21 The FAST1™ intraosseous device. (*Image courtesy of Teleflex Inc. © 2020 Teleflex Inc. All rights reserved*)

insert the infusion tube into the sternum. The infusion tube is then left in the sternum and attached to an IV extension set [77]. This device is shown in Fig. 7.21.

Pyng released the *FASTResponder*™ in 2013, a modified version of the FAST1™ device. Another version of the FASTResponder™, termed the *FASTCombat*™, became available around the same time, in "combat colors." In 2016, Pyng released the *FASTTactical*™ sternal IO device, which is analogous to the FAST1™ but includes a rigid tube packaging to protect the device from damage [78]. The FASTResponder™ is shown in Fig. 7.22.

At the time of this writing, the FAST1™ appears to be primarily marketed to military users, while the FASTResponder™ is being marketed to civilian users. FASTTactical™ is available to both military and civilian providers [78].

Becton, Dickinson and Company has more recently released the BD™ manual Intraosseous Vascular Access System, which uses needle cannulae of variable lengths attached to a color-coded manual driver handle (pink 15 mm, blue 25 mm, yellow 45 mm). During placement, the catheter is advanced through the soft tissues and into the marrow space by manually rotating the device clockwise and counterclockwise while applying gentle downward pressure. This is a

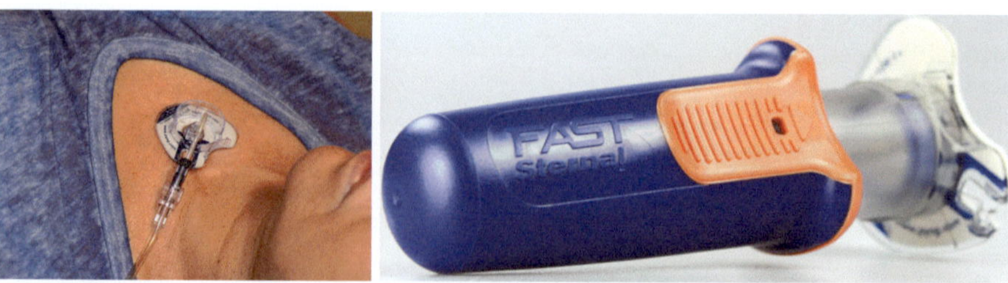

Fig. 7.22 The FASTResponder™ intraosseous device. (*Image courtesy of Teleflex Inc. © 2020 Teleflex Inc. All rights reserved*)

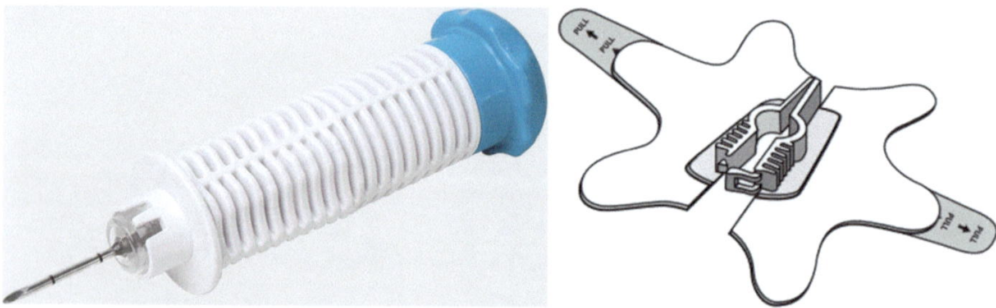

Fig. 7.23 The BD™ Intraosseous Vascular Access System, shown with 15 mm needle and manual driver handle (left), securement device (right). (*Image courtesy of Becton, Dickinson and Company Inc. © 2020 Becton, Dickinson and Company Inc. All rights reserved*)

single-use device, and the kit comes with a securement device and extension tubing set with needle-free valve. The securement device clamps around the needle hub, allowing for it to be applied before or after the extension tubing has been attached. The BD™ Intraosseous Vascular Access System is shown in Fig. 7.23.

Semiautomatic Intraosseous Devices

The deployment of intraosseous devices for adult subjects has been made easier by the advent of mechanically driven (i.e., semiautomatic) techniques. These devices, unlike manual IO needles, do not rely exclusively on force provided by the clinician. Consequently, these devices may be easier to deploy in the hardened bones of adult subjects but may also introduce a greater risk of iatrogenic injury if the delivered force is excessive or the device is deployed inappropriately.

At present, mechanically driven IO devices are generally of two types: *battery-powered drills* and *spring-loaded devices*. The battery-powered drill devices may offer superior user control over the insertion process, as they allow the provider to control and adjust the depth of insertion. However, these devices rely upon a battery for the energy required to drive the insertion and thus may be exposed to the risk of battery depletion, which can cause slowing or failure of insertion due to binding of the motor or even motor failure. With these devices, the IO needle and driver device are usually packaged (and sold) separately, and the driver device (e.g., "drill") is reusable but requires sterilization between patient uses.

The EZ-IO™ system is an FDA-approved device for proximal tibia, proximal humerus, and distal tibia insertion in adult and pediatric patients, as well as distal femur insertion in pediatric patients [4]. The EZ-IO™ is a battery-powered device with three needle sizes that are 15 gauge and differ in length (15, 25, and 45 mm) [79]. This device was the first battery-powered IO device to appear on the market [4]. Pediatric subjects are defined as those weighing 3 to 39 kg, regardless of age [4]. The IO catheters for this device are color-coded, including 15 mm (pink), 25 mm (blue), and 45 mm (yellow) sizes. In October 2020, the device received FDA 510(k) clearance to expand the indications for use to allow for up to 48-hour (previously 24-hour) dwell time when alternate IV access is not available or reliably established in patients aged 12 years and above. The EZ-IO™ system is shown in Fig. 7.24.

The BD™ Intraosseous Vascular Access system is a newer competitor in the field, with similar mechanism for placement, including a "drill" placement device and individual needles (Fig. 7.25).

Spring-loaded devices, on the other hand, use the potential energy from an internal coiled metal spring to drive the IO needle into the bone. These devices incorporate the "driver" inside the same housing as the IO needle, obviating the need to sterilize a separate driver after use. These devices generally come prepackaged inside a sterile wrapping and are more lightweight than even the smallest battery-powered drills. However, the depth and the force of insertion are preset in these devices, with different devices recommended for different applications (according to patient age or weight, with insertion site according to soft tissue depth, etc.). Consequently, spring-loaded IO devices must be selected carefully for the right application, as inappropriate device selection may result in excessive force or depth being used with the insertion. Spring-loaded devices compress the soft tissues during deployment and therefore may not require the longer needle length required with other IO devices.

The *B.I.G.™ (Bone Injection Gun)* device is approved by the FDA for proximal humerus and proximal tibia insertion in adults and children [4]. This device is FDA-approved for proximal tibial and humeral insertions [4]. This device is a single-use spring-loaded IO device with both pediatric and adult gauges. The insertion angle is 90 degrees from the site of insertion [4]. The pediatric catheter is 18 gauge, and the adult catheter is 15 gauge in diameter [78]. The pediatric B.I.G.™ catheter is recommended for patients aged less than 12 years old [4]. The international version of the B.I.G.™ has a dial for selecting variable predetermined needle lengths, although the US version is sold as a fixed-depth device. This device is shown in Fig. 7.26.

The *NIO™* (PerSys Medical) device is FDA-approved for proximal humerus and proximal tibial insertion. It is a semiautomated single-use device that has both pediatric and adult versions [68]. The NIO™ adult is for subjects aged 12 years of age or older. The pediatric device is intended for ages 3–11 years [69]. These devices

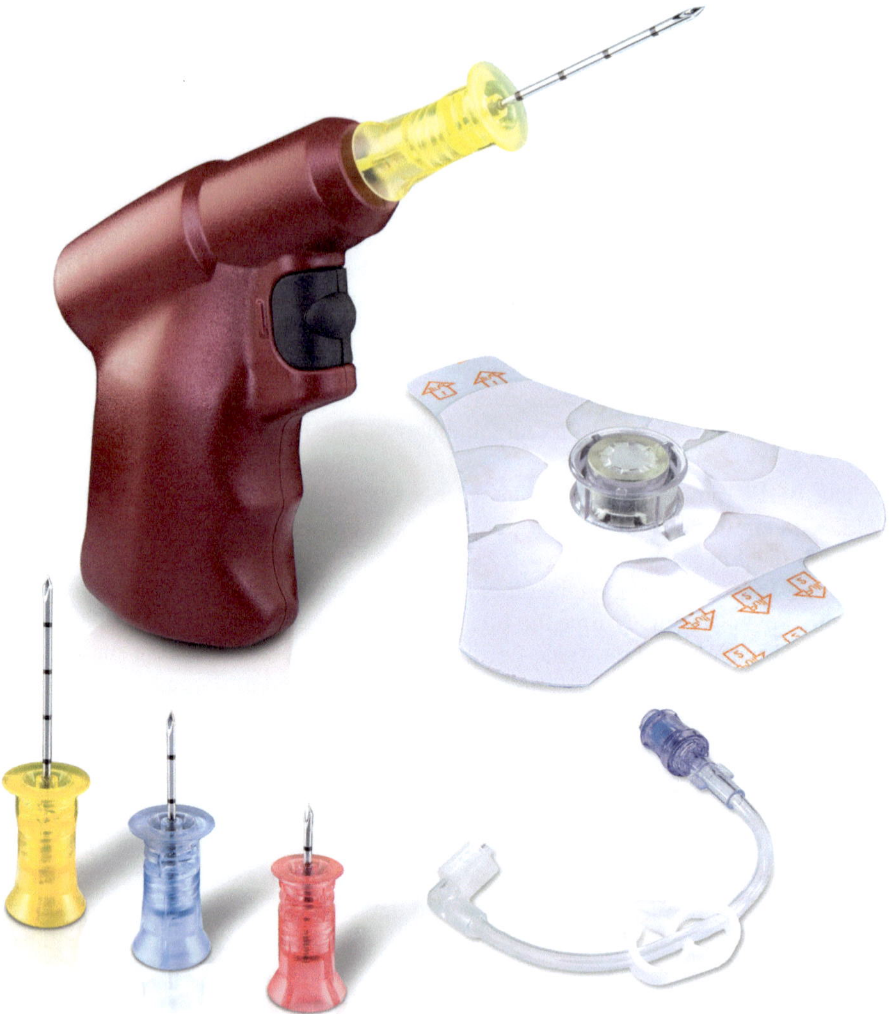

Fig. 7.24 The EZ-IO™ intraosseous system, including stabilizer and extension tubing. (*Image courtesy of Teleflex Inc. © 2020 Teleflex Inc. All rights reserved*)

have a 5-year shelf-life. The NIO™ for adults and pediatric subjects is shown in Fig. 7.27.

PerSys Medical has more recently introduced the *NIO™ Infant* device, which is indicated for patients between gestational age 36 weeks (weight ≥2.3 kg) and 3 years old. This device features an innovative Stepped Needle® design, which provides gradated penetration into the bone marrow cavity to prevent over-penetration. It also includes a safety needle cap and unique fixation dressing, allowing for universal securement. This device is shown in Fig. 7.28.

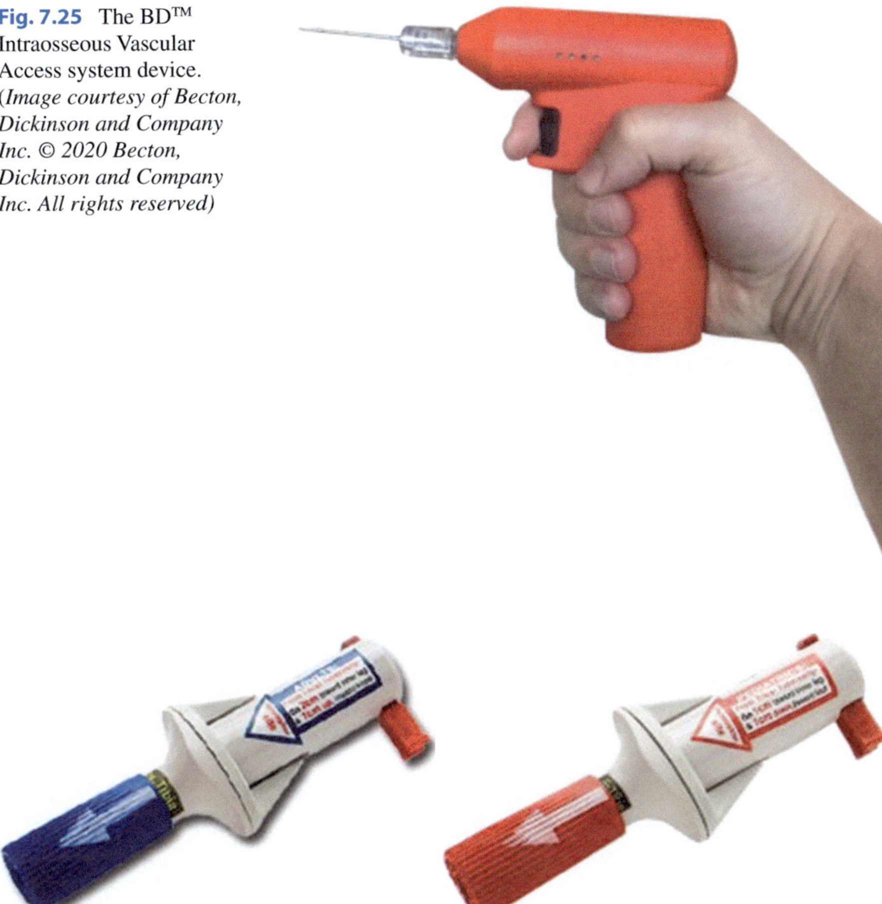

Fig. 7.25 The BD™ Intraosseous Vascular Access system device. (*Image courtesy of Becton, Dickinson and Company Inc. © 2020 Becton, Dickinson and Company Inc. All rights reserved*)

Fig. 7.26 The BIG™ (Bone Injection Gun) for adult (blue) and pediatric subjects (red). (*Images courtesy of PerSys Medical Inc. © 2020 PerSys Medical Inc. All rights reserved*)

Confirmation of Proper Placement

Although the ability to aspirate bone marrow through an IO catheter immediately after placement does suggest that the tip of the device is within the medullary cavity, the inability to aspirate bone marrow is not a reliable indicator of inappropriate tip position. Bony spicules or particulate matter within the medullary space can prevent aspiration of blood and other marrow contents without preventing infusion through the device. Given the risks of infiltration or extravasation associated with catheter malposition, most notably subsequent soft tissue necrosis and compartment syndrome, alternative strategies have been sought to confirm proper catheter placement prior to the initiation of infusion.

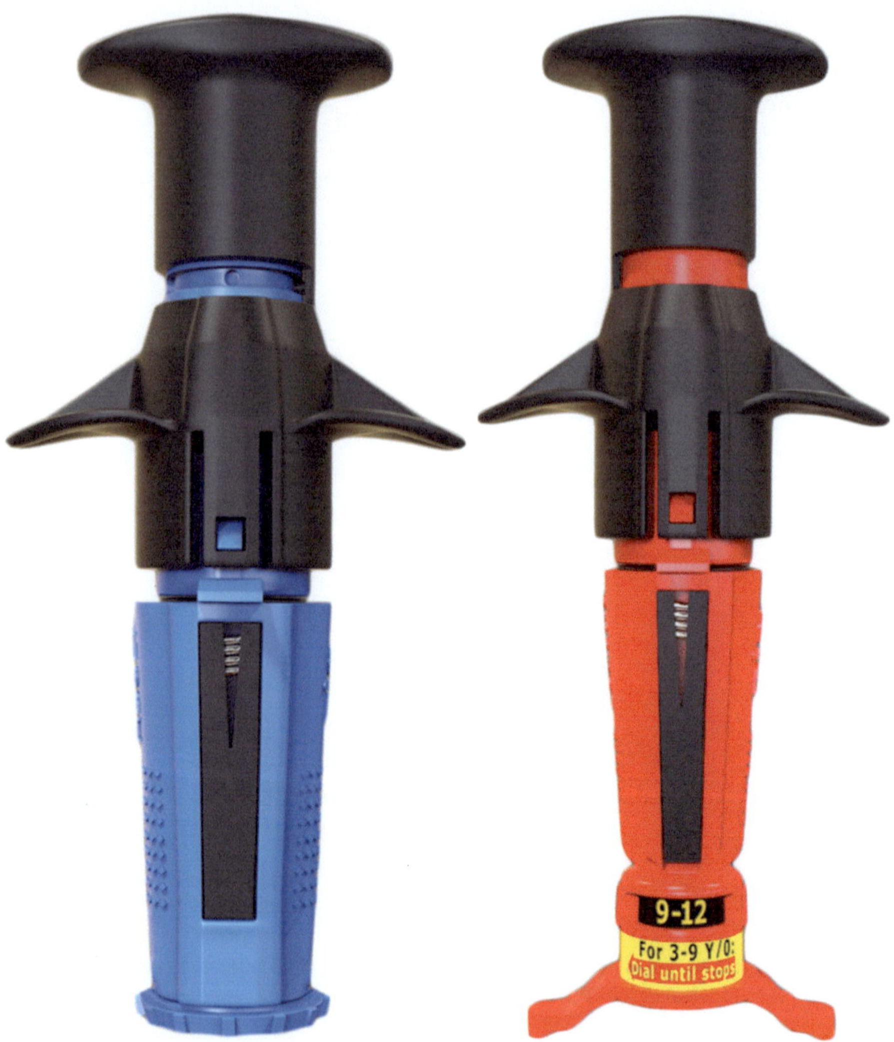

Fig. 7.27 The NIO™ intraosseous device for adult (blue) and pediatric (red) subjects. (*Images courtesy of PerSys Medical Inc. © 2020 PerSys Medical Inc. All rights reserved*)

Ultrasound visualization of the insertion site, including color flow Doppler imaging of the intramedullary space during a 10 mL syringe infusion, has been proposed as a potential solution [19, 80, 81]. The absence of turbulent intramedullary flow (or the presence of flow in the adjacent soft tissues) during a "test" 10 mL syringe infusion has been shown to detect catheter tip position in the soft tissues [19, 80, 81]. Catheters that are properly positioned, with their tip inside the medullary cavity, should generate detectable intramedullary color flow Doppler signals when rapid IO infusion is performed. Real-time ultrasound imaging of the target bone and

Fig. 7.28 The NIO™ Infant intraosseous device. (*Image courtesy of PerSys Medical Inc. © 2020 PerSys Medical Inc. All rights reserved*)

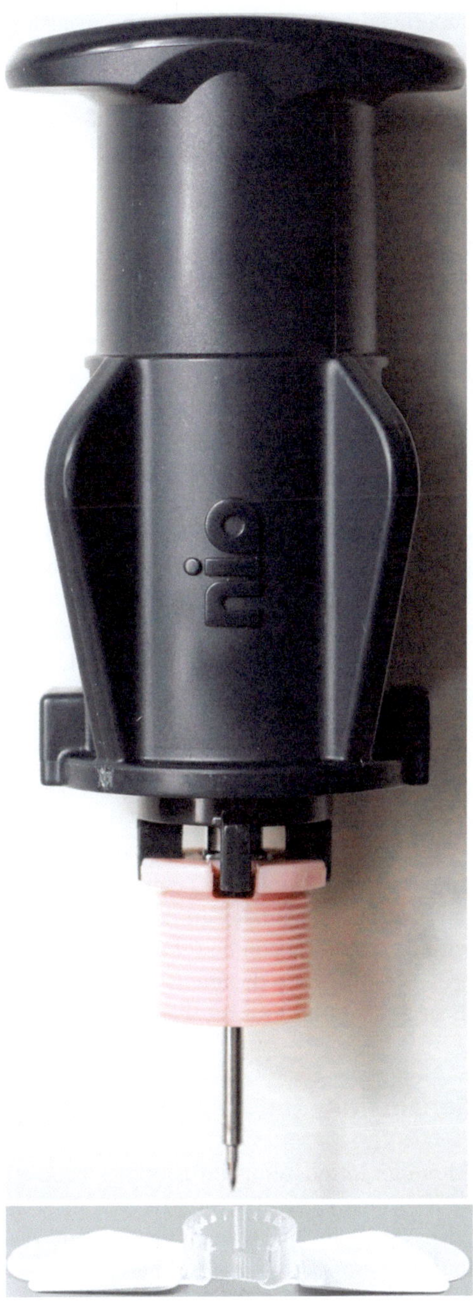

superficial soft tissues during the insertion attempt can also be used to aid in the identification of the proper insertion site.

The so-called "squeeze test" may also be of benefit to providers when ultrasound confirmation is not available [82, 83]. Although this technique was developed in piglets [82], its use has been reported in the care of human patients [83]. Because compression of the soft tissues increases soft tissue compartment pressure but does not substantially increase intramedullary pressure, direct manual compression ("squeezing") of the soft tissues around an IO insertion site is expected to increase resistance to flow (and reduce fluid flow rates) when the catheter has been placed incorrectly resulting in infusion into the soft tissue compartment. Alternatively, the flow through a properly placed IO catheter (with tip in the medullary space) does not appear to be adversely affected [82, 83].

Since IO cannulae are composed of surgical steel, they do appear on plain X-ray films, and X-ray may be adequate to confirm that the catheter tip has penetrated the bony cortex [84]. However, reliance upon X-ray films to confirm IO placement introduces additional cost and radiation exposure, and single-view X-rays may not exclude the possibility of both *trans* and *cis* (i.e., "through-and-through") cortical penetration. Complete penetration through both cortices can be especially problematic in pediatric subjects due to the small caliber of the medullary space and less resistance to penetration with their relatively softer bones. The target space for pediatric IO placement can be quite small. For example, the medullary cavity diameter at the proximal tibia is 7 mm ± 3 mm for infants, <1 year., 4 mm for newborn, and 2 mm in neonates [85, 86]. At least one institution has developed a computed tomography protocol to confirm proper IO placement, with claims by the authors that this approach is easier and faster and leads to less radiation and procedure time than plain film imaging [87].

Devices are also beginning to be developed to help providers to identify the proper insertion site for IO catheter placement. One such device is the Tib-Finder™ intraosseous placement guide, which is placed on the patient's leg and interfaces with the patient's patella ("kneecap") to suggest the correct IO insertion site to the provider [88]. The designers of this device are currently working on the development of a similar tool for the humeral insertion site.

Conclusion

Although intraosseous infusion has been employed for most of a century, the value of IO infusion has become increasingly apparent for patients who present to the emergency care provider with difficult vascular access. Intraosseous access has a long and storied history and has been proven over time to be safe and effective at achieving vascular access when intravenous access is delayed or impossible. Limitations in the use of IO access are mostly focused upon the pain associated with its use, and this limitation must be considered in its use in the clinical environment. Despite its limitations, IO access should be considered by emergency care providers who are unable to establish intravenous access rapidly. Emergency care providers must be aware of the potential IO insertion sites available to them and should not hesitate to utilize this approach when other options are not available. Although the proximal tibial IO insertion site is generally preferred by providers, this site offers suboptimal access in low-flow states such as cardiac arrest. Providers should consider humeral and sternal IO options when immediate resuscitation is required, especially when proximal intravenous access is not available. Modern devices allow easy access to the IO medullary space, and powered IO devices should be selected over manual devices, when available. Future research should seek to assess the present assumption that medications administered through the IO route are equally efficacious to those infused through IV devices. This is especially important to the future of cardiac arrest research. Providers should consider IO access whenever they are unable to establish IV access rapidly. Additional research is needed to determine the most effective means of achieving analgesia for IO infusion, as pain is a major limitation to the use of IO infusion for sensate patients.

Key Concepts
- Intraosseous catheters are a useful adjunct for the experienced clinician in treating patients with difficult vascular access, especially clinically unstable patients.
- Intraosseous access utilizes a non-collapsible space to deliver fluids and medications and therefore may be a more reliable route for patients with cardiovascular collapse and profound hypovolemia than direct intravenous access.
- While the proximal tibia and proximal humerus are the most commonly utilized IO insertion sites, other insertion sites may offer distinct advantages.
- The "depot effect" and other physiological factors could theoretically lead to delayed or diminished response to certain medications infused through the IO route, but very few medications have been extensively studied.
- Pain with infusion remains a challenge for providers who wish to utilize the IO route in awake patients. Other complications appear to be rare and generally preventable with proper insertion technique and close monitoring of the insertion site.
- Providers should carefully consider the advantages and disadvantages of intraosseous cannulation as they relate to the specific needs of their patient.

References

1. Staub NC, Cecil K. Drinker: pioneer lymphologist. Lymphology. 1979;12(3):115–7.
2. Drinker CK, Drinker KR. A method for maintaining an artificial circulation through the tibia of the dog, with a demonstration of the vasomotor control of the marrow vessels. Am J Physio. 1916;40(4):514–21.

3. Drinker CK, Drinker KR, Lund CC. The circulation in the mammalian bone-marrow. Am J Physio. 1922;62(1):1–92.
4. Paxton JH. Intraosseous vascular access: a review. Trauma. 2012;14(3):195–232.
5. Doan CA. The circulation of the bone marrow. Contribut Embryol. 1922;14:27–45.
6. Massa DJ, Lundy JS, Faulconer A, Ridley RW. A plastic needle. Proc Staff Meet Mayo Clin. 1950;25(14):413–5.
7. Orlowski J. My kingdom for an intravenous line. Am J Dis Child. 1984;138:803.
8. American Heart Association and American Academy of Pediatrics: Textbook of pediatric advanced life support. American Heart Association, Dallas, TX. USA. 1988. p. 43–4.
9. American Heart Association. Advanced cardiac life support guidelines. Management of cardiac arrest. Circulation. 2005;112-IV, 57–66.
10. American Heart Association. American Heart Association (AHA) guidelines for cardio- pulmonary resuscitation (CPR) and emergency cardiovascular care (ECC) of pediatric and neonatal patients: pediatric advanced life support. Pediatrics. 2006;117:e1005–28.
11. Neumar RW, Otto CW, Link MS, et al. Part 8: adult advanced cardiovascular life support: 2010 American Heart Association guidelines for cardiopulmonary resuscitation and emergency cardiovascular care. Circulation. 2010;122(suppl 3):S729–67.
12. Link MS, Berkow LC, Kudenchuk PJ, et al. Part 7: adult advanced cardiovascular life support: 2015 American Heart Association guidelines update for cardiopulmonary resuscitation and emergency cardiovascular care. Circulation. 2015;132(suppl 2):S444–64.
13. Panchal AR, Berg KM, Kudenchuk PJ, et al. 2018 American Heart Association focused update on advanced cardiovascular life support use of antiarrhythmic drugs during and immediately after cardiac arrest: an update to the American Heart Association guidelines for cardiopulmonary resuscitation and emergency cardiovascular care. Circulation. 2018;138(23):e740–9.
14. Subcommittee on Advanced Trauma Life Support (ATLS), American College of Surgeons (ACS), Committee on Trauma, 2017–2018. Advanced Trauma Life Support Course for Physicians. Chicago: Committee on Trauma, American College of Surgeons; 2018. p. 52.
15. Standring S. Gray's anatomy: the anatomic basis of clinical practice. 40th ed. Jordan Hill, GBP: Churchill Livingstone; 2008.
16. Hall SJ. Basic biomechanics. 6th ed. New York: McGraw-Hill; 2012.
17. LaRoche M. Intraosseous circulation from physiology to disease. Joint Bone Spine. 2002;69:262–9.
18. Tocantins LM, O'Neill JF. Complications of intra-osseous therapy. Ann Surg. 1945;122(2):266–77.
19. Bustamante S, Cheruku S. Ultrasound to improve target site identification for proximal humerus intraosseous vascular access. Anesth Analg. 2016;123(5):1335–7.
20. Byars DV, Tsuchitani SN, Yates J, et al. A multijurisdictional experience with the EZ-IO intraosseous device in the prehospital setting. Am J Emerg Med. 2013;31(12):1712–3.
21. Dev SP, Stefan RA, Saun T, et al. Insertion of an intraosseous needle in adults. N Engl J Med. 2014;370(24):e35(2).
22. Paxton JH, Knuth TE, Klausner HA. Proximal humerus intraosseous infusion: a preferred emergency venous access. J Trauma. 2009;67(3):606–11.
23. Chreiman KM, Dumas RP, Seamon MJ, et al. The intraosseous have it: a prospective observational study of vascular access success rates in patients in extremis using video review. J Trauma Acute Care Surg. 2018;84(4):558–63.
24. Philbeck T, Miller L, Montez D. 407: pain management during intraosseous infusion through the proximal humerus. Ann Emerg Med. 2009;54(3):S128.
25. De Lorenzo RA, Ward JA, Jordan BS, et al. Relationships of intraosseous and systemic pressure waveforms in a swine model. Acad Emerg Med. 2014;21(8):899–904.
26. Hoskins SL, do Nascimento P, Lima RM, et al. Pharmacokinetics of intraosseous and central venous drug delivery during cardiopulmonary resuscitation. Resuscitation. 2012;83(1):107–12.
27. Bakir F. Fatal sternal puncture. Dis Chest. 1963;44(4):435–9.
28. Iwama H, Katsumi A, Shinohara K, et al. Clavicular approach to intraosseous infusion in adults. Fukushima J Med Sci. 1994;40(1):1–8.

29. Iwama H, Katsumi A. Emergency fields, obtaining intravascular access for cardiopulmonary arrest patients is occasionally difficult and time-consuming. J Trauma. 1996;41(5):931–2.
30. Lairet J, Bebarta V, Lariet K, et al. A comparison of proximal tibia, distal femur, and proximal Humerus infusion rates using the EZ-IO intraosseous device on the adult swine model. J Prehosp Emerg Care. 2013;17(2):280–4.
31. McCarthy G, O'Donnell C, O'Brien M. Successful intraosseous infusion in the critically ill patient does not require a medullary cavity. Resuscitation. 2003;56(2):183–6.
32. Bradburn S, Gill S. World Federation of Societies of Anaesthesia [Internet]. [Place unknown]: Creative Commons Attribution-Non-Commercial-No Derivatives 4.0 International;2015. Cited 2020 May 22. Available from: https://www.wfsahq.org/components/com_virtual_library/media/16e6c27236edb7c17558cc17a04e6a5f-317-Understanding-and-Establishing-Intraosseous-Access.pdf.
33. DeBoer S, Russell T, Seaver M, et al. Infant intraosseous infusion. Neonatal Netw. 2008;27(1):25–32.
34. Tocantins LM. Rapid absorption of substances injected into the bone marrow. Exp Biol Med. 1940;45(1):292–6.
35. Feinstein BA, Stubbs BA, Rea T, et al. Intraosseous compared to intravenous drug resuscitation in out-of-hospital cardiac arrest. Resuscitation. 2017;117:91–6.
36. Kuhn GJ, White BC, Swetnam RE, et al. Peripheral vs central circulation times during CPR: a pilot study. Ann Emerg Med. 1981;10(8):417–9.
37. Pasley J, Miller C, DuBose JJ, et al. Intraosseous infusion rates under high pressure: a cadaveric comparison of anatomic sites. J Trauma Acute Care Surg. 2015;78(2):295–9.
38. Ngo A, Oh J, Chen Y, Yong D, et al. Intraosseous vascular access in adults using the EZ-IO in an emergency department. Int J Emerg Med. 2009;2(3):155–60.
39. McCarthy G, Buss P. The calcaneum as a site for intraosseous infusion. J Accid Emerg Med. 1998;15:421–9.
40. Lewis P, Wright C. Saving the critically injured trauma patient: a retrospective analysis of 1,000 uses of intraosseous access. Emerg Med J. 2014;32:463–7.
41. Santos D, Carron PN, Yersin B, et al. EZ-IO® intraosseous device implementation in a pre-hospital emergency service: a prospective study and review of the literature. Resuscitation. 2013;84(4):440–5.
42. Hallas P, Brabrand M, Folkestad L. Complication with intraosseous access: Scandinavian users' experience. West J Emerg Med. 2013;14(5):440–3.
43. Glaeser PW, Hellmich TR, Szewczuga D, et al. Five-year experience in prehospital intraosseous infusions in children and adults. Ann Emerg Med. 1993;22(7):1119–24.
44. LaSpada J, Kissoon N, Melker R, et al. Extravasation rates and complications of intraosseous needles during gravity and pressure infusion. Crit Care Med. 1995;23(12):2023–8.
45. La Fleche FR, Slepin MJ, Vargas J, et al. Iatrogenic bilateral tibial fractures after intraosseous infusion attempts in a 3-month-old infant. Ann Emerg Med. 1989;18(10):1099–101.
46. Strausbaugh SD, Manley LK, Hickey RW, et al. Circumferential pressure as a rapid method to assess intraosseous needle placement. Pediatr Emerg Care. 1995;11(5):274–6.
47. Adams T, Blouin D, Johnson D. Effects of tibial and humerus intraosseous and intravenous vasopressin in porcine cardiac arrest model. Am J Disaster Med. 2016;11(3):211–8.
48. Andropoulos DB, Solfer SJ, Schreiber MD. Plasma epinephrine concentrations after intraosseous and central venous injection during cardiopulmonary resuscitation in the lamb. J Pediatr. 1990;116(2):312–5.
49. Blouin D, Gegel BT, Johnson D, Garcia-Blanco JC. Effects of intravenous, sternal, and humerus intraosseous administration of Hextend on time of administration and hemodynamics in a hypovolemic swine model. Am J Disaster Med. 2016;11(3):183–92.
50. Cornell M, Kelbaugh J, Todd B, Christianson K, et al. Pharmacokinetics of sternal intraosseous atropine administration in normovolemic and hypovolemic swine. Am J Disaster Med. 2016;11(4):233–6.

51. Smith S, Borgkvist B, Kist T, Annelin J, et al. The effects of sternal intraosseous and intravenous administration of amiodarone in a hypovolemic swine cardiac arrest model. Am J Disaster Med. 2016;11(4):271–7.
52. Vallier DJ, Torrence AD, Stevens R 3rd, et al. The effects of sternal and intravenous vasopressin administration on pharmacokinetics. Am J Disaster Med. 2016;11(3):203–9.
53. Wenzel V, Lindner K, Augenstein S, et al. Intraosseous vasopressin improves coronary perfusion pressure rapidly during cardiopulmonary resuscitation in pigs. Crit Care Med. 1999;27(8):1565–9.
54. Buck M, Wiggins B, Sesler JM. Intraosseous drug administration in children and adults during cardiopulmonary resuscitation. Ann Pharmacother. 2007;41(10):1679–86.
55. Tocantins LM, O'Neill JF, Jones HW. Infusions of blood and other fluids via the bone marrow. J Am Med Assoc. 1941;117(15):1229.
56. Dubick M, Holcomb J. A review of intraosseous vascular access: current status and military application. Mil Med. 2000;165(7):552–9.
57. Ong MEH, Chan YH, Oh JJ, et al. An observational, prospective study comparing tibial and humeral intraosseous access using the EZ-IO. Am J Emerg Med. 2009;27(1):8–15.
58. Lange J, Boysen SR, Bentley A, et al. Intraosseous catheter flow rates and ease of placement at various sites in canine cadavers. Front Vet Sci. 2019;6:312.
59. Warren D, Kissoon N, Sommerauer J, et al. Comparison of fluid infusion rates among peripheral intravenous and humerus, femur, malleolus, and tibial intraosseous sites in normovolemic and hypovolemic piglets. Ann Emerg Med. 1993;22(2):183–6.
60. Tan BKK, Chong S, Koh ZX, Ong MEH. EZ-IO in the ED: an observational, prospective study comparing flow rates with proximal and distal tibia intraosseous access in adults. Am J Emerg Med. 2012;30(8):1602–6.
61. Jun H, Haruyama AZ, Chang KSG, Yamamoto LG. Comparison of a new screw-tipped intraosseous needle versus a standard bone marrow aspiration needle for infusion. Am J Emerg Med. 2000;18(2):135–9.
62. Brenner T, Bernhard M, Helm M, et al. Comparison of two intraosseous infusion systems for adult emergency medical use. Resuscitation. 2008;78(3):314–9.
63. Shavit I, Hoffmann Y, Galbraith R, et al. Comparison of two mechanical intraosseous infusion devices: a pilot, randomized crossover trial. Resuscitation. 2009;80(9):1029–33.
64. Leidel BA, Kirchhoff C, Braunstein V, et al. Comparison of two intraosseous access devices in adult patients under resuscitation in the emergency department: a prospective, randomized study. Resuscitation. 2010;81(8):994–9.
65. Kurowski A, Timler D, Evrin T, et al. Comparison of 3 different intraosseous access devices for adult during resuscitation. Randomized crossover manikin study. Am J Emerg Med. 2014;32(12):1490–3.
66. Sunde GA, Heradstveit BE, Vikenes BH, et al. Emergency intraosseous access in a helicopter emergency medical service: a retrospective study. Scand J Trauma Resusc Emerg Med. 2010;18(1):52.
67. Byars DV, Tsuchitani SN, Erwin E, et al. Evaluation of success rate and access time for an adult sternal intraosseous device deployed in the prehospital setting. Prehosp Disaster Med. 2011;26(2):127–9.
68. Szarpak L, Truszewski Z, Smereka J, et al. A randomized cadaver study comparing first-attempt success between tibial and humeral intraosseous insertions using NIO device by paramedics. Medicine. 2016;95(20):e3724.
69. Bielski K, Szarpak L, Smereka J, et al. Comparison of four different intraosseous access devices during simulated pediatric resuscitation: a randomized crossover manikin trial. Eur J Pediatr. 2017;176(7):865–71.
70. Banerjee S, Singhi SC, Singh S, et al. The intraosseous route is a suitable alternative to intravenous route for fluid resuscitation in severely dehydrated children. Indian Pediatr. 1994;31(12):1511–20.

71. Halm B, Yamamoto LG. Comparing ease of intraosseous needle placement: Jamshidi versus Cook. Am J Emerg Med. 1998;16(4):420–1.
72. Jamshidi K, Swaim WR. Bone marrow biopsy with unaltered architecture: a new biopsy device. J Lab Clin Med. 1971;77:335–42.
73. Shaltot A, Michell PA, Betts JA, et al. Jamshidi needle biopsy of bone lesions. Clin Radiol. 1982;33(2):193–6.
74. Parapia LA. Trepanning or trephines: a history of bone marrow biopsy. Brit J Haematol. 2007;139:14–9.
75. Teleflex, Inc. [Internet]. Vascular Access: EZ-IO® T.A.L.O.N.™ Needle Set. Cited 2020 June 9. Available from: https://teleflex.com/usa/en/product-areas/military-federal/intraosseous-access/ez-io-talon-needle-set/index.html.
76. SAM Medical [Internet]. SAM IO: Intraosseous Access System. Cited 20 July 2020. Available from: https://www.sammedical.com/products/sam-io.
77. Blumberg SM, Gorn M, Crain EF. Intraosseous infusion: a review of methods and novel devices. Pediat Emerg Care. 2008;24(1):50–6.
78. PYNG Medical (Internet). FASTTactical Sternal IO. Cited 20 July 2020. Available from: http://www.pyng.com/fasttactical/.
79. Anson JA. Vascular access in resuscitation. Anesthesiology. 2014;120(4):1015–31.
80. Tsung JW, Blaivas M, Stone MB. Feasibility of point-of-care color Doppler ultrasound confirmation of intraosseous needle placement during resuscitation. Resuscitation. 2009;80(6):665–8.
81. Abramson TM, Alreshaid L, Kang T, Mailhot T, Omer T. FascIOtomy: ultrasound evaluation of an intraosseous needle causing compartment syndrome. Clin Pract Cases Emerg Med. 2018;2(4):323–5.
82. Lee BK, Jeung KW, Lee HY, Lee SJ, Bae SJ, Lim YD, Moon KS, Heo T, Min YI. Confirmation of intraosseous cannula placement based on pressure measured at the cannula during squeezing the extremity in a piglet model. Resuscitation. 2014;85:143–7.
83. [Internet] Academic Life in Emergency Medicine (ALIEM) website. Avila J, Smith B, Hennings J. "Trick of the trade: Squeeze test for confirmation of IO placement." Cited 2021 April 17. Available from: https://www.aliem.com/trick-of-the-trade-squeeze-test-for-confirmation-of-io-placement/.
84. Garcia CT, Cohen DM. Intraosseous needle: use of the miniature C-arm imaging device to confirm placement. Pediatr Emerg Care. 1996;12:94–7.
85. Fuchs Z, Scaal M, Haverkamp H, Koerber F, Persigehl T, Eifinger F. Anatomical investigations on intraosseous access in stillborns – comparison on different devices and techniques. Resuscitation. 2018;127:79–82.
86. Rodriguez JI, Palacios J, Rodriguez S. Transverse bone growth and cortical bone mass in the human prenatal period. Biol Neonate. 1992;62:23–31.
87. Baadh AS, Singh A, Choi A, Baadh PK, Katz DS, Harcke HT. Intraosseous vascular access in radiology: review of clinical status. Am J Radiol. 2016;207:241–7.
88. Slocum AH, Reinitz SD, Jariwala SH, van Citters DW. Design, development, and validation of an intra-osseous needle placement guide. J Med Devices. 2017;11:1–8. https://doi.org/10.1115/1.4037442.

Special Populations: Pediatrics

Jennifer R. Noble, Jordan Schneider, and James H. Paxton

Introduction

Obtaining emergent vascular access for pediatric patients poses additional challenges beyond those routinely encountered with adult patients, including anatomical differences, difficulties restraining patient movement during cannulation procedures, and parental anxiety [1]. Anatomical considerations for pediatric subjects include greater head-to-body size ratio, excess superficial soft tissue, increased tissue softness, and smaller, more compressible vasculature. These differences impact both landmark identification and cannulation success rates for pediatric patients [1, 2]. Practical concerns relating to these anatomical differences will lead providers to consider the benefits and risks of vascular access differently for pediatric subjects. This chapter summarizes the key considerations when attempting emergent vascular access for pediatric patients, with a special focus on how pediatric venous access techniques differ from those used with adult subjects.

The type and gauge of vascular access device (VAD) recommended for pediatric subjects differs according to the age of the patient. It is important to remember that pediatric patients have smaller blood vessels than adults, which influences the gauge of catheter recommended. A balance should be sought between providing adequate

J. R. Noble (✉)
Department of Pediatrics, Division of Pediatric Emergency Medicine, Children's Hospital of Michigan, Detroit, MI, USA
e-mail: JNoble@med.wayne.edu

J. Schneider
Department of Pediatrics, Division of Critical Care Medicine, Children's Hospital of Michigan, Detroit, MI, USA
e-mail: JSCHNEID@dmc.org

J. H. Paxton
Department of Emergency Medicine, Wayne State University School of Medicine, Detroit, MI, USA
e-mail: james.paxton@wayne.edu

© Springer Nature Switzerland AG 2021
J. H. Paxton (ed.), *Emergent Vascular Access*,
https://doi.org/10.1007/978-3-030-77177-5_8

capacity for flow and avoiding complications related to an excessively large cannula. In general, a cross-sectional *catheter-to-vein ratio (CVR)* of <50% is recommended for pediatric patients and <33% for neonates [3–5]. Larger CVRs may predispose to venous thrombosis and phlebitis [3, 4], while exceedingly small-caliber catheters are predisposed to catheter occlusion [5].

Certain definitions for the various classifications of pediatric subjects must be familiar to the emergent access provider. *Neonates* are generally defined as pediatric subjects within the first 28 days of extrauterine life, while *infants* are those subjects less than 1 year of age [6]. Children born prematurely (<37 weeks' gestation) or with low birth weight (<2500 grams) generally have decreased whole-body energy stores, despite greater metabolic needs when compared to full-term, average-weight newborns. Additionally, extracellular water makes up a larger proportion of body weight in infants (70–80%) compared to adults (60%) [7]. Circulating blood volume is approximately 89–105 mL/kg in premature newborns, drops to 82–86 mL/kg in term births, and declines to 70 mL/kg in adults [8]. Although infants have more circulating blood volume per unit of body weight than adults, their absolute blood volume remains quite small. These factors combine to make neonates and infants more vulnerable to hypovolemia than older children and adults [9]. Although the absolute volumes of fluid required to restore euvolemia may be less in pediatric subjects, they remain more sensitive to fluid loss than adults, underscoring the need for rapid vascular access to meet their infusion needs.

Pediatric Vascular Access Devices

Many options are available to providers when attempting emergent vascular access for pediatric subjects, including intraosseous (IO), peripheral intravenous (PIV), midline (MLC), peripherally inserted central catheter (PICC), and central venous catheter (CVC) devices. These approaches to vascular access are discussed in greater depth in the corresponding chapters of this text. Table 8.1 compares the types of vascular access device (VAD) most commonly utilized for pediatric subjects, including the relative advantages and disadvantages of each technique.

Intraosseous (IO) Catheter

The intraosseous route is ideal for critically-ill children, as the medullary space of long bones provides a non-collapsible vascular access route, even in the presence of severe hypovolemia and hypotension. This starkly contrasts with the peripheral venous system, which typically collapses in shock states, complicating peripheral (or even central) venous cannulation. As mentioned in Chap. 7, a wide range of IO access systems exist, including manual and mechanically powered devices.

Most designated IO catheters are 20-gauge in diameter, but the length of IO catheter required for individual patients will vary according to the patient's body weight and the anatomic site selected for cannulation. In general, a 15-mm IO needle is

Table 8.1 Comparison of different vascular access devices used for pediatric resuscitation

Type of access	Common sites	Advantages	Disadvantages
Intraosseous (IO) catheter	Femur, proximal tibia, distal tibia	Easily and rapidly placed, accesses a non-collapsible space	Short-term use, can only infuse PIV-compatible solutions, risk of extravasation and related complications
Peripheral intravenous (PIV) catheter	Dorsal plexus of hand or foot, saphenous vein, antecubital veins, external jugular vein, scalp veins	Simple, cost-efficient, minimal complications, may be placed rapidly	Short-term use, infiltration risk, can be difficult to place in some patients, blood draws can be difficult
Midline catheter (MLC)	Deep peripheral veins of the upper extremity	Longer dwell times than IO/PIV, more easily inserted than CVC, no radiographic confirmation required	Blood draws can be difficult, can only infuse PIV-compatible solutions
Peripherally inserted central catheter (PICC)	Cephalic vein, brachial vein, basilic vein	Blood sampling possible, patient can be sent home with PICC, central-only solutions can be given, can monitor CVP and mixed venous oxygen saturation	Need specialized training to place, radiographic confirmation needed, patient care education required if going home with PICC
Central venous catheter (CVC)	Internal jugular vein, femoral vein, subclavian vein	Multiple lumens, easy blood sampling, can monitor CVP and mixed venous oxygen saturation, central-only solutions can be given, can be placed faster than PICC	Need specialized training to place, cannot be sent home, limited dwell times due to infection risk, highest risk of life-threatening complications

utilized at all body sites for patients weighing 3 to 39 kg, regardless of age. Manufacturers do not generally endorse the use of IO for patients with body weight <3 kg, although the use of IO catheters in neonatal subjects has been well-described in the medical literature [10]. The long bones of pediatric patients are softer and less calcified than those of adults, which may allow alternate IO infusion devices (e.g., butterfly needle, short spinal tap needle) to penetrate the bony cortex and cannulate the IO space for purposes of IO infusion [10, 11]. Pediatric patients with excessive soft tissue thickness at the selected insertion site may require the use of a 25-mm-long IO catheter, although care should be taken to avoid excessive insertion depths to reduce the risk of extravasation. The use of excessive force with IO insertion must be avoided in pediatric subjects, as pediatric long bones are poorly calcified and prone to fracture when excessive force is applied. In addition, the smaller size of the intramedullary space inherently reduces the volume-accepting capacity of the IO space, and the veins that drain this space are of smaller caliber and therefore less able to accommodate large volumes of infusion.

These differences would seem to increase the risk that excessive infusion pressure and volume could lead to extravasation of fluid into the soft tissues surrounding the IO insertion site. Given the smaller size of extremity soft tissue compartments relative to the volume infused, it follows that excessive volume infusion through an

Table 8.2 Comparison of anatomic sites for intraosseous catheter insertion in children and adults

Location	Adult (≥40 kg)	Child (3–39 kg)
Proximal humerus	Yes	Not recommended
Sternum	Yes	Not recommended
Iliac crest	Yes	Not recommended
Distal femur	Yes	Yes
Proximal tibia	Yes	Yes
Distal tibia	Yes	Yes

IO catheter may be more likely to lead to increased compartmental pressures and produce compartment syndrome. The risk of simultaneous iatrogenic *cis* and *trans* penetration of the target bone (i.e., penetration through both sides of the bone) would also seem to be increased with pediatric IO placement due to small medullary size, further increasing the risk of extravasation with IO infusion. While monitoring IO insertion sites for signs of extravasation is important for any patient of any age, the risk of compartment syndrome due to IO extravasation in the pediatric population may be greater than that for adult subjects. Thus, a heightened awareness of this risk is paramount when placing IO catheters in children.

The anatomic locations recommended for IO catheter placement in children are more restrictive than those endorsed for adults. Recommended sites for IO placement in infants and children with body weight <40 kg include the proximal tibia, distal tibia, and distal femur [11]. Chapter 7 of this book describes IO placement, including the wide range of devices available to the emergency care provider. A comparison of recommended IO catheter insertion sites for adult and pediatric subjects is provided in Table 8.2.

Landmark-Based Peripheral Intravenous (PIV) Catheter

Peripheral intravenous (PIV) access has traditionally been considered the preferred approach for rapid delivery of isotonic solutions in pediatric patients with undifferentiated hypotension and shock. Large-bore PIV catheters are preferred to central venous catheter (CVC) placement, due to more rapid placement times, shorter cannula lengths, and lower rates of complications [12, 13]. The shorter length characteristic of PIV catheters allows for less resistance to forward flow, facilitating higher fluid infusion rates [14]. Peripheral veins in the scalp, hands, feet, and antecubital region may be the only accessible PIV insertion sites in infants, due to increased body fat relative to older children and adults. The gauge of catheter selected depends upon the age of the patient and the site selected. Among neonates, 24- or 26-gauge catheters are most often used, although any catheter in the 20- to 28-gauge range may be considered [5, 9]. The 22- to 24-gauge over-the-needle-type PIV catheters are most commonly used in children [9].

Placement of PIV devices in pediatric subjects differs from that in adults, although some similarities are found. As with adults, the nondominant hand is preferred for cannulation, although younger children may not have a dominant hand.

Areas of flexion (e.g., wrist) should be avoided [4]. Distal veins in the upper extremities should be considered before more proximal or lower extremity venous targets. In contrast to adult patients, lower extremity veins are often considered in pediatric subjects. Due to decreased compliance with vascular access attempts, it is generally recommended to consider the use of arm boards when the hand veins are targeted in pediatric subjects, to minimize movement of the extremity after venous access has been established.

The *dorsal arch veins* of the hand are often the first area targeted in pediatric patients, although care must be taken to avoid the dorsal digital arteries. Collateral circulation exists between the deep and superficial arterial arches of the hand at most digits, which appears to minimize the risk of ischemia when the dorsal digital arteries are injured during vascular access attempts. However, the thumb may be at a higher risk of VAD-related ischemia, as both the dorsal and palmar arteries may arise from the *princeps pollicis artery* of the thumb (a branch of the radial artery), which is dorsal and superficial to the first web space muscles in 10–15% of infants [15]. The *cephalic vein* at the anatomic snuffbox of the wrist is a common target for pediatric patients. This vein is often quite large and generally available. Veins at the volar (palmar) aspect of the wrist are small in pediatric patients and not as durable as dorsal hand or antecubital veins. Since central venous access is often attempted in pediatric subjects at the antecubital fossa, this site is not recommended for first consideration in pediatric PIV access attempts.

When treating a conscious pediatric inpatient, vascular access attempts should be conducted outside of the child's room whenever possible, leaving the child's room their "safe space." Regardless of where the attempt is made, providers should ensure that additional staff are on hand to help in distracting the patient or otherwise facilitating the attempt. Providers should use developmentally supportive measures to minimize stress, such as a pacifier, talking softly, swaddling with the parent [16], or avoiding sudden moves [7]. When parents are available to assist the provider, it is recommended to have the child face the parent [16].

Infants should be covered with a blanket to minimize cold stress during the attempt. Providers should consider placing the extremity on an arm board before venipuncture attempts on the dorsal hand. Transillumination devices (as mentioned in Chap. 10) placed beneath the extremity can help to improve vein visualization. The oral administration of 2 mL of a 25% sucrose solution by syringe or on a pacifier immediately prior to the procedure may help to decrease pain perception [16]. Providers should also consider use of a topical anesthetic cream at the planned insertion site, although this application should occur up to 1 hour before venipuncture to maximize the effect. Providers should use only hypoallergenic or paper tape to secure the catheter and should apply warm water to the catheter during the removal attempt to facilitate easy removal.

The major superficial *scalp veins* can be used for vascular access in children up to age 18 months of age, after which time this route becomes more challenging due to the maturation of the hair follicles and toughening of the epidermis [9]. The four scalp veins most commonly used for PIV access are the *temporal, frontal, posterior auricular*, and *occipital veins*. Unlike most peripheral veins, scalp veins do not contain valves [7]. The patient's head is maintained in a dependent position during the attempt to promote venous distension. The four most common scalp veins used for venous access are illustrated in Fig. 8.1. Image also shows a rubber band across the forehead to engorge the veins, as well as a common technique for securing the butterfly needle to the scalp with adhesive tape.

The use of scalp veins for venous access may be foreign to those providers who are accustomed to treating adult patients, as this is not a recommended access site for adults. However, scalp veins are frequently accessible in infant subjects due to their larger relative head size in comparison with body size. In general, this access site is considered when other access sites for peripheral IV cannulation have been exhausted or determined to be inaccessible. When considering the scalp veins for cannulation, the provider should locate the commonly accessed scalp veins (as above), with preference for a vein behind the hairline to avoid visible scarring due to PIV placement. It may be necessary to shave the area of interest to increase visualization of the target vein and facilitate dressing adherence to the scalp. Elastic band placement around the head above the level of the ears and eyes may help to engorge the target veins prior to cannulation. A butterfly needle (23-, 25-, or 27-gauge) or 22- or 24-gauge over-the-needle PIV catheter is typically used for this procedure.

When placing a scalp PIV, the patient should be restrained in the supine position, with an assistant available to stabilize the patient's head during the

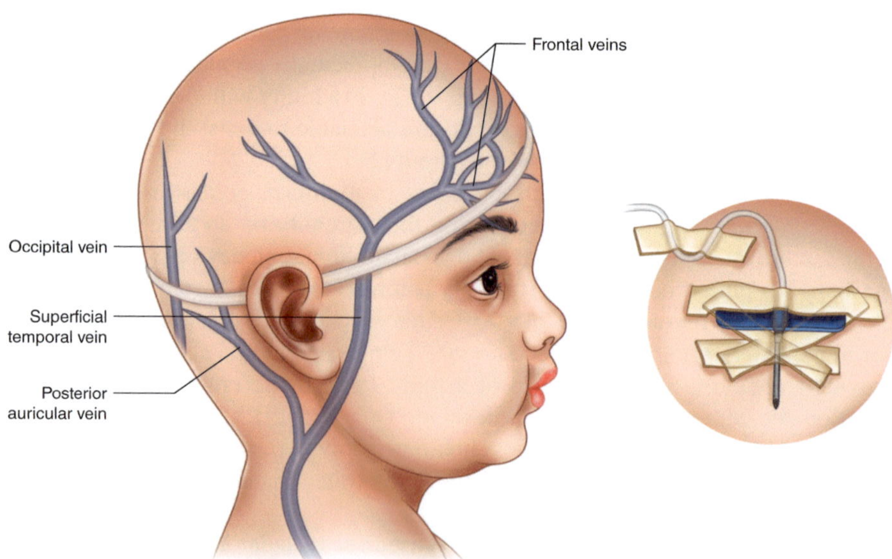

Fig. 8.1 Scalp veins commonly available for peripheral intravenous cannulation in infants

procedure to prevent patient movement during placement. The optimal vein selected will have a straight segment long enough to accommodate the length of PIV catheter intended to dwell within the vein. It is important to assess target vessels for the presence of pulsation, which would suggest that the vessel is arterial and not appropriate for cannulation. An elastic band (e.g., rubber band) may be placed around the head above the level of the eyes and ears to enhance engorgement of the vessel. This will increase the diameter of the vessel and enhance visualization. It may be helpful to place a piece of tape around the rubber band to provide a tab to grasp and lift when removal of the elastic band is desired after cannulation.

Topical antiseptic solution should be applied to the insertion site and allowed to dry prior to cannulation. The needle should penetrate the scalp 5 mm from the desired venous cannulation site, with an angle of insertion of about 30 degrees. The needle should be inserted in the direction of blood flow. Once the needle has penetrated the target vein, the elastic band should be released and the catheter flushed with 0.5 mL of saline to confirm intravascular placement. If the fluid extravasates with formation of a wheal at the site, this is evidence of extravasation and suboptimal cannulation, and the insertion should be attempted at a different site. Once the catheter has been appropriately placed, the device should be anchored to the scalp with tape and measures taken to avoid accidental dislodgement. Complications include accidental arterial cannulation, ecchymosis and hematoma at the insertion site, and infection.

Additional peripheral venous cannulation sites should also be considered. The *external jugular (EJ)* vein is generally visible in pediatric subjects and lies superficial to the skin surface, over the sternocleidomastoid muscle [1]. Although this vein drains into the central circulation, the EJ vein turns sharply under the clavicle, preventing central venous cannulation from this site [1]. This vein's superficial depth usually allows for direct compression in the event of iatrogenic hematoma [2]. However, pediatric patients with excessive neck fat or short neck may not have a visible EJ vein. The use of this insertion site is *not recommended in pediatric subjects if the vein is not superficially visible* [1].

Cannulation of the pedal (foot) veins is often attempted in pediatric subjects, although pedal vein cannulation is not recommended in adult patients. Peripheral venous cannulation of the foot is targeted at the *dorsal venous arch* and *venous plexus*, including the long saphenous vein, short saphenous vein, and lateral/medial marginal veins. These pedal veins, along with the other common pediatric peripheral venous targets of the hands and feet, are illustrated in Fig. 8.2.

In an undifferentiated pediatric population, PIV catheter insertion appears to be most often successful when performed at the cephalic vein in the proximal forearm using US guidance, or at the antecubital fossa [17, 18]. Peripheral IV cannulae placed in the forearm also appear to be more durable than those placed in the scalp, hand, or leg [19]. Catheters inserted at the bend of the arm or the lower extremity appear to be more likely to infiltrate or fail to infuse [20].

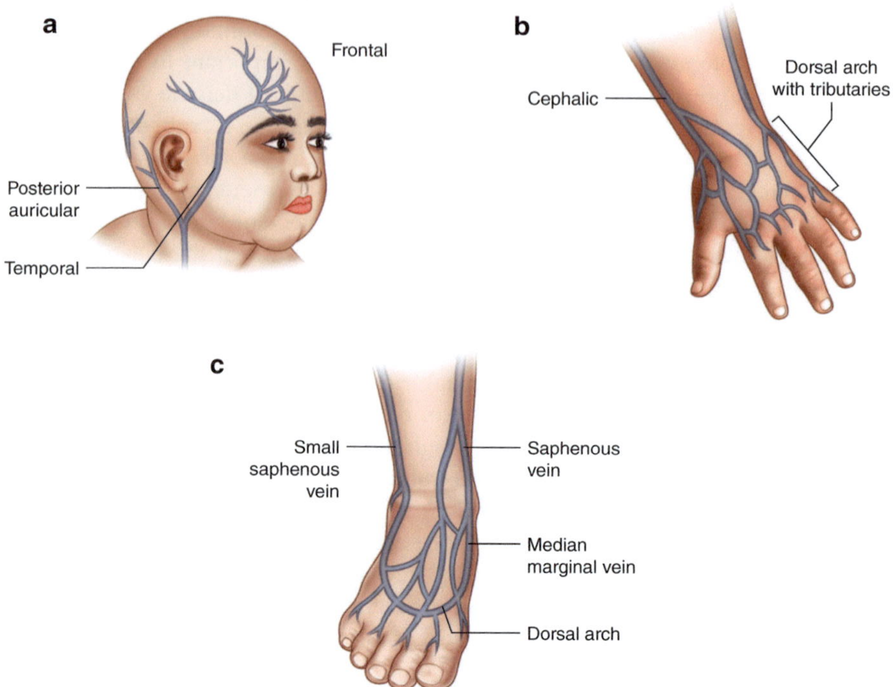

Fig. 8.2 Common sites for landmark-based PIV cannulation in infants and children

Ultrasound-Guided Peripheral Intravenous (US-PIV) Catheter

The success rate for ultrasound-guided PIV (US-PIV) placement is highly variable in children, and the use of US guidance *does not improve first-attempt success rates* for PIV catheterization in a general pediatric population [21]. However, US-PIV placement may be of special value in pediatric patients with difficult venous access, including those who have already failed multiple previous landmark-based PIV attempts [22], obese subjects, and chronically ill patients with a history of frequent hospitalizations requiring IV insertion [23]. Among pediatric patients (including infants) with difficult vascular access, the use of US guidance is associated with faster peripheral venous cannulation, with fewer attempts and needle redirections [24–27]. These benefits have been demonstrated with both emergency nurse and emergency physician providers [25]. Considering the additional challenges inherent to the pediatric population, US visualization of anatomy may be of use by allowing providers to better evaluate and identify the most appropriate venous access points, to more safely insert peripheral and central venous catheters, and to immediately identify complications [13, 28–31]. The complication rate for PIV access has been shown to positively correlate with the number of vascular access attempts made;

thus, the use of ultrasound to decrease the number of required attempts may reasonably be expected to reduce complication rates for pediatric patients [28].

The *brachial vein*, *cephalic vein*, and *basilic vein* of the upper arm are the vessels most commonly targeted with US-PIV placement in pediatric subjects [2]. Ultrasound guidance is most useful for pediatric patients with small-caliber veins or excessive peripheral fat, especially at the antecubital veins [2, 32]. The use of ultrasound-guided peripheral venous catheters may be especially valuable to pediatric subjects requiring infusions lasting longer than 5 days [33, 34].

The IV catheters used for US-PIV placement are generally longer than standard PIV catheters; as with adults, short PIV catheters may not be long enough to cannulate deeper arm veins [2]. However, the use of longer PIV catheters, especially those with small internal diameters, is associated with greater resistance to flow [14]. Pressure-assisted flow and/or micropuncture catheters may be required if rapid fluid administration is needed, to compensate for this additional vascular resistance [14].

The degree of venous and arterial compression may be different during US-PIV insertion in pediatric patients when compared to adult subjects, as the vasculature of pediatric subjects is more easily collapsed with soft tissue compression [2]. Generous use of ultrasound gel appears to help mitigate excessive probe pressures [35].

Central Venous Catheter (CVC)

The approach to CVC placement for pediatric patients mirrors that of adult patients, which is already described in Chaps. 5 and 6 of this text. It should be noted that PIV or intraosseous (IO) access is generally preferred to central venous access during initial pediatric resuscitative efforts, although the decision to place a CVC should be guided by the patient's specific medical condition and therapeutic needs. The common indications for the use of CVC are listed as follows [36]:

- Short-term administration of intravenous medications requiring continuous administration or frequent blood collection
- Prolonged administration of intravenous medications
- Administration of parenteral nutrition or hyperosmolar solutions
- Administration of total plasma exchanges, red blood cell exchanges, erythrocytapheresis, and clotting factors
- Administration of cyclical chemotherapy

Ultrasound guidance is recommended for central venous catheter (CVC) placement in all pediatric patients [2]. Existing evidence suggests that ultrasound-guided central venous catheter (US-CVC) placement in pediatric populations has a success rate of up to 98% [29]. The complication rate for pediatric US-CVC placement in a general pediatric population is quite low, reported to be around 5% [29]. However, complications rates have been shown to be higher in infants than in older children, especially among infants less than 2.5 kg in body weight, at around 28% [30].

Locations for CVC placement in the pediatric population include the *femoral (FEM) vein, internal jugular (IJ) vein, subclavian (SC) vein,* and *peripherally inserted central catheters (PICC)* in the *basilic vein* or *brachial vein* of the upper extremity. While the preferred insertion sites for CVC lines are the IJ and SC veins in adults, these veins may be prohibitively difficult to cannulate in pediatric subjects. Consequently, the FEM vein is often considered first-line for CVC cannulation in pediatric subjects [2, 37]. This vein is easily accessed under emergent conditions and is less prone to difficulties in line placement with pediatric subjects.

Many factors should be taken into consideration during selection of a CVC insertion site, including the patient's preexisting medical conditions, venous anatomy, the indication and urgency of the need for venous access, provider experience, and available devices [2]. Patient age, weight, and height are important determinants of catheter length and caliber among pediatric patients [38–43]. Table 8.3 provides a comparison of the mean IJ, SC, and FEM central vein diameters associated with different age categories.

Previous studies have shown that the internal diameter of the IJ vein in neonates and infants may be smaller than the diameter of the standard "big-radius" curved J-tip Seldinger guidewire, leading to difficulties in cannulating the IJ and SC veins with a standard guidewire [46]. Furthermore, the use of Trendelenburg positioning does not appear to increase IJ diameter in children less than 6 years old [46]. The diameter of CVC device recommended depends greatly upon the age of the patient. For example, 3-Fr catheters are recommended for FEM CVC placement in patients <1 year old, with 4- or 5-Fr catheters used in young children [42].

Although the extrapolation of evidence from studies of adult populations to pediatric subjects is controversial, pediatric-specific studies have confirmed that the carina remains an appropriate anatomical and radiological landmark for determining whether the tip of an IJ or SC catheter is placed properly in infants and small children [48].

In general, complications of CVC placement in children mirror those encountered in the adult population. Early complications include pneumothorax, hemothorax, cardiac tamponade, arterial puncture, hematoma formation, air embolism, and cardiac arrhythmia [1]. Late complications include erosion of the vessel wall, vein thrombosis (including potential occlusion of the lumen), catheter rupture, dislodgement or migration of the catheter, and catheter-associated infections of the soft tissues or bloodstream [1]. These risks may be further increased in infants and other

Table 8.3 Mean central vein diameter (mm), according to age [38–47]

Central vein	Neonates	Infant	Child (<6 yo)	Adolescent	Adult
Internal jugular (IJ) vein	5.5	8.9	10.5	11.9	11.3
Subclavian (SC) vein	5.6	5.5	6.9	8.5	11
Femoral (FEM) vein	3.8	4.5	7.3	7.8	8.9

pediatric patients with extremity or vascular abnormalities [1]. The risk of catheter-associated infection appears to be increased with increased proximity of the insertion site, as well as the use of a polyurethane catheter in infants [49]. Younger pediatric subjects appear to have a higher risk of iatrogenic vertebral artery puncture with IJ attempts due to the relative proximity of this artery to the IJ vein [50].

The *femoral (FEM) vein* is often the first choice of insertion site for emergent CVC access in pediatric subjects, as it is associated with easily recognizable landmarks [49] and can be cannulated quickly during emergent resuscitation [1]. Contraindications to FEM CVC placement include vascular malformation of the lower extremity, congenital malformation of the lower extremity, femoral hernia, abdominal tumor, trauma, or abdominal ascites [1]. Ultrasound-guided CVC placement at the FEM site is associated with a higher first-attempt success rate and fewer needle passes in pediatric patients when compared to other CVC sites [49]. Reported disadvantages of the FEM site include a high risk of contamination, difficulty securing the catheter, and patient discomfort [1]. However, the complication rate associated with FEM CVC insertion is similar to that for other central venous sites in the pediatric population (including infants) [51, 52]. Although the FEM insertion site is generally discouraged for adult patients due to concerns of increased infection risk, the rate of bloodstream infection associated with FEM CVCs in children is approximately 3.7%, lower than that for other CVC insertion sites (7.3%) [52].

The *internal jugular (IJ) vein* is associated with the highest procedural success rate for CVC placement among pediatric patients (86% vs. 65% at other CVC sites), but this site may also be associated with a higher risk of complications in children [33]. Like the FEM insertion site, placement of an IJ CVC does not interfere with cardiopulmonary resuscitation efforts in pediatric patients [2]. Unlike subclavian insertions, the insertion site for IJ cannulation is well-exposed and allows for direct compression of the site to avoid hematoma formation or excessive bleeding following a failed attempt [2]. Despite the relative safety of IJ placement, ultrasound guidance is recommended for placement of IJ CVCs in pediatric patients [2]. Certain characteristics common to pediatric subjects, including excessive neck fat and short neck size, may complicate use of the IJ insertion site [33]. Reported complications following IJ CVC placement include carotid artery puncture, pneumothorax, thoracic duct injury (especially if performed on the left side), sympathetic nerve injury, neuropathy, venous thrombosis, and infection [53]. As with adults, the IJ vein is typically easier to cannulate on the patient's right side, since the IJ vein usually joins with the SC vein at a straighter angle on this side [54]. The pleural dome is also lower on the right, theoretically decreasing the risk of pneumothorax [1]. In addition, the thoracic duct is significantly larger on the left side; on the right, it is generally smaller and often congenitally absent [1].

The *subclavian (SC) vein* is not a common choice of site for emergent central vascular access in pediatric patients [2, 49]. The SC vein is generally smaller and arches more superiorly in infants than in adults, and the percutaneous entry site for this venous access point may be more difficult to identify [1, 49]. Additionally, while subclavian vein catheters are associated with a low risk for infectious complications in adults, this has not been definitively established in children [55].

Successful placement of a subclavian CVC for pediatric patients, especially infants, requires an advanced skill set, due to the presence of increased subcutaneous fat obscuring external landmarks and obstructed views of the target vessel due to shadowing from the clavicle [1]. Proper positioning of the patient during the access attempt is essential. Placement of a towel roll between the shoulders may help to elevate the chest and expose the relevant anatomy [55]. Malpositioning is a common problem with pediatric SC lines, including catheter migration [55]. Complications known to be associated with SC CVC placement include pneumothorax, bleeding, cardiac tamponade, dysrhythmia, thoracic duct injuries, air embolism, and neuropathy [1]. In children, the SC CVC insertion site is associated with the highest rate of fatal complications, when compared to the FEM or IJ insertion sites [53, 56, 57].

Axillary (AX) vein CVC placement can be performed using US guidance and appears to be associated with higher first-attempt placement success rate (46% vs. 40%) and shorter median time to placement (156 sec vs. 180 sec) than landmark-based SC CVC placement [58]. Ultrasound-guided supraclavicular *brachiocephalic (BC) vein* CVC placement appears to be more successful on the first attempt than IJ CVC, with reduced puncture attempts and cannulation time in critically ill children [59].

A comparison of the three most common CVC insertion sites, including their relative advantages, disadvantages, and characteristic complications, are provided in Table 8.4.

Table 8.4 Comparison of CVC insertion sites for pediatric patients

Central vein	Advantages	Disadvantages	Complications
Internal jugular (IJ)	Direct route to SVC (RIJ), larger lumen diameter, removed from the resuscitation field, directly compressible	Takes longer, requires more operator experience, more difficult in pts. <1 year with short, fat necks; more difficult in patients with tracheostomies or who are not intubated	Carotid artery puncture, pneumothorax, thoracic duct injury, infection, bleeding, thrombosis
Subclavian (SC)	Less collapsible, easier to secure, lower infection rates (in older children)	Requires operator experience, no access to control bleeding, higher risk of pneumothorax/ hemothorax during placement, not commonly placed under US guidance	Pneumothorax, hemothorax, thoracic duct injury, tamponade, catheter malposition, infection, bleeding, thrombosis
Femoral (FEM)	Requires the least operator experience, fastest, remote from the resuscitation field, available for direct compression	Risk of contamination, may be more uncomfortable for patients	Femoral artery puncture, intraperitoneal/ retroperitoneal catheter malposition, infection, bleeding, thrombosis

Peripherally Inserted Central Catheter (PICC)

A peripherally inserted central catheter (PICC) is an intermediate-term vascular access inserted in a vein of the deep arm (e.g., basilic, brachial, or cephalic), with the tip positioned at the junction of superior vena cava and right atrium. Insertion of a PICC line is typically not a viable option for emergent vascular access in children or adults. Placement of these lines requires specific resources (e.g., equipment, expertise, time, and patient compliance) that may not be available to the unstable patient. When they are placed in children, the *basilic vein* appears to be the preferred insertion site, although many other options are available [3, 4].

In older children, ultrasound-guided Seldinger technique is used [60]. In neonates, cubital or saphenous veins are cannulated utilizing a sheath-over-needle apparatus. Fluoroscopy is typically used to confirm proper placement [61]. Complications of forearm venous cannulations in pediatric patients include infection, hematoma, infiltration, and superficial and deep vein thrombosis [62–64]. Placement of PICC lines in the lower extremity is suggested in patients with congenital cardiac conditions, due to lower associated risk of complications [5]. The rate of complications associated with PICC line insertion has been shown to decrease with advancing age in children [20].

Umbilical Vein/Artery Catheterization (UVC/UAC)

Although most commonly performed in the delivery room, *umbilical vein catheterization (UVC)* and *umbilical artery catheterization (UAC)* remain a viable option for emergent vascular access in newborns within the first 7–14 days of life [65–67]. It should be reserved for cases in which alternate access is impossible or inadequate, as UVC is associated with a high rate of complications, including infection and thrombosis [65–68].

Although direct peripheral intravenous access remains the preferred vascular access route for neonates, UVC is associated with greater placement success rates than peripheral venous access techniques in the setting of emergent neonatal resuscitation [66]. The umbilical vein can be used for exchange transfusions, central venous pressure monitoring, fluid infusion, and medication administration [66]. However, both UVC and UAC are contraindicated in patients with gastroschisis, omphalitis, omphalocele, peritonitis, necrotizing enterocolitis, or compromised lower extremity blood flow.

At term birth, the umbilical cord is approximately 1.8 cm in diameter, containing two umbilical arteries and one umbilical vein [69]. The umbilical arteries are distinguished from the veins by their smaller (4 mm vs. 8 mm) internal diameter and thicker vessel walls. As illustrated in Fig. 8.3, the umbilical vein is usually situated at the 12 o'clock position on the stump, with the paired umbilical arteries on the opposite side of the cord. The three umbilical vessels are surrounded within the cord by Wharton's jelly, a mucoid connective tissue that performs the role of the *tunica adventitia*, which is not present in umbilical vessels [70]. Thus, this substance

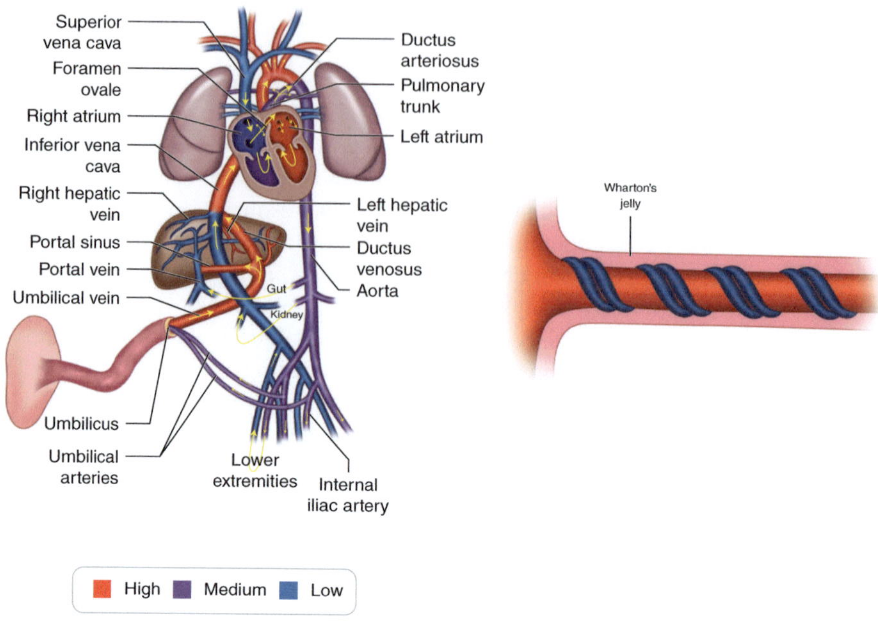

Fig. 8.3 Neonatal vascular anatomy, including oxygenation levels of blood in the umbilical cord and associated vessels

provides structural support for the vessels and aids in their contraction, to prevent kinking of the vessels in utero.

Prior to birth, the uterine placenta provides the fetus with oxygen, so the blood coming from the fetus into the placenta is moderately deoxygenated, and the blood coming from the placenta to the fetus via the umbilical veins is oxygen-rich. The umbilical vein anastomoses with the fetal venous system via the *ductus venosus*, which bypasses the hepatic vasculature to drain directly into the inferior vena cava (IVC). The ductus venosus begins to close within days of birth and is functionally closed in most newborns by age 1 week [71]. This limits the use of the umbilical vein for direct infusion into the IVC to the first 1–2 weeks after birth. The two umbilical arteries anastomose with the corresponding internal iliac arteries, which derive from the common iliac arteries arising from the terminal aorta [72]. Figure 8.3 shows the normal fetal anatomy, including major blood vessels of the fetus and neonate. As this figure shows, blood entering the fetus from the placenta is highly oxygenated, while blood leaving the fetus via the umbilical arteries has a mid-level oxygen saturation.

Cannulation of the UVC is performed as follows [73]. The umbilical stump is first scrubbed with a bactericidal solution, and a loop of umbilical tape (or purse-string suture) is placed around the cord at its junction with the skin surface. Povidone-iodine solution is recommended for UVC and UAC, as the use of chlorhexidine solution is associated with increased risk of chemical burns to the skin, especially in preterm neonates [4].

The cord is then transected with a No. 11 blade scalpel approximately 1 cm above the skin surface, and the vessels are identified. The umbilical vein may continue to bleed after cutting, although the arteries tend not to bleed. The umbilical vein can be dilated gently with non-teethed curved Iris forceps, as needed. The catheter is then inserted to a depth of 1–2 cm beyond the point at which good blood flow is detected. The standard umbilical vein catheter sizes range from 3.5 Fr (for preterm neonates, <3500 grams) to 5 Fr (for term neonates, >3500 grams) [73]. The usual depth of insertion for a term newborn is 4–5 cm [73]. Once free backflow of blood is verified, the catheter is anchored to the umbilical cord with the umbilical tape or purse-string suture. If resistance is met, the stump can be pulled inferiorly (i.e., toward the patient's feet) so that the catheter is being directed more superiorly (i.e., toward the patient's head). This may reduce the angle of insertion and alleviate obstruction from the surrounding soft tissues. An overly tight umbilical tape (or purse-strong suture) may also be suspected if difficulty is encountered when attempting to advance the catheter.

If central venous monitoring is desired, the catheter should be inserted further (usually 10–12 cm) until it reaches the IVC. Proper tip position (within the IVC, just distal to the right atrium) is confirmed radiologically but usually corresponds to an insertion depth equal to two-thirds of the distance from the patient's shoulder to the umbilicus. Visualization of injected saline through the UVC with ultrasound can be used to confirm proper UVC tip position and identify inadvertent malpositioning within the hepatic portal circulation [4, 74]. A tape bridge may be used to secure the catheter to the patient's abdomen after placement. Figure 8.4 shows the three stages of UVC placement, including cord transection (a), catheter insertion (b), and subsequent stabilization of the line with a tape bridge (c).

Umbilical artery catheterization (UAC) can be used to facilitate continuous arterial blood pressure monitoring, blood gas sampling, and exchange transfusions in neonates. The placement technique mirrors that of umbilical vein catheterization, although curved Iris forceps may be needed to dilate the arteries as they are usually smaller and more muscular than the vein. After cannulation of the umbilical artery, the catheter is flushed with heparinized saline to avoid inadvertent introduction of

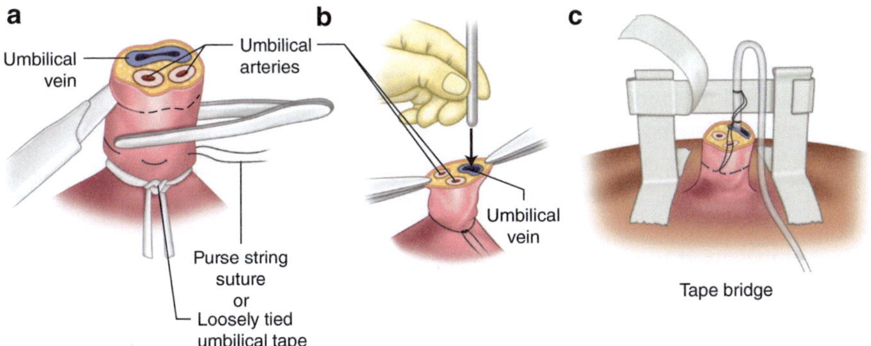

Fig. 8.4 Three stages of umbilical vein catheterization

air bubbles. Lidocaine 2% for intravascular use may be trickled on the artery to prevent arterial spasm. The radiological position of the catheter tip on post-placement chest X-ray should be between the sixth and ninth thoracic vertebrae. This "high position" of umbilical artery catheter (i.e., between T6 and T9 vertebral levels) is preferred over the "low position" (L3 to L4 level), as it is associated with fewer complications [4]. The formula used to calculate the required insertion depth for umbilical artery catheters is *depth (cm) = 9 + (3 × weight in kg)* [61].

Umbilical venous catheters should be removed as soon as they no longer needed (ideally within 7–10 days) but can be used for up to 14 days if managed appropriately [4]. Umbilical artery catheters should be removed as soon as no longer needed or when providers note any sign of vascular insufficiency to the lower extremities. An umbilical artery catheter should not be left in place for more than 5 days [75]. Removal of umbilical catheters should be done over several minutes, to reduce the risk of bleeding and to allow vasospasm (in the case of UACs) [4].

Arterial Catheters

Arterial catheters are generally used for invasive continuous blood pressure monitoring or when frequent arterial blood gas analysis is required. In newborns <2 weeks of age, the umbilical artery can be used, as described above. In infants and children, the *radial artery, femoral artery*, and *posterior tibial artery* are commonly used. The technique is like that used for adults, as described in Chap. 13. However, US guidance for radial artery cannulation has been shown to improve first-attempt success rates and reduce complications when compared to the palpation or Doppler US methods traditionally used with adults [61].

Methods to Enhance Placement Success

Establishing emergent vascular access in unstable (or merely uncooperative) pediatric patients offers many unique challenges to the care provider. These challenges include the need to engage the child's cooperation with VAD placement, increased potential for psychological trauma, smaller veins, and increased subcutaneous fat, making both palpation and visualization of veins more difficult [76]. Earlier in this chapter, several methods were described to help minimize the anxiety and psychological trauma associated with vascular access device placement in children. Many of the techniques described for vein identification and cannulation among patients with difficult vascular access described Chap. 10 may also be applied to pediatric patients.

Techniques used to facilitate PIV placement through improved visualization of the veins include local warming, transillumination, the application of epidermal nitroglycerin, and the use of ultrasound guidance. Pain perception can also be mitigated in pediatric and adult subjects through topical medications. Moderate-quality evidence suggests that the use of a *vapocoolant* (e.g., topical anesthetic skin refrigerants, PainEase®) immediately before intravenous cannulation reduces pain during the procedure and does not increase the difficulty of cannulation or cause serious adverse effects but is associated with mild discomfort during application [77]. Local anesthetic techniques, including the application of a *eutectic mixture of lidocaine and prilocaine (EMLA)* to the insertion site, may help alleviate patient discomfort but must be placed at the insertion site well in advance, as this topical anesthetic requires 20–30 minutes to achieve its full effect [78].

Providers may need to briefly restrain pediatric subjects during the access attempt or immobilize the target extremity during and after line placement. Shielding of the VAD insertion site may be helpful in preventing the child from pulling on the infusion tubing and dislodging the VAD after placement. Traditional examples of protective devices for VAD insertion sites include taping the tubing to the skin, wrapping the extremity loosely with gauze, taping a small paper cup over the insertion site, or taping the extremity to an arm board or sandbag to reduce movement of the extremity. Although these techniques and devices may protect the VAD, patient safety remains a chief concern and care should be taken to avoid injury to the patient with their use. When using gauze or other wrappings, it is important to ensure that the VAD and insertion site remain accessible to care providers and that the dressings allow for adequate visualization of the extremity to identify complications of intravenous infusion such as extravasation and compartment syndrome.

Decision-Making for Pediatric Subjects

Decision-making regarding VAD selection in children mirrors that of adults, although differences exist. As with adults, *landmark-based PIV catheterization should be considered first* in pediatric subjects, if it is deemed both possible and adequate to treat the patient's condition [21, 24, 27, 32, 79, 80]. Target veins should be visible or palpable to the provider, and "blind" attempts should not be made. *US-PIV placement should be considered after two failed landmark-based PIV insertion attempts* in stable patients, as the US-guided approach appears to be associated with higher rates of cannulation success when compared to additional landmark-based attempts past this milestone [24].

Acceptable PIV insertion sites among pediatric trauma patients should be those in uninjured extremities, with preference for the antecubital, external jugular (in patients without suspected cervical spine injury), and saphenous veins. In the hemodynamically unstable (e.g., hypovolemic) pediatric patient, the size and length of PIV catheter must be optimized for high-volume infusion. That said, the gauge of PIV catheter required may be highly variable within the pediatric population. An adequately gauged "volume line" for an infant may not be adequate for older children [76].

Unstable patients, especially those in extremis or experiencing cardiac arrest may be best served by placement of an intraosseous catheter. Both the Pediatric Advanced Life Support (PALS) and Advanced Trauma Life Support (ATLS) guidelines appear to support consideration of IO line placement if adequate PIV access cannot be established within three attempts or 90 seconds, whichever is sooner [81, 82]. Although IO flow rates may be highly variable in pediatric patients, flow through the catheter can be improved with the application of a pressure bag or the use of syringe injection [76]. Intraosseous catheters should not be placed in extremities with confirmed or suspected fracture or significant soft tissue injury, due to increased risk of extravasation and resulting compartment syndrome.

Conclusions

Pediatric vascular access can be challenging under emergent conditions, especially for infants and newborns. Even providers who are adept at line placement in adults may be intimidated by the prospect of establishing emergent vascular access in a young child. Many important anatomic differences exist between pediatric and adult patients, and these differences must be considered in determining the best techniques for emergent pediatric vascular access. When choosing a vascular access site, the practical and anatomical differences of pediatric patients must be considered in addition to the patient's presenting and preexisting medical conditions, risk of infection, available equipment, and urgency of the need for access.

Key Concepts

- Speed and efficacy are of the utmost importance when establishing venous access, and the well-trained pediatric provider will understand the various devices and approaches that can help to facilitate safe, fast, and effective vascular access.
- Ultrasound can serve as a valuable adjunct to traditional PIV catheter insertion techniques, although this modality may not offer the same advantages as with adult subjects.
- Landmark-based PIV insertion should be attempted first in pediatric patients, although alternative strategies for vascular access should be considered when landmark-based PIV methods fail.
- Ultrasound guidance should be used for pediatric CVC placement, to reduce the risk of line-related complications.
- Umbilical vein catheterization can provide emergent vascular access for newborns up until 2 weeks of age.

References

1. Lavelle JM. Central Venous Cannulation. In: King C, editor. Textbook of pediatric emergency procedures. 2nd ed. Philadelphia: Lippincott Williams and Wilkins; 2008. p. 247–70.
2. AIUM practice guideline for the use of ultrasound to guide vascular access procedures. J Ultrasound Med. 2013;32(1):191–215.
3. Doellman D, Buckner JK, Hudson GJ, et al. Best practice guidelines in the care and maintenance of pediatric central venous catheters. 2nd ed. Association for Vascular Access: Herriman; 2015.
4. Gorski LA, Hadaway L, Hagle ME, et al. Infusion therapy standards of practice. J Infus Nurs. 2021;44(suppl 1):S1–S224. https://doi.org/10.1097/NAN.0000000000000396.
5. Wyckoff MM, Sharpe EL. Peripherally inserted central catheters: guidelines for practice. 3rd ed. National Association of Neonatal Issues: Chicago; 2015.
6. Gorski LA, Phillips LD. Phillips's manual of I.V. Therapeutics. 7th ed. Philadelphia: FA Davis Company; 2018.
7. Doellman D. Pediatrics. In: Alexander M, Corrigan A, Gorski L, Phillips L, editors. Core curriculum for infusion nursing. 4th ed. Philadelphia: Lippincott, Williams & Wilkins; 2014.
8. Sisson TRC, Lund CJ, Whalen LE, Telek A. The blood volume of infants II. The premature infant during the first year of life. J Pediatr. 1959;55(4):430–46.
9. Frey AM, Pettit J. Infusion therapy in children. In: Alexander M, Corrigan A, Gorski L, Hankins J, Perucca R, editors. Infusion nursing: an evidence-based practice. 3rd ed. St. Louis: Saunders / Elsevier; 2010.
10. Scrivens A, Reynolds PR, Emery FE, et al. Use of intraosseous needles in neonates: a systematic review. Neonatology. 2019;116:305–14.
11. Sá RA, Melo CL, Dantas RB, Delfim LV. Vascular access through the intraosseous route in pediatric emergencies. Rev Bras ter Intensiva. 2012;24(4):407–14.
12. Pittiruti M, Hamilton H, Biffi R, MacFie J, Pertkiewicz M. ESPEN Guidelines on Parenteral Nutrition: central venous catheters (access, care, diagnosis and therapy of complications). Clin Nutrit (Edinburgh, Scotland). 2009;28(4):365–77.
13. Pittiruti M. Ultrasound guided central vascular access in neonates, infants and children. Curr Drug Targets. 2012;13(7):961–9.
14. Kamata M, Walia H, Hakim M, Tumin D, Tobias JD. An in vitro assessment of the efficacy of various IV cannulas for the rapid IV fluid administration. Ped Crit Care Med. 2017;18(5):e224–8.
15. Wehbé MA, Moore JH. Digital ischemia in the neonate following intravenous therapy. Pediatrics. 1985;76(1):99–103.
16. Cohen LL. Behavioral approaches to anxiety and pain management for pediatric venous access. Pediatrics. 2008;122:S134–9.
17. Takeshita J, Nakayama Y, Nakajima Y, et al. Optimal site for ultrasound-guided venous catheterisation in paediatric patients: an observational study to investigate predictors for catheterisation success and a randomised controlled study to determine the most successful site. Crit Care. 2015;19:15–23.
18. Qian SY, Horn MT, Barnes R, Armstrong D. The use of 8-cm 22G Seldinger catheters for intravenous access in children with cystic fibrosis. J Vasc Access. 2014;15(5):415–7.
19. Birhane E, Kidanu K, Kassa M, et al. Lifespan and associated features of peripheral intravenous cannula admitted in public hospitals of Mekelle city, Tigray, Ethiopia, 2016. BMC Nurs. 2017;16:33.
20. Unbeck M, Forberg U, Ygge BM, Ehrenberg A, Petzold M, Johansson E. Peripheral venous catheter related complications are common among paediatric and neonatal patients. Acta Paediatr (Oslo, Norway:1992). 2015;104(6):566–74.

21. Curtis SJ, Craig WR, Logue E, Vandermeer B, Hanson A, Klassen T. Ultrasound or near-infrared vascular imaging to guide peripheral intravenous catheterization in children: a pragmatic randomized controlled trial. Can Med Assoc J. 2015;187(8):563–70.
22. O'Neill MB. Validating the difficult intravenous access clinical prediction rule. Ped Emerg Care. 2012;28(12):1314–6.
23. Kost S. Ultrasound-assisted venous access. In: King C, editor. Textbook of pediatric emergency procedures. 2nd ed. Philadelphia: Lippincott Williams and Wilkins; 2008. p. 1255–61.
24. Egan G, Healy D, O'Neill H, Clarke-Moloney M, Grace PA, Walsh SR. Ultrasound guidance for difficult peripheral venous access: systematic review and meta-analysis. Emerg Med J. 2013;30(7):521–6.
25. Benkhadra M, Collignon M, Fournel I, et al. Ultrasound guidance allows faster peripheral IV cannulation in children under 3 years of age with difficult venous access: a prospective randomized study. Paediatr Anaesth. 2012;22(5):449–54.
26. Doniger SJ, Ishimine P, Fox JC, Kanegaye JT. Randomized controlled trial of ultrasound-guided peripheral intravenous catheter placement versus traditional techniques in difficult-access pediatric patients. Ped Emerg Care. 2009;25(3):154–9.
27. Heinrichs J, Fritze Z, Vandermeer B, Klassen T, Curtis S. Ultrasonographically guided peripheral intravenous cannulation of children and adults: a systematic review and meta-analysis. Ann Emerg Med. 2013;61(4):444–54.
28. Bruzoni M, Slater BJ, Wall J, et al. A prospective randomized trial of ultrasound- vs landmark-guided central venous access in the pediatric population. J Am Coll Surg. 2013;216(5):939–43.
29. Donaldson JS, Morello FP, Junewick JJ, et al. Peripherally inserted central venous catheters: US-guided vascular access in pediatric patients. Radiology. 1995;197(2):542–4.
30. Goutail-Flaud MF, Sfez M, Berg A, et al. Central venous catheter-related complications in newborns and infants: a 587-case survey. J Pediatr Surg. 1991;26(6):645–50.
31. Kanter RK, Zimmerman JJ, Strauss RH, Stoeckel KA. Pediatric emergency intravenous access. Evaluation of a protocol. Am J Dis Child. 1986;140(2):132–4.
32. Schnadower D, Lin S, Perera P, Smerling A, Dayan P. A pilot study of ultrasound analysis before pediatric peripheral vein cannulation attempt. Acad Emerg Med. 2007;14(5):483–5.
33. Nicolson SC, Sweeney MF, Moore RA, Jobes DR. Comparison of internal and external jugular cannulation of the central circulation in the pediatric patient. Crit Care Med. 1985;13(9):747–9.
34. Paladini A, Chiaretti A, Sellasie KW, et al. Ultrasound-guided placement of long peripheral cannulas in children over the age of 10 years admitted to the emergency department: a pilot study. BMJ Paediatr Open. 2018;2(1):e000244.
35. Levy JCJ, Abo A, Rempell R, Deanehan JK. Ultrasound. In: Shaw KN, Bachur R, editors. Fleisher & Ludwig's textbook of pediatric emergency medicine. 7th ed. Philadelphia: Wolters Kluwer; 2016.
36. Ares G, Hunter CJ. Central venous access in children: indications, devices, and risks. Curr Opinion Ped. 2017;29(3):340–6.
37. Pafitanis G, Spyridon K, Theodorakopoulou E, Mason K, Ygropoulou O, Mousafiri O. A case report of abdominal compartment syndrome caused by malposition of a femoral venous catheter. Int J Surg Case Rep. 2015;12:84–6.
38. Choi YH, Cheon JE, Shin SH, et al. Optimal insertion lengths of right and left internal jugular central venous catheters in children. Pediatr Radiol. 2015;45(8):1206–11.
39. Karazincir S, Akoğlu E, Balci A, Sangün O, Okuyucu S, Ozbakiş C, et al. Dimensions of internal jugular veins in Turkish children aged between 0 and 6 years in resting state and during Valsalva maneuver. Int J Pediatr Otorhinolaryngol. 2007;71(8):1247–50.
40. Keiler J, Seidel R, Wree A. The femoral vein diameter and its correlation with sex, age and body mass index - an anatomical parameter with clinical relevance. Phlebology. 2019;34(1):58–69.
41. Tartière D, Seguin P, Juhel C, Laviolle B, Mallédant Y. Estimation of the diameter and cross-sectional area of the internal jugular veins in adult patients. Crit Care (London, England). 2009;13(6):R197.
42. Warkentine FH, Clyde Pierce M, Lorenz D, Kim IK. The anatomic relationship of femoral vein to femoral artery in euvolemic pediatric patients by ultrasonography: implications for pediatric femoral central venous access. Acad Emerg Med. 2008;15(5):426–30.

43. Yildirim I, Yüksel M, Okur N, Okur E, Kýliç MA. The sizes of internal jugular veins in Turkish children aged between 7 and 12 years. Int J Pediatr Otorhinolaryngol. 2004;68(8):1059–62.

44. Breschan C, Platzer M, Jost R, et al. Size of internal jugular vs subclavian vein in small infants: an observational, anatomical evaluation with ultrasound. Br J Anaesth. 2010;105(2):179–84.

45. Souza Neto EP, Grousson S, Duflo F, et al. Ultrasonographic anatomic variations of the major veins in paediatric patients. Brit J Anaesth. 2014;112(5):879–84.

46. Sayin MM, Mercan A, Koner O, et al. Internal jugular vein diameter in pediatric patients: are the J-shaped guidewire diameters bigger than internal jugular vein? An evaluation with ultrasound. Pediatr Anesth. 2008;18(8):745–51.

47. Fortune JB, Feustel P. Effect of patient position on size and location of the subclavian vein for percutaneous puncture. Arch Surg. 2003;138(9):996–1000.

48. Albrecht K, Breitmeier D, Panning B, Troger HD, Nave H. The carina as a landmark for central venous catheter placement in small children. Eur J Pediatr. 2006;165(4):264–6.

49. Practice guidelines for central venous access 2020: an updated report by the American Society of Anesthesiologists task force on central venous access. Anesthesiology. 2020;132(1):8–43.

50. Jung CW, Jailov G, Song IK, et al. Position and relative size of the vertebral artery according to age: implications for internal jugular vein access. Paediatr Anaesth. 2017;27(10):997–1002.

51. Gaballah M, Krishnamurthy G, Keller MS, et al. US-guided placement and tip position confirmation for lower-extremity central venous access in neonates and infants with comparison versus conventional insertion. J Vasc Interv Radiol. 2014;25(4):548–55.

52. Stenzel JP, Green TP, Fuhrman BP, Carlson PE, Marchessault RP. Percutaneous femoral venous catheterizations: a prospective study of complications. J Pediatr. 1989;114(3):411–5.

53. Prince SR, Sullivan RL, Hackel A. Percutaneous catheterization of the internal jugular vein in infants and children. Anesthesiology. 1976;44(2):170–4.

54. Cote CJ, Jobes DR, Schwartz AJ, Ellison N. Two approaches to cannulation of a child's internal jugular vein. Anesthesiology. 1979;50(4):371–3.

55. Trieschmann U, Cate UT, Sreeram N. Central venous catheters in children and neonates – what is important? Images Paediatr Cardiol. 2007;9(4):1–8.

56. Filston HC, Grant JP. A safer system for percutaneous subclavian venous catheterization in newborn infants. J Pediatr Surg. 1979;14(5):564–70.

57. Isaev Iu V, Bulatsev SM, Skorinova GI. Horner's syndrome as a complication during catheterization of subclavian vein in young children. Vestn Khir Im I I Grek. 1990;145(10):80–1.

58. Kim EH, Lee JH, Song IK, et al. Real-time ultrasound-guided axillary vein cannulation in children: a randomised controlled trial. Anaesthesia. 2017;72(12):1516–22.

59. Oulego-Erroz I, Muñoz-Lozón A, Alonso-Quintela P, et al. Comparison of ultrasound guided brachiocephalic and internal jugular vein cannulation in critically ill children. J Crit Care. 2016;35:133–7.

60. Motz P, Von Saint Andre Von Arnim A, Iyer RS, Chabra S, Likes M, Dighe M Point-of-care ultrasound for peripherally inserted central catheter monitoring: a pilot study. J Perinat Med 2019;47(9):991–996.

61. Naik VM, Mantha SSP, Rayani BK. Vascular access in children. Indian J Anaesth. 2019;63(9):737–45.

62. Metz RI, Lucking SE, Chaten FC, Williams TM, Mickell JJ. Percutaneous catheterization of the axillary vein in infants and children. Pediatrics. 1990;85(4):531–3.

63. Newman BM, Jewett TC Jr, Karp MP, Cooney DR. Percutaneous central venous catheterization in children: first line choice for venous access. J Pediatr Surg. 1986;21(8):685–8.

64. Shime N, Hosokawa K, MacLaren G. Ultrasound imaging reduces failure rates of percutaneous central venous catheterization in children. Pediatr Crit Care Med. 2015;16(8):718–25.

65. Abe KK, Blum GT, Yamamoto LG. Intraosseous is faster and easier than umbilical venous catheterization in newborn emergency vascular access models. Amer J Emerg Med. 2000;18(2):126–9.

66. Loisel DB, Smith MM, MacDonald MG, Martin GR. Intravenous access in newborn infants: impact of extended umbilical venous catheter use on requirement for peripheral venous lines. J Perinatol. 1996;16(6):461–6.
67. Rajani AK, Chitkara R, Oehlert J, Halamek LP. Comparison of umbilical venous and intraosseous access during simulated neonatal resuscitation. Pediatrics. 2011;128(4):e954–8.
68. Patterson RS, Chopra V, Brown E, et al. Selection and insertion of vascular access devices in pediatrics: a systematic review. Pediatrics. 2020;145(suppl3):S243–68.
69. Weissman A, Jakobi P, Bronshtein M, Goldstein I. Sonographic measurements of the umbilical cord and vessels during normal pregnancies. J Ultrasound Med. 1994;13:11–4.
70. Davies JE, Walker JT, Keating A. Concise review: Wharton's jelly: the rich, but enigmatic, source of mesenchymal stromal cells. Stem Cells Translat Med. 2017;6:1620–30.
71. Kondo M, Itoh S, Kunikata T, et al. Time of closure of ductus venosus in term and preterm neonates. Arch Dis Child Neonatal Ed. 2001;85:F57–9.
72. Murphy PJ. The fetal circulation. Cont Ed Anaesth Crit Care Pain. 2005;5(4):107–12.
73. Lewis K, Spirnak PW. Umbilical vein catheterization. In: StatPearls [Internet]. Treasure Island: StatPearls Publishing; 2021. Accessed 15 March 2021
74. Kishigami M, Shimokaze T, Enomoto M, Shibasaki J, Toyoshima K. Ultrasound-guided umbilical venous catheter insertion with alignment of the umbilical vein and ductus venosus. J Ultrasound Med. 2020;39(2):379–83.
75. O'Grady NP, Alexander M, Burns LA, et al. Guidelines for the prevention of intravascular catheter-related infections. Am J Infect Control. 2011;39(4 Supp):S1–S34.
76. Greene N, Bhananker S, Ramaiah R. Vascular access, fluid resuscitation, and blood transfusion in pediatric trauma. Int J Crit Ill Inj Sci. 2012;2(3):135–42.
77. Griffith RJ, Jordan V, Herd D, Reed PW, Dalziel SR. Vapocoolants (cold spray) for pain treatment during intravenous cannulation. Cochrane Database Syst Rev. 2016;4:CD009484.
78. Fetzer SJ. Reducing venipuncture and intravenous insertion pain with eutectic mixture of local anesthetic: a meta-analysis. Nurs Res. 2002;51(2):119–24.
79. Brannam L, Blaivas M, Lyon M, Flake M. Emergency nurses' utilization of ultrasound guidance for placement of peripheral intravenous lines in difficult-access patients. Acad Emerg Med. 2004;11(12):1361–3.
80. Stein J, George B, River G, Hebig A, McDermott D. Ultrasonographically-guided peripheral intravenous cannulation in emergency department patients with difficult intravenous access: a randomized trial. Ann Emerg Med. 2009;54(1):33–40.
81. Topjian AA, Raymond TT, Atkins D, et al. Part 4: Pediatric basic and advanced life support: 2020 American Heart Association guidelines for cardiopulmonary resuscitation and emergency cardiovascular care. Circulation. 2020;142(16 Suppl 2):S469–523.
82. American College of Surgeons (ACS). Committee on Trauma. Advanced trauma life support: student course manual. 10th ed. Chicago: American College of Surgeons; 2018. p. 186–212.

Special Populations: Cardiac Arrest

Sarah Meram, Theodore Falcon, and James H. Paxton

Introduction

Cardiac arrest (CA) is unlike any other medical condition. Patients presenting in the absence of native cardiac function, by definition, have minimal perfusion to vital organs without any assurances of return of spontaneous circulation (ROSC). The role of the emergent vascular access provider in treating this condition is therefore to *establish vascular access for the purpose of introducing medications into the circulation that will stimulate the resumption of native cardiac activity while supporting continued organ perfusion.* Timing is key for this intervention. Delayed administration of the necessary medications and fluids required for adequate organ perfusion will likely lead to worse outcomes for these patients. This chapter will address some of the common obstacles that prevent emergent vascular access in patients experiencing cardiac arrest, including solutions to these obstacles. Providers should prioritize the rapid establishment of a vascular access device (VAD) for these patients, *assuming that early access is always preferred to delayed or deferred access.* Providers should recognize that delays in obtaining vascular access for patients experiencing cardiac arrest directly contributes to increased mortality and morbidity for these patients.

Cardiac arrest can affect patients of any age, race, gender, or ethnicity, in any location, and at any time. As reported by the American Heart Association (AHA) Advanced Cardiovascular Life Support (ACLS) guidelines, approximately 356,000 incidences of out-of-hospital cardiac arrest (OHCA) were reported in the United

S. Meram (✉) · J. H. Paxton
Department of Emergency Medicine, Wayne State University School of Medicine, Detroit, MI, USA
e-mail: smera@med.wayne.edu; james.paxton@wayne.edu

T. Falcon
Department of Emergency Medicine, Wayne State University, Nursing Development & Research, Henry Ford Health System, Detroit, MI, USA
e-mail: tfalcon@med.wayne.edu

© Springer Nature Switzerland AG 2021
J. H. Paxton (ed.), *Emergent Vascular Access*,
https://doi.org/10.1007/978-3-030-77177-5_9

States in 2018, with only about 10.4% of these patients surviving to hospital discharge [1]. The likelihood of permanent brain and other irreversible organ damage increases with extended duration of reduced organ perfusion following cardiac arrest. Therefore, decreasing the time between onset of cardiac arrest and the initiation of external chest compressions is essential to the appropriate management of cardiac arrest. A high priority is also placed on obtaining immediate vascular access, as the prompt administration of vasopressors and other medications following OHCA appears to improve patient survival when compared to chest compressions alone [1–3].

Pathophysiology of Cardiac Arrest

The heart is the central organ of blood flow. Its primary function is to circulate blood throughout the body. Blood is collected through the venous system and deposited in the right atrium and then into the right ventricle, where it is pushed through the lungs, where oxygenation of the blood occurs. In the lungs, carbon dioxide is removed and oxygen is bound. Oxygenated blood is then deposited in the left atrium before traveling to the left ventricle, where it is pumped into the arterial system to provide oxygenation to the body's tissues. This pumping action is essential to survival. During cardiac arrest, the heart stops effectively pumping oxygenated blood, which leads to hypoxemia as vital organs are deprived of oxygenated blood flow. Oxygen deprivation leads to injury to the brain, kidneys, heart, and other vital organs.

As depicted in Fig. 9.1, patients may have regular, organized cardiac rhythm prior to the precipitating event (e.g., acute myocardial infarction or acute respiratory arrest) that leads to cardiac arrest. However, following this precipitating event, most patients will experience a predictable stage-wise decompensation in cardiac function, progressing from an organized dysrhythmia (e.g., ventricular tachycardia, or VT) into a disorganized rhythm (e.g., ventricular fibrillation, or VF). Once the dysrhythmia has adequately disrupted the heart's ability to contract in an organized fashion, the patient's pulse will begin to disappear. By the time that the patient is experiencing ventricular fibrillation, the pulse is typically absent. However, the pulse can already be absent in the VT phase, and this is referred to as pulseless

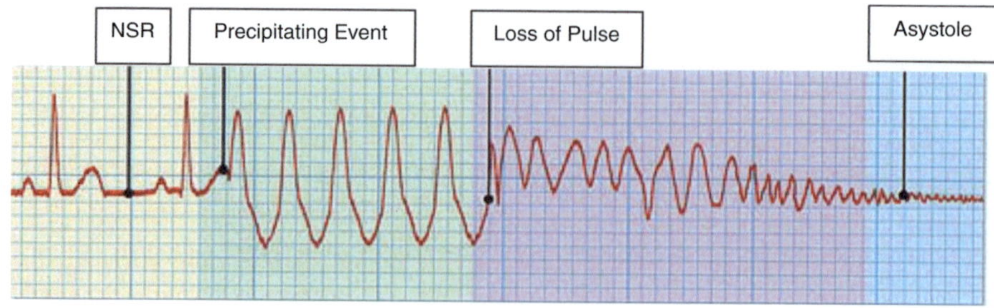

Fig. 9.1 Progression of life-threatening dysrhythmias following cardiac arrest

ventricular tachycardia (pVT). Patients who have pVT/VF are generally very responsive to electrical defibrillation, so these rhythms are categorized as "shockable rhythms." Patients who present with a shockable rhythm as their initial cardiac rhythm will generally have a better prognosis than patients who present with a non-shockable rhythm (e.g., asystole or other pulseless rhythms) [4]. A table of the shockable and non-shockable cardiac rhythms is presented in Fig. 9.2.

Torsades de pointes (TdP) is a specific type of polymorphic ventricular tachycardia seen in patients with a long QT interval. This phrase translates from the French as, "twisting of the points." It is characterized by rapid, irregular QRS complexes, which appear to be twisting around the electrocardiogram (ECG) baseline, as shown in Fig. 9.3. This specific form of VT may respond favorably to magnesium sulfate infusion, which is why it is important that the emergency care provider recognize it.

The *presence or absence of a palpable pulse* is the most important finding in the management of OHCA patients. The absence of a pulse mandates immediate recognition and action, as does the return of a pulse when management is ultimately successful. It should be noted that the "pulse" referenced here is a detectable arterial pulse using the provider's hands. Thus, patients may be experiencing some degree of organized cardiac contraction (e.g., cardiac activity on ultrasound) even when a pulse is absent. Similarly, the patient may have a normal sinus rhythm (NSR) or other organized cardiac rhythms without a pulse – this is called pulseless electrical activity (PEA). Although PEA is often portrayed as a pulseless sinus rhythm, it can be any non-shockable rhythm. All non-shockable pulseless rhythms are treated the same, unless there is evidence of organized cardiac contraction or forward flow on ultrasound imaging.

Although cardiopulmonary resuscitation (CPR) has been the subject of aggressive research since the 1950s, modern resuscitation theory is largely built upon the "three-phase" model introduced by Weisfeldt in 2002 [5]. This model for our understanding of the pathophysiology of cardiac arrest begins at ventricular fibrillation

Shockable rhythms	Non-shockable rhythms
Ventricular fibrillation (VF)	Asystole
Ventricular tachycardia (VT)	Pulseless electrical activity (PEA)

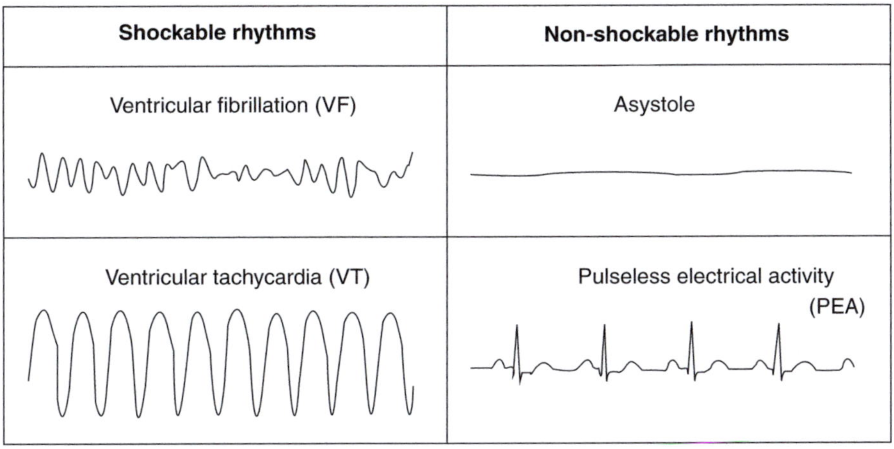

Fig. 9.2 Shockable and non-shockable cardiac rhythms associated with cardiac arrest

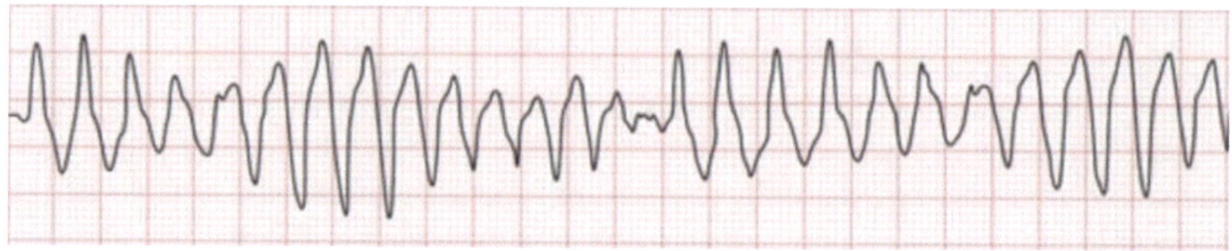

Fig. 9.3 *Torsades de pointes* (polymorphic VT) waveform

(VF) and pulseless ventricular tachycardia (pVT), soon followed by three discrete time periods or phases following the moment of cardiac arrest (i.e., when systemic perfusion is lost). The "electrical" *phase* begins at the precise moment of cardiac arrest and lasts about 5 minutes [5]. During this initial phase, immediate electrical defibrillation should be the priority for emergency providers, and survival appears to be very good (about 60%) for patients in this phase who are treated promptly with defibrillation. Those patients who are not adequately defibrillated within the first 5 minutes following cardiac arrest will progress to the "circulatory" *phase*, which appears to begin 5–10 minutes after the onset of VF. Patients who present during this second phase will require a brief period (e.g., 1–3 minutes) of aggressive chest compression to restore circulation prior to defibrillation attempts. In this phase, the blood remains adequately oxygenated with a tolerable acid-base balance, permitting stabilization of the myocardium with restoration of blood flow to the coronary arteries through chest compressions alone. Unfortunately, very few cardiac arrest patients present to the emergency provider within 10–15 minutes following the onset of cardiac arrest. Consequently, most patients who present to the emergency department have already entered the third phase, the so-called "metabolic" phase, before receiving any specific intervention. Patients in the metabolic phase of cardiac arrest may require drug administration to restore homeostasis, especially correction of metabolic acidosis (with sodium bicarbonate) and other pharmacologic measures, including epinephrine infusion, to restore homeostasis. Chest compressions and electrical defibrillation alone cannot restore native cardiac function for patients presenting in the metabolic phase. These patients invariably appear to require vascular access for the infusion of medications to restore biochemical homeostasis before traditional measures can succeed. Unfortunately, the vast majority of patients treated for cardiac arrest are first encountered by medical providers in the metabolic phase. In this phase, vascular access is an even higher priority, since these patients are unlikely to survive without the administration of resuscitative medications.

Weisfeldt's three-phase model helps to explain why patients presenting to the emergency care provider with an initially shockable rhythm have a three times higher survival rate (37%) than patients presenting with asystole or PEA (12%) [4]. This differential is likely due to the fact that patients presenting with VT/VF are in an earlier phase of their disease process. Unfortunately, delayed reperfusion following ischemic injury leads to metabolic acidosis and a higher concentration of pro-inflammatory mediators, which will prevent epinephrine and other cardioactive/

vasoactive medications from working. In vitro studies with myocardial cells suggest that delayed reperfusion worsens outcomes [6, 7]. Thus, the timing of vascular access and medication infusion are paramount to patient survival, as most patients presenting to emergency care providers have already progressed to the metabolic phase of injury. Minutes wasted by failed vascular access attempts readily translate to decreased survival for cardiac arrest patients.

In the 1970s, approximately 60% of all OHCA patients treated in the United States presented with VF/VT, but this proportion has declined to only 25–30% over the last few decades [8]. The cause of this change is unclear and may be due to reporting bias or to later (i.e., more advanced) presentations for out-of-hospital cardiac arrest patients. Whatever the cause, almost three-fourths of OHCA patients receiving care in the United States today present with asystole or PEA (e.g., non-shockable rhythms) as the initial documented cardiac rhythm. Since these patients are presenting in the metabolic phase of cardiac arrest, these patients will not respond favorably to defibrillation and chest compressions alone. Patients with OHCA require immediate intervention (including the infusion of medications) to stabilize their condition, and their likelihood of survival decreases with increasing delay from time of arrest to time of first intervention. Assuming that present trends continue, we suggest that emergent vascular access will play an increasingly important role in the care of OHCA patients into the future.

Many other outcomes are important in the setting of cardiac arrest, beyond mere survival. It has been well-established that OHCA patients have a very low rate of survival-to-hospital discharge. Only about 30% of subjects presenting with VT/VF survive to hospital discharge, and this percentage is much lower for those presenting in PEA or asystole (e.g., 2–5%) [8]. Although it has recently been suggested that epinephrine infusion may not improve survival to hospital discharge following OHCA [9], there seems to be consensus within the medical literature that some medications are needed to supplement the effects of high-quality CPR and early defibrillation, even if the optimal medications and doses are not yet understood. Even if epinephrine is ultimately demonstrated to not be the optimal resuscitative medication, it is still likely that most patients presenting to the emergency care provider during the metabolic phase of cardiac arrest will still require some medication or fluid to aid in the restoration of metabolic homeostasis. As more effective medications are discovered to treat cardiac arrest, immediate vascular access will undoubtedly remain an essential requirement for patient survival [10].

In 1991, the AHA introduced the "Chain of Survival" model, meant to guide the effective and efficient treatment of cardiac arrest [11]. This model was originally intended for use by emergency medical services (EMS) but has subsequently been adapted to apply to all healthcare providers who treat cardiac arrest patients. The Chain of Survival includes five time-sensitive and co-dependent factors, including early vascular access, early CPR, early defibrillation, early ACLS, and early post-resuscitative care, as described in Table 9.1.

The first goal of ACLS intervention is to restore native cardiac function, generally referred to as return of spontaneous circulation (ROSC). The *achievement of ROSC*

Table 9.1 The American Heart Association (AHA) "Chain of Survival" [11]

Early access	All pre-EMS arrival efforts of care. This includes identifying the event as "sudden cardiac death" (SCD) and initiating emergency medical protocols
Early CPR	Initiation of immediate cardiopulmonary resuscitation
Early defibrillation	Electrical shock to restore spontaneous heart rhythm (if the patient presents with a "shockable rhythm")
Early ACLS	Drug therapies and airway management intended to achieve spontaneous heart rhythm
Early post-resuscitative care	To restore and conserve cognitive function and prevent secondary organ damage

may be considered to be an essential first step toward restoring homeostasis and organ perfusion. However, ROSC can be short-lived, especially if the underlying cause of the cardiac arrest is not adequately corrected. Therefore, transient ROSC may not necessarily be associated with improved survival or other important clinical outcomes. While minimal organ perfusion may be provided with external chest compressions, patients cannot survive without eventually realizing ROSC. It is imperative that organ perfusion be restored as soon as possible following cardiac arrest, and perfusion to the vital organs must be maintained to prevent necrotic tissue damage.

As transient ROSC appears to have limited clinical value, sustained ROSC should be the provider's initial goal during the earliest stages of OHCA resuscitation. We suggest that *sustained ROSC* (commonly defined as lasting >20 minutes) represents a more clinically relevant outcome for cardiac arrest patients than transient ROSC. Consequently, any intervention that is associated with sustained ROSC should be valued above interventions that produce a more transient ROSC. While interventions associated with sustained ROSC may not ultimately be associated with improved survival-to-hospital discharge, achievement of sustained ROSC is at least a marker that should be considered evidence of improved outcome as compared to unsustained ROSC. Clearly, *survival-to-hospital discharge with good neurological outcome* is the gold standard for a favorable cardiac arrest outcome. However, this outcome depends upon myriad factors beyond the control of the vascular access provider, including decisions about goals of care and withdrawal of care that may be made days or weeks after successful ROSC. We suggest that the emergency vascular access provider should prioritize the realization of sustained ROSC above other outcomes in the emergent setting, understanding that this outcome does not necessarily translate to improved long-term survival.

Consequently, we suggest that *the goal of the emergency vascular access provider should be to provide emergent vascular access leading to sustained ROSC for out-of-hospital cardiac arrest patients*, understanding that more ambitious outcomes may be, at least in part, dependent upon subsequent management by the inpatient team. Restoring native cardiac function appears to be an essential first step toward enabling survival-to-hospital discharge with good neurologic function. Unfortunately, whether this gold standard outcome is actually realized relies upon many decisions and events that extend well beyond the scope of the frontline vascular access provider.

Medications in Cardiac Arrest

Understanding that early medication administration is not guaranteed to elicit improved outcomes for patients, responsibility for establishing the earliest possible vascular access should remain a priority for emergency care providers treating patients in cardiac arrest. Many routes for possible medication infusion are available to the emergency care provider, and these will be discussed in later portions of this chapter. In this section, we will discuss the potential roles of various medications currently recommended by the AHA for the restoration of metabolic homeostasis following cardiac arrest. These medications include *epinephrine, amiodarone, lidocaine, magnesium sulfate*, and *sodium bicarbonate* and are listed in Table 9.2. Current ACLS recommendations do not require dosing adjustment according to route of administration, and all of these medications can be given by the intraosseous (IO), peripheral intravenous (PIV), or central venous catheter (CVC) routes.

Table 9.2 Medications recommended by Advanced Cardiac Life Support (ACLS) guidelines for the management of OHCA [12, 13]

Drug	Indication	Drug class	Mechanism	Dosing
Epinephrine	Pulseless arrest	α-adrenergic agonist	Vasoconstriction (increases venous return and preload)	1 mg every 3–5 minutes
Vasopressin	Pulseless arrest	Non-adrenergic vasoconstrictor	Vasoconstriction (increases venous return and preload)	40 units to *replace* the first or second dose of epinephrine, one time only
Amiodarone	Refractory or recurrent lethal arrhythmia	Non-selective cation blocker (Class III-A recommendation)	Sodium, potassium, and calcium channel antagonism (anti-arrhythmic properties)	300 mg bolus followed by 150 mg 3–5 minutes later
Lidocaine	Refractory or recurrent lethal arrhythmia	Anti-arrhythmic (Class II-B recommendation)	Sodium channel blocker (anti-arrhythmic properties)	1–1.5 mg/kg (increase dosage by 0.5 mg/kg in 5-minute intervals until a max dose of 3 mg/kg is reached)
Magnesium sulfate	Hypomagnesemia or *torsade de pointes* cardiac arrest	Electrolyte supplementation/ anti-arrhythmic (Class II-B recommendation)	Sodium and potassium transport co-factor (anti-arrhythmic properties)	1–2 gm bolus diluted via 10 mL D_5W
Sodium bicarbonate	Metabolic acidosis	Alkalizing agent (Class III recommendation)	Increases blood pH (reduces acidosis)	1 mEq/kg

Generally, resuscitation drugs should be delivered within the first 10 seconds of a new round of CPR [12, 13]. Due to reduced cardiac output and the inefficiency of venous return during cardiac arrest, resuscitative medications may require up to 90–120 seconds to reach central circulation, depending upon the route of administration.

Epinephrine (Adrenaline)

The early administration of epinephrine for the treatment of cardiac arrest has been shown to increase the likelihood of achieving ROSC, although it may not lead to improved 30-day outcomes [14]. Nonetheless, epinephrine is currently recommended as a first-line medication to stimulate ROSC in patients presenting with a non-shockable rhythm (Class 1 recommendation) in the most recent AHA guidelines update [13]. Despite widespread adoption of the use of epinephrine to treat cardiac arrest, the dosing, timing, and frequency of epinephrine administration for cardiac arrest remain controversial. Although high-dose (e.g., 5–10 mg) bolus doses of epinephrine have been recommended in the past, the current recommendation is for epinephrine to be provided in aliquots of 1 mg every 3–5 minutes [13].

There is evidence in a canine model that subsequent doses of epinephrine exert a lessening effect on myocardial contractility without diminishing the drug's effect on arterial blood pressure. This phenomenon is termed "differential tachyphylaxis" and may have implications for the use of epinephrine in the treatment of cardiac arrest [15]. The potential benefit of epinephrine infusion appears to be integrally linked to the timing of its administration. In a rat model, one study showed that 100% of subjects survived if CPR was initiated within 2 minutes of cardiac arrest, regardless of the use of epinephrine. However, when CPR was 6 minutes after cardiac arrest, only 32% of subjects achieved ROSC with compressions alone, while 81% of subjects receiving epinephrine achieved ROSC [16].

While epinephrine use does appear to increase the rate of ROSC in cardiac arrest patients presenting with unshockable rhythms, this benefit may not universally translate to improved survival-to-hospital discharge, favorable neurologic outcomes, or other desirable outcomes. In 1998, the OTAC Study Group reported an association between the use of epinephrine and increased mortality for in-hospital cardiac arrest (IHCA) patients, although this study excluded anyone who presented more than 15 minutes after the onset of cardiac arrest, and the mean time from onset of CPR to first dose of epinephrine was more than 5 minutes (5.14 ± 6.9 min) even in those who survived to 1 hour [17]. In fact, the authors found similar poor outcomes for all of the other studied ACLS drugs (i.e., atropine, bicarbonate, calcium, lidocaine, bretylium) [17]. It seems unlikely that these results can be directly translated to an out-of-hospital cardiac arrest population, especially when the "down time" (i.e., time from the onset of cardiac arrest to the initiation of chest compressions and other interventions) is unknown.

Results from the PARAMEDIC-2 trial suggest that the use of epinephrine in OHCA patients leads to improved ROSC and 30-day survival (when compared to placebo) but is not associated with improved survival with favorable neurologic outcomes, since more survivors from the epinephrine group in this study experienced severe neurologic impairment [3]. Thus, it seems that epinephrine has a time-dependent effect, with little benefit seen in the first few minutes following cardiac arrest, followed by a period of unknown duration in which it may increase the likelihood of ROSC but may not offer long-term survival benefit or increase the likelihood of survival with a favorable neurologic outcome. It remains to be discovered whether the unfavorable outcomes associated with the use of epinephrine in OHCA are related to uncorrectable ischemic injuries or, perhaps more likely, are due to inadequacies in current post-cardiac arrest management.

While the importance of epinephrine infusion to realization of ROSC appears to be increased with prolonged durations of cardiac arrest, a paradoxical myocardial epinephrine response also appears to exist, with epinephrine infusion given later in the treatment of OHCA also contributing to greater post-ROSC myocardial suppression [16].

In his original investigation of the IO route for epinephrine administration in animal models, Macht noted that aqueous solutions of epinephrine were absorbed just as quickly via IO as PIV routes. Effects on heart rate and blood pressure were also similar in duration. However, suspensions of epinephrine in oil showed a significantly longer duration of pressor effect. He speculated that these oil emulsions remained in the marrow for a long time and "act as reservoirs for a drug that is slowly liberated and dispensed by the oil." [18]

Spivey and colleagues [19] observed that IO epinephrine at standard IV doses (0.01 mg/ kg) had no significant effect on diastolic or mean blood pressure in an anaesthetized swine model. Higher doses (0.1 mg/kg) produced a more pronounced effect on blood pressure. One recent study showed that early IO epinephrine leads to better neurological outcomes than delayed IV epinephrine in a swine model of prolonged ventricular fibrillation [20].

Although studies in human subjects are lacking, animal models have been developed which appear to suggest a difference in the timing and maximum concentration of epinephrine realizable from PIV versus IO infusion of epinephrine. While no difference has been shown between the appearance of epinephrine administered via sternal IO and PIV into the central circulation, tibial IO delivery of the drug appears to be delayed when compared to these more proximal infusion sites [21]. Furthermore, the maximum concentration of epinephrine realized with IV infusion of 1 mg epinephrine appears to be 5.87 and 2.86 times greater than with tibial IO and sternal IO infusion, respectively [21]. The results of this and other studies suggest that larger doses of epinephrine may be warranted with IO infusion [22], although current ACLS recommendations assume that the 1 mg IO dose is equivalent to the 1 mg IV dose.

Vasopressin

This medication is recommended as an alternative vasopressor to epinephrine, currently recommended to replace the first or second dose of epinephrine.

Amiodarone

During resuscitative efforts, amiodarone may terminate lethal arrhythmias unresponsive to high-quality CPR and electrical defibrillation. In two randomized, double-blind, placebo-controlled trials – the ARREST [23] and ALIVE trials [24] – amiodarone demonstrated improved survival-to-hospital admission when compared to lidocaine and placebo, respectively, for the use of shock refractory ventricular fibrillation (VF) or pulseless ventricular tachycardia (pVT) in OHCA. Although these trials did not show improvement in favorable neurological outcome or survival-to-hospital discharge, they were not powered to assess for these outcomes.

One recent secondary analysis of a randomized, placebo-controlled trial of anti-arrhythmic drug infusion to terminate shock-refractory VF/pVT in the prehospital setting suggested improved hospital discharge survival and other important clinical outcomes among patients who received IV amiodarone or lidocaine, when compared to those who received IO infusion of the same dose of medication [25]. Of note, the vast majority of subjects in this study received tibia 1 IO cannulation, and all subjects received standard drug dosing regardless of route of infusion.

Lidocaine

Lidocaine has not been shown to be associated with improved neurological outcomes or survival in OHCA due to refractory ventricular fibrillation or pulseless VT, when compared to amiodarone or placebo [23]. However, it may be considered if amiodarone is not available.

Magnesium Sulfate

The use of magnesium sulfate for the treatment of a presenting *torsades de pointes* rhythm has been shown to be effective, as reported in two trials [26, 27]. However, the routine administration of magnesium sulfate during cardiac arrest is not recommended unless this cardiac rhythm is identified.

Sodium Bicarbonate

Sodium bicarbonate may help to restore metabolic homeostasis by reducing the metabolic acidosis caused by inadequate peripheral blood flow during cardiac arrest. Analysis of results from the Brain Resuscitation Clinical Trial III showed that earlier and more frequent use of sodium bicarbonate was associated with higher rates of early resuscitation and better long-term outcomes [28]. Early restoration of oxygen content, tissue perfusion, and cardiac output with a combination of high-quality chest compressions and effective ventilation may also help to restore the acid-base imbalance. However, providers should be aware that high-quality chest compressions alone only achieve a blood pressure about one-third of the native blood pressure, and this may be inadequate to ensure optimal perfusion of the vital organs. Thus, even patients receiving appropriate optimal chest compressions may not realize normalization of their blood acid-base balance with external cardiac compressions alone.

While normal blood pH is between 7.35 and 7.45, cardiac arrest patients often present with profound acidosis (pH < 7.35). Depending upon the etiology of the cardiac arrest, the acidosis could be due to respiratory causes (e.g., hypoventilation with carbon dioxide retention), metabolic causes (e.g., lactic acid accumulation due to hypoxic shunting toward anaerobic metabolism), or both. Unfortunately, profound acidosis (pH < 6.80) causes severe direct myocardial depression [29] and limits the ability of epinephrine to increase myocardial contractile force [15]. In fact, the effect of exogenous (and likely endogenous) epinephrine on contractile force becomes progressively worse as the pH descends [15]. Thus, reversing acidosis early in the course of the patient's management should be a goal of early cardiac arrest resuscitation. Although sodium bicarbonate infusion can increase the pH transiently, permanent correction of the acidosis will depend on a variety of factors, including ROSC, the restoration of adequate intravascular fluid volume, reversal of carbon dioxide retention, and correction of ongoing tissue ischemia.

Intravenous fluids (e.g., lactated Ringer's or normal saline solution) should also be considered a medication for purposes of OHCA management, as patients with hypovolemia may require rehydration in order to restore homeostasis. It is also likely that IV fluids help to restore normal acid-base balance, thereby improving the serum pH and increasing the likelihood that exogenous epinephrine and other cardioactive medications are able to exert their effects.

Several pharmacokinetic studies in animal models have shown that medications given via IO had the same efficacy as medications given with the IV route [30]. However, other studies have suggested that epinephrine dosing may need to be higher with IO infusion than with PIV infusion [19]. Whatever the proper dose, many previous studies have suggested efficacy for the IO infusion of epinephrine [31–40].

Other medications that have been given via the IO route for the treatment of cardiac arrest include *atropine* [32, 33, 35, 36, 39], *calcium chloride* [34, 35, 38], *dextrose* [35], and *lidocaine* [35, 37].

Location Matters

Burgert et al. conducted a randomized study to assess pharmacokinetics of epinephrine administered using tibial IO, sternal IO, and peripheral IV in a porcine model of cardiac arrest [21]. This group found that the more distal the insertion site, the slower the epinephrine reached maximum concentrations. Similarly, Vorhees et al. found in a dog CPR model that there is extensive central blood flow redistribution during CPR, resulting in significant reductions in arterial blood flow to the abdominal organs [41]. Extrapolating these findings to the extremities of man, one would expect that perfusion to the distal parts of the extremities (especially the lower extremities) should be lower (with less venous return) than the more proximal portions of the extremities. In other words, the closer a VAD is placed to the heart and central vessels, the more medication will likely find its way to the heart. It has been well-established that cardiac output and resulting systolic blood pressure are only about *one-third* of normal levels during CPR [42, 43]. Thus, peripheral veins (and the IO spaces drained by them) are likely to be poorly perfused with reduced venous return during CPR. This disadvantage is likely progressively worsened as the insertion site is moved more distally from the central circulation.

Previous studies performed on human subjects echo these findings from animal studies. In one study comparing peripheral to central venous infusion of Cardio-Green® dye in adult human cardiac arrest victims undergoing CPR, the authors sampled blood from the right femoral artery every 30 seconds during 5 minutes of closed chest compressions [44]. They found that dye injections given through an antecubital PIV were associated with no dye appearance at the femoral artery until more than 60 seconds after infusion. In fact, the concentration of dye recovered following antecubital PIV infusion was negligible even at the conclusion of the 5-minute study period. Conversely, the concentration of dye noted 30 seconds after central venous infusion was four times greater than the highest concentration ever achieved following PIV infusion [44]. These findings led the study authors to conclude that central venous infusion of ACLS medications is far superior to PIV infusion, suggesting that central venous access should be the standard of care for CA management. However, since the blood sampling site in this study was located at the femoral artery (well below the diaphragm), the lack of dye appearance in the PIV samples may represent the combined effect of impaired venous return from the upper extremity as well as impaired perfusion of the lower extremities during CPR.

Selection of Vascular Access Device

The current ACLS guidelines for the establishment of emergent vascular access for OHCA patients appears to be based primarily upon anecdotal evidence, with PIV access prioritized as the gold standard for immediate access, as "the pharmacokinetic properties, acute effects, and clinical efficacy of emergency drugs have primarily been described when given intravenously" [1]. This seemingly historical basis for the preference of PIV infusion of medications, combined with conflicting evidence on the equivalency of IO versus PIV infusion dosing, has led to significant disagreement within the scientific community on whether or not IO infusion is truly equivalent to IV dosing of commonly utilized OHCA medications.

In the absence of adequate conflicting evidence, the IO infusion of equivalent doses of resuscitative medications has been endorsed, "if attempts at intravenous accesss are unsuccessful or not feasible" [1]. But this guidance fails to provide the emergent vascular access specialist with usable guidance on precisely when and how IO or other alternative vascular access methods should be utilized when PIV access appears to be unobtainable. At present, emergent vascular access specialists

Table 9.3 Comparison of different VADs commonly used for OHCA management

	PIV	CVC	IO
Insertion	Varying degree of difficulty	Time-consuming; may require advanced level provider	Rapid, simple insertion
Medication Delivery	All ACLS meds	All ACLS meds	All ACLS meds
Dosing	Standard	Standard	Presumed standard
Duration of use	Long term	Long term	Short term (<48 hrs)
Representative Complications	Delayed placement, extravasation	Delayed placement, pneumothorax, hematoma, arterial placement	Dislodgement, extravasation

are left to decide for themselves when this apparent threshold marking the inability to obtain PIV access has been realized.

Despite this lack of guidance, we suggest that many factors should be taken into account during the selection of a VAD for OHCA management. These factors include *speed* of placement, anticipated *success* of placement, likely *complications*, *adequacy* of the line for present and *future vascular access needs*, and potential need for *dosing adjustments*. Table 9.3 provides a brief comparison of the various VAD options available to the emergency care provider when establishing emergent vascular access for OHCA.

Speed of Access

The first priority to consider in selecting a VAD for OHCA is how quickly the provider can achieve successful placement. When feasible, it is suggested that *multiple care providers attempt VAD placement simultaneously* on the same patient. Although this approach may be more labor-intensive, a simultaneous collateral approach to obtaining vascular access is likely to yield useable vascular access more rapidly than a linear single-provider technique. This competitive approach may also yield multiple useable VADs for the patient, allowing the delivery of multiple drugs or fluid boluses simultaneously. In general, IO access appears to be most rapidly accomplished in the setting of OHCA management, requiring less than 2 minutes, as compared to PIV or CVC placement [24, 45, 46].

First-Attempt Success Rates

A randomized, controlled trial comparing the effectiveness of PIV with proximal tibial IO (PTIO) and proximal humeral IO (PHIO) insertion demonstrated that PTIO insertion is more likely to be successful on the first attempt (91% PTIO, 51% PHIO, 43% PIV) with time to successful placement significantly shorter for this approach (4.6 min, versus 7.0 min for PHIO, and 5.8 min with PIV) [47]. However, utilizing current ACLS guidelines for medication dosing, patients who receive a

PIV versus an IO insertion appear to be more likely to achieve ROSC (55.5% vs. 43.6%, $p < 0.001$) and likely have improved survival-to-hospital discharge rates (22.8% vs. 14.9%, $p = 0.003$) when compared to those who receive PTIO insertion [48]. Thus, the clinical benefits of improved first-attempt success rates for PTIO insertion may be compromised by the apparent reduced efficacy of standard IV/IO dosing for resuscitative medications.

Future Directions for OHCA Research

The urgent need for head-to-head prospective comparisons between PIV and IO access for OHCA patients cannot be overstated. At present, guidelines for the establishment of vascular access in OHCA appear to be based almost entirely upon anecdotal and profoundly limited data. Prospective studies comparing important clinical outcomes for patients randomized to PIV or IO at the time of prehospital or early emergency department presentation for OHCA will be required to clearly identify any potential advantage to one vascular access technique or another. Considering the conflicting evidence that exists for the equivalency of PIV and IO dosing, additional research is also needed to determine if IO dosing should reasonably be assumed to be equivalent to PIV dosing. Current evidence suggests consistently that IO dosing may need to be greater than PIV dosing, especially if providers wish to continue utilizing subdiaphragmatic IO insertion sites. The importance of simultaneous crystalloid fluid infusion during OHCA resuscitation to improve the circulation of medications infused from the lower extremities also appears to be warranted. We suggest that supradiaphragmatic (i.e., humeral, sternal) IO insertion sites should be prioritized in such studies and that they should be compared with upper extremity PIV insertion sites.

An Algorithmic Approach to VAD Placement for OHCA

Given the relative dearth of clear guidance on the timing and preference of vascular access techniques currently offered by authorities on the topic, the emergency vascular access specialist is left, to some degree, to weigh the relative indications and contraindications of each vascular access technique on its own merits with each vascular access episode. *Peripheral intravenous access appears to be the optimal form of vascular access, when it is viewed to be readily available and adequate for therapy by the provider.* That said, the provider must determine for him or herself whether PIV access is actually feasible, and this assessment appears to depend upon a myriad of considerations. Given the immediate need for vascular access in the setting of OHCA, we propose that the inability to immediately (e.g., within 30 seconds) achieve PIV access should imply the need to consider IO insertion, preferably at the proximal humeral or sternal IO insertion site. Proximal tibial IO insertion (or other lower extremity IO insertion sites) should be considered suboptimal to more proximal IO insertion sites and should only be considered when more proximal IO or PIV insertion sites are not felt to be available for cannulation.

Conclusions

Out-of-hospital cardiac arrest is a unique clinical condition, which requires careful attention to the need for immediate vascular access to allow for stabilization and resuscitation of the patient. Although current ACLS recommendations do not provide adequate guidance for VAD selection in this context, the peripheral intravenous route is currently endorsed as the gold standard for emergent vascular access with OHCA. When PIV access is not felt to be immediately available, other forms of vascular access, including IO and CVC placement, should be considered. Dosing considerations remain unclear, especially whether IO dosing is truly equivalent to PIV dosing for commonly utilized resuscitative medications. Future prospective research comparing IO to PIV cannulation in the prehospital and early emergency department setting is needed to determine whether the route of vascular access selected for OHCA management is likely to influence important clinical OHCA outcomes.

Key Points
- The gold standard technique for obtaining emergent vascular access in the setting of OHCA remains peripheral intravenous cannulation.
- Intraosseous cannulation should be considered when PIV cannulation is deemed to be inadequate or unavailable by the emergency care provider.
- Current IO dosing may be inadequate, when compared to standard PIV dosing, at achieving adequate serum concentrations of epinephrine and other commonly used medications.
  - Cardiac arrest management is highly time-sensitive, underscoring the need for early and rapid venous access.
  - Sternal and proximal humeral IO catheters provide superior access to the central circulation during cardiac arrest, when compared to peripheral (e.g., tibial) IO access sites.
  - Volume infusion of crystalloid fluids with pressure bag likely improves the delivery and distribution of resuscitative medications during cardiac arrest, especially when introduced via the IO or PIV route.
- Emergent vascular access providers should utilize their own clinical acumen in assessing the need for PIV versus other forms of vascular access in the treatment of OHCA.

References

1. Panchal AR, Bartos JA, Cabanas JG, et al. Part 3: adult basic and advanced life support. 2020 American Heart Association guidelines for cardiopulmonary resuscitation and emergency cardiovascular care. Circulation. 2020;142(Suppl2):S366–468.
2. Jacobs IG, Finn JC, Jelinek GA, et al. Effect of adrenaline on survival in out-of-hospital cardiac arrest: a randomised double-blind placebo-controlled trial. Resuscitation. 2011;82:1138–43.

3. Perkins GD, Ji C, Deakin CD, et al. A randomized trial of epinephrine in out-of-hospital cardiac arrest. N Engl J Med. 2018;379:711–21.

4. Halperin HR, Tsitlik JE, Gelfand M, et al. A preliminary study of cardiopulmonary resuscitation by circumferential compression of the chest with use of a pneumatic vest. N Engl J Med. 1993;329:762–8.

5. Weisfeldt ML, Becker LB. Resuscitation after cardiac arrest: a 3-phase time-sensitive model. JAMA. 2002;288:3035–8.

6. Hoek TLV, Becker LB, Shao Z, et al. Reactive oxygen species released from mitochondria during brief hypoxia induce preconditioning in cardiomyocytes. J Biol Chem. 1998;273:18092–8.

7. Hoek TLV, Becker LB, Shao ZH, et al. Preconditioning in cardiomyocytes protects by attenuating oxidant stress at reperfusion. Circ Res. 2000;86:541–8.

8. Cobb LA, Fahrenbruch CE, Olsufka M, Copass MK. Changing incidence of out-of-hospital ventricular fibrillation, 1980–2000. JAMA. 2002;288:3008–13.

9. Nolan JP, Perkins GD. Is there a role for adrenaline during cardiopulmonary resuscitation? Curr Opin Crit Care. 2013;19:169–74.

10. Kudenchuk PJ, Sandroni C, Drinhaus HR, et al. Breakthrough in cardiac arrest: reports from the 4th Paris international conference. Ann Intensive Care. 2015;5:22.

11. Cummins RO, Ornato JP, Thies WH, et al. Improving survival from sudden cardiac arrest: the "chain of survival" concept. A statement for health professionals from the Advanced Cardiac Life Support Subcommittee and the Emergency Cardiac Care Committee, American Heart Association. Circulation. 1991 May;83(5):1832–47.

12. Link MS, Berkow LC, Kudenchuk PJ, et al. Part 7: Adult Advanced Cardiovascular Life Support. 2015 American heart Association Guidelines Update for cardiopulmonary resuscitation and emergency cardiovascular care. Circulation. 2015;132(suppl 2):S444–64.

13. Panchal AR, Berg KM, Hirsch KG, et al. 2019 American Heart Association Focused Update on Advanced Cardiovascular Life Support: use of advanced airways, vasopressors, and extracorporeal cardiopulmonary resuscitation during cardiac arrest: an update to the American Heart Association guidelines for cardiopulmonary resuscitation and emergency cardiovascular care. Circulation. 2019;140:e881–94.

14. Hagihara A, Hasegawa M, Abe T, et al. Prehospital epinephrine use and survival among patients with out-of-hospital cardiac arrest. JAMA. 2012;307(11):1161–8.

15. Bendixen HH, Laver MB, Flacke WE. Influence of respiratory acidosis on circulatory effect of epinephrine in dogs. Circ Research. 1963;13(1):64.

16. Angelos MG, Butke RL, Panchal AR, et al. Cardiovascular reponse to epinephrine varies with increasing duration of cardiac arrest. Resuscitation. 2008;77:101–10.

17. Van Walraven C, Stiell IG, Wells GA, et al. Do advanced cardiac life support drugs increase resuscitation rates from in-hospital cardiac arrest? The OTAC Study Group. Ann Emerg Med. 1998;32(5):544–53.

18. Macht DI. Studies on intraosseous injection of epinephrine. Am J Physiol. 1943:269–72.

19. Spivey WH, Crespo SG, Fuhs LR, Schoffstall JM. Plasma catecholamine levels after intraosseous epinephrine administration in a cardiac arrest model. Ann Emerg Med. 1992;21(2):127–31.

20. Zuercher M, Kern KB, Indik JH, et al. Epinephrine improves 24-hour survival in a swine model of prolonged ventricular fibrillation demonstrating that early intraosseous is superior to delayed intravenous administration. Anesth Analg. 2011;112:884–90.

21. Burgert J, Gegel B, Loughren M, et al. Comparison of tibial intraosseous, sternal intraosseous, and intravenous routes of administration on pharmacokinetics of epinephrine during cardiac arrest: a pilot study. AANA J. 2012;80(4):S6–S10.

22. Burgert J, Gegel BT, Johnson D. The pharmacokinetics of intravenous, tibial intraosseous and sternal intraosseous epinephrine during cardiopulmonary resuscitation in a swine model of cardiac arrest. Minerva Med. 2014;105(2 Suppl 1):35.

23. Dorian P, Cass D, Schwartz B, et al. Amiodarone as compared with lidocaine for shock-resistant ventricular fibrillation. N Engl J Med. 2002;346(12):884–990.

24. Daya MR, Leroux BG, Dorian P, et al. Survival after intravenous versus intraosseous amiodarone, lidocaine, or placebo in out-of-hospital shock-refractory cardiac arrest. Circulation. 2020;141(3):188–98.

25. Kudenchuk PJ, Cobb LA, Copass MK, et al. Amiodarone for resuscitation after out-of-hospital cardiac arrest due to ventricular fibrillation. N Engl J Med. 1999;341(12):871–8.
26. Tzivoni D, Banai S, Schuger C, et al. Treatment of torsade de pointes with magnesium sulfate. Circulation. 1988;77:392–7.
27. Manz M, Pfeiffer D, Jung W, Lueritz B. Intravenous treatment with magnesium in recurrent persistent ventricular tachycardia. N Trends Arrhythmias. 1991;7:437–42.
28. Bar-Joseph G, Abramson NS, Kelsey SF, et al. Brain Resuscitation Clinical Trial III (BRCT III) Study Group: improved resuscitation outcome in emergency medical systems with increased usage of sodium bicarbonate during cardiopulmonary resuscitation. Acta Anaesthesiol Scand. 2005;49(1):6–15.
29. Thrower WB, Darby TD, Aldinger EE. Studies of the relationship between sympatho-adrenal function, acid-base derangements and ventricular contractile force. Surg Forum. 1960;10:535.
30. Von Hoff DD, Kuhn JG, Burris HA III, Miller LJ. Does intraosseous equal intravenous? A pharmacokinetic study. Am J Emerg Med. 2008;26(1):31–8.
31. Berg RA. Emergency infusion of catecholamines into bone marrow. Am J Dis Child. 1984;138(9):810–1.
32. McNamara RM, Spivey WH, Unger HD, Malone DR. Emergency applications of intraosseous infusion. J Emerg Med. 1987;5:97–101.
33. Spivey WH. Intraosseous infusions. J Pediatr. 1987;111:639–43.
34. Brunette DD, Fischer R. Intravenous access in pediatric cardiac arrest. Am J Emerg Med. 1998;6:577–9.
35. Glaeser PW, Hellmich TR, Szewczuga D, Losek JD, Smith DS. Five-year experience in pre-hospital intraosseous infusions in children and adults. Ann Emerg Med. 1993;22:1119–24.
36. Guy J, Haley K, Zuspan SJ. Use of intraosseous infusion in the pediatric trauma patient. J Ped Surg. 1993;28(2):158–61.
37. Davidoff J, Fowler R, Gordon D, et al. Clinical evaluation of a novel intraosseous device for adults: prospective, 250–patient, multi-center trial. JEMS. 2005;30(10):s20–3.
38. Fiorito BA, Mirza F, Doran TM, et al. Intraosseous access in the setting of pediatric critical care transport. Pediatr Crit Care Med. 2005;6(1):50–3.
39. Valdes M, Araujo P, de Andres C, et al. Intraosseous administration of thrombolysis in out-of-hospital massive pulmonary thromboembolism. Emerg Med J. 2010;27(8):641–4.
40. Gazin N, Auger H, Jabre P, et al. Efficacy and safety of the EZ-IO intraosseous device: out-of-hospital implementation of a management algorithm for difficult vascular access. Resuscitation. 2011;82:126–9.
41. Vorhees WD, Babbs CF, Tacker WA. Regional blood flow during CPR in dogs. Crit Care Med. 1980;8:134.
42. Del Guercio LRM, Coomarswamy RP, State D. Cardiac output and other hemodynamic variables during external cardiac massage in man. N Engl J Med. 1963;269:1398.
43. Oriol A, Smith HJ. Hemodynamic observations during cardiac massage. J Can Med Assoc. 1968;98:841.
44. Kuhn GJ, White BC, Swetnam RE, et al. Peripheral vs central circulation times during CPR: a pilot study. Ann Emerg Med. 1981;10(8):417–9.
45. Leidel BA, Kirchhoff C, Bogner V, et al. Comparison of intraosseous versus central venous vascular access in adults under resuscitation in the emergency department with inaccessible peripheral veins. Resuscitation. 2012;83(1):40–5.
46. Paxton JH, Knuth TE, Klausner HA. Proximal humerus intraosseous infusion: a preferred emergency venous access. J Trauma. 2009;67(3):606–11.
47. Reades R, Studnek JR, Vandeventer S, Garrett J. Intraosseous versus intravenous vascular access during out-of-hospital cardiac arrest: a randomized controlled trial. Ann Emerg Med. 2011;58(6):509–16.
48. Feinstein BA, Stubbs BA, Rea T, et al. Intraosseous compared to intravenous drug resuscitation in out-of-hospital cardiac arrest. Resuscitation. 2017;117:91–6.

Difficult Vascular Access

10

James H. Paxton, Bethanie Ann Szydlowski,
and Call G. Coddington

Introduction

Establishing and maintaining venous access is one of the most common, and arguably most important, practices in modern healthcare. Whether in the prehospital setting, the medical floor, or the intensive care unit, ready access to the venous circulatory system is essential for the administration of potentially life-saving intravenous fluids and medication. However, obtaining an emergent intravenous line can be difficult. This chapter will address common challenges that emergency care providers face in establishing venous access, including means by which these obstacles can be overcome.

Definition of DVA

Although *difficult vascular access (DVA)* lacks a universal definition, many authors have attempted to provide it. Fields et al. defined DVA as "at least 2 failed IV attempts, together with a lack of palpable or visible veins," characterizing DVA patients as frequently requiring "rescue" methods of vascular access, including ultrasound guidance, intraosseous access, or the cannulation of veins in atypical

J. H. Paxton (✉)
Department of Emergency Medicine, Wayne State University School of Medicine, Detroit, MI, USA
e-mail: james.paxton@wayne.edu

B. A. Szydlowski
Medline Industries, Inc., Mundelein, IL, USA
e-mail: BSzydlowski@medline.com

C. G. Coddington
Michigan State University College of Osteopathic Medicine, East Lansing, MI, USA
e-mail: codding9@msu.edu

© Springer Nature Switzerland AG 2021
J. H. Paxton (ed.), *Emergent Vascular Access*,
https://doi.org/10.1007/978-3-030-77177-5_10

peripheral locations such as the external jugular vein [1]. Another author has defined DVA as the presence of "non-visible and non-palpable veins, requiring a highly-experienced operator with the use of technological aids to insert a vascular device" [2]. Others consider DVA to be present when the provider realizes "three failed IV attempts or the anticipation of special interventions to secure vascular access" [3, 4]. Despite this lack of a strict definition, emergency care providers do appear to agree that DVA is a multifaceted problem, characterized by the need to consider nontraditional methods for venous access, especially after multiple failed attempts using standard techniques.

While an estimated 70–80% of all hospitalized patients ultimately require venous cannulation, most will not present a significant vascular access challenge to the experienced provider [3]. However, *patients presenting in extremis may not be able to tolerate delays in IV catheter insertion*. For this reason, we propose that any agreed-upon definition of "difficult vascular access" must account for the importance of *timing*. Under non-emergent conditions, adequate peripheral IV placement requires an average of 2.5 to 16 minutes to achieve [5, 6]. However, the management of critically ill patients often requires greater efficiency in the administration of IV fluids, blood products, and medications. When managing patients in the emergent setting, the wise clinician will *establish certain a priori expectations about the number and duration of failed IV attempts* that should be tolerated before considering alternative vascular access techniques.

Given the great importance of timing to the establishment of emergent vascular access, we propose that DVA be characterized in the emergent setting as *venous access efforts involving at least two failed PIV attempts over the course of at least 2 minutes, necessitating the use of alternative methods, including intraosseous or ultrasound-guided techniques*. Of course, the patient's vascular access history, clinical condition, and acuity of need for emergent infusion of fluids and medications, rather than any strict definition, should dictate the parameters of acceptable delay in obtaining venous access.

Risk Factors for Difficult Vascular Access

Difficult vascular access is not simply a feature of at-risk patients. Rather, it is a condition produced by *time constraints*, further influenced by *patient-specific*, *provider-specific*, and *environmental factors*. These factors are all interlinked with, and interdependent upon, the timing and acuity of the need for venous access. A systematic approach is suggested in exploring these relationships – one which highlights how DVA exists as a function of these four interrelated factors.

Instances of DVA may be attributed to any combination of the four named risk factors (i.e., timing, patient-specific, provider-specific, and environmental factors), or they can appear to relate to a single factor alone. But in the emergent setting, timing is *always* a central concern. The time required to obtain venous access is paramount in the management of deteriorating patients, because failure to rapidly obtain usable venous access generally translates to delays in administering potentially life-saving fluids and medications. As Fig. 10.1 illustrates, the time required for venous access both influences and is influenced by the other three DVA risk factors. Minimizing or eliminating each of these factors in the care of the emergent patient will help to decrease time-to-cannulation and streamline efforts toward patient resuscitation and stabilization.

Of the named factors, we suggest that *time constraints* may have the greatest effect on the appearance and severity of DVA. Under non-emergent conditions, with more time available to consider and investigate vascular access options, the influence of the other three DVA factors may appear to be insignificant. Factors such as provider inexperience, lack of visible patient veins, or environmental distractions can all be corrected or addressed given adequate time. But the critically ill patient's need for immediate vascular access imparts a sense of urgency to providers. This urgency may reveal deficits in provider competence under pressure or may expose other obstacles that might appear insurmountable in the "heat of the moment." Thus, difficult or failed attempts to provide emergent venous access can teach us to improve our techniques, by revealing deficiencies or flaws in our approach. In this way, patients with DVA may be the "canaries in the coal mine" for providers, as they reveal our competence, and sometimes our incompetence, in securing venous access for the undifferentiated patient. In addition to the personal challenge that DVA patients present to care providers, these patients can also present a challenge to institutions, by diverting time, attention, and other resources away from other

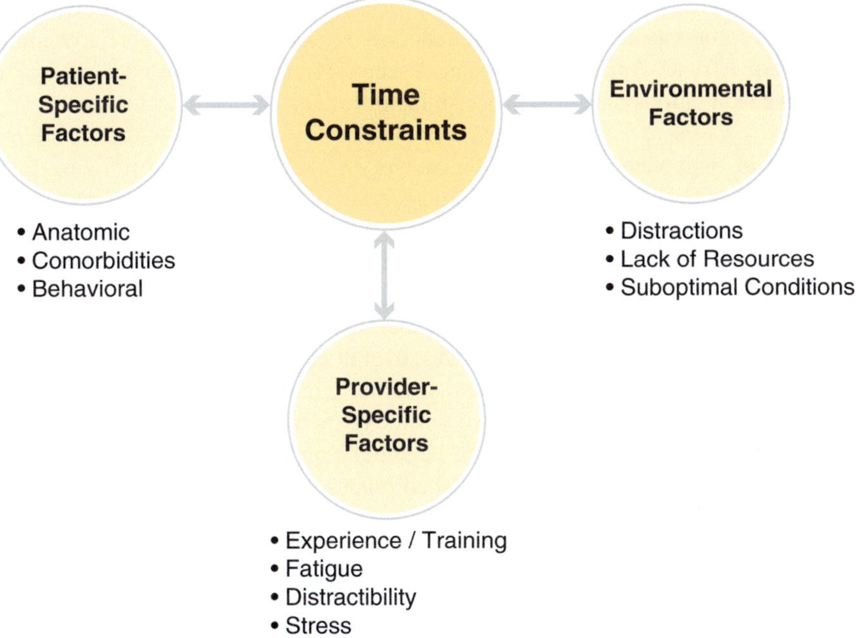

Fig. 10.1 Factors contributing to difficult vascular access

patients. This can lead to increased morbidity, expense, and other costs to all patients in the care environment, not just those patients experiencing DVA [7].

Patient-Specific Causes of DVA

Specific patient characteristics may predict the presence of DVA and should be considered. Traits such as obesity, skin color, age, gender, and anatomic variation (among others) have all been shown to be associated with DVA. Chronically ill patients who have been subjected to repeated vascular access attempts accumulate anatomic and physiologic changes to their veins and surrounding soft tissues that can influence future access attempts. Even presumably healthy individuals presenting under emergent conditions can challenge providers with unique vascular anatomy or other unexpected patient-specific factors. Of course, certain patient characteristics may be more likely to predict DVA than others. Poor vein visibility and palpability have been shown to be a major predictor of PIV insertion failure [8–12]. Other patient-specific factors, such as previous cannulation failure, obesity, and small vein caliber, have also been shown to exhibit statistically significant DVA odds ratios in individual studies [8–12].

Vein Visibility

Poor vein visibility is often cited as a major contributor to DVA [1, 2, 8, 9, 13, 14]. Dark skin color appears to contribute to decreased vein visibility, especially among patients of African-American or Asian descent [15, 16]. The presence of dark or extensive skin tattoos may also be a risk factor for DVA for similar reasons.

Many *vascular access support devices (VASDs)* have been developed to address the issue of poor vein visibility. One category of VASDs is those utilizing light-emitting diode (LED) transillumination or infrared light to highlight venous topography. These devices allow the provider to visualize deep or obscured veins that would normally remain hidden. Despite claims of their effectiveness, VASDs are not routinely used in clinical practice [17, 18]. This lack of widespread interest may be due, in part, to conflicting evidence of their usefulness. While VASDs do appear to improve first-attempt PIV success rates, overall efficacy within the general population appears to be equal to standard external landmarking techniques [19–24]. These devices may be more effective with DVA pediatric patients than with non-DVA patients [25]. Unfortunately, the potential benefits of VASDs for adult DVA patients remain unclear, as most published reports have focused on their use with infants and children [21, 24, 26].

Near-infrared (NIR) light or transillumination devices are a common type of VASD used to enhance vein visibility [27]. The AccuVein® AV500 (Accuvein, Inc.) (Fig. 10.2) and VeinViewer® (Christie Medical Holdings) NIR devices are well-suited for emergency care providers, as they do not require a dark environment for their use and are handheld and easily portable [21, 24, 27, 28].

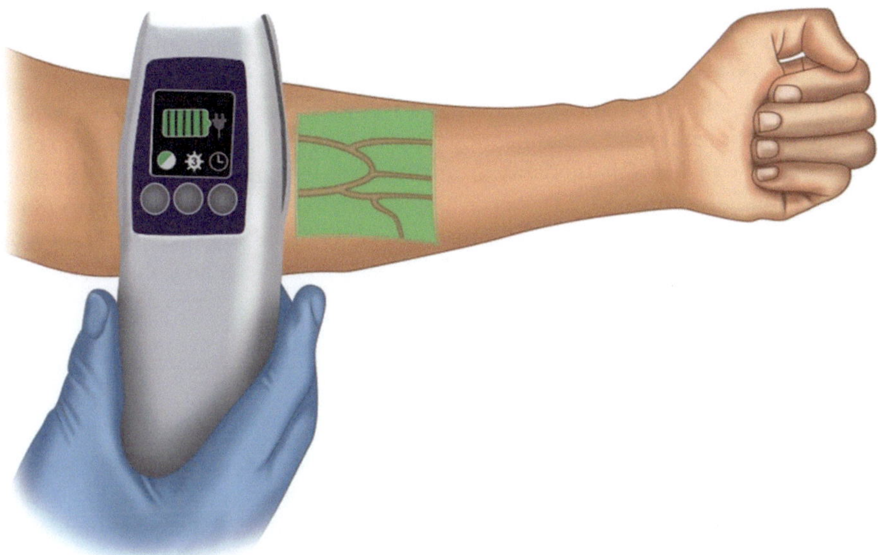

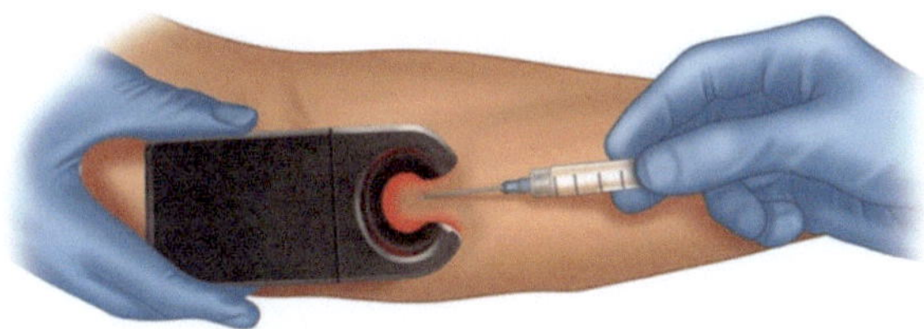

Fig. 10.2 AccuVein AV500®. (Image courtesy of Accuvein, Inc. © 2020 Accuvein, Inc. All rights reserved)

Fig. 10.3 Veinlite LED+®. (Image courtesy of TransLite, LLC. © 2020 TransLite, LLC. All rights reserved)

Light-emitting diode (LED) or white light transillumination devices, such as the Veinlite® (TransLite, LLC), Illumivein® (Easy-RN, LLC), and Venoscope® (Venoscope) systems, allow the provider to evaluate vein diameter and depth more easily than with infrared light, and their ease of use allegedly precludes the need for practical training [21, 24, 27, 28]. The Veinlite LED+® (Fig. 10.3) has been shown to enhance clinical PIV cannulation success rates and can be operated without the need for a second provider [21, 24]. When using the Veinlite LED+®, providers place the device directly on the skin and scan side-to-side, perpendicular to the direction of venous flow [29]. Once a target vein is identified, the device should be rotated 90 degrees so that the mouth of the device surrounds the desired vein [29]. During cannulation, the clinician holds the device in the nondominant hand and presses the device against the patient's skin. This gentle traction helps to prevent the vein from rolling while simultaneously raising the vein closer to the skin surface [27, 29]. Cannulation is then achieved using a needle-syringe complex held in the provider's dominant hand.

Ultrasound (US) guidance is another useful adjunct to peripheral line placement in the emergent setting [2, 30, 31]. The use of ultrasound to identify target vessels allows for the visualization of both arteries and veins beneath the skin and may improve first-attempt IV success rates [32]. This modality can be utilized for either central or peripheral venous cannulation [32, 33]. Several authors suggest that clinicians should consider this modality as an effective first-line solution after repeated IV insertion failures [2, 30, 31]. According to the Michigan Appropriateness Guide for Intravenous Catheters (MAGIC) recommendations, ultrasound should be used for peripheral IV catheter placement in DVA patients and can be utilized as a route for PICC introduction later in therapy, as needed [34].

Venous Cutdown

Venous cutdown (Fig. 10.4) is an invasive procedure involving the cannulation of a target vein using direct visualization following placement of a skin incision overlying the target insertion site. Venous cutdown of a central (e.g., external jugular) or

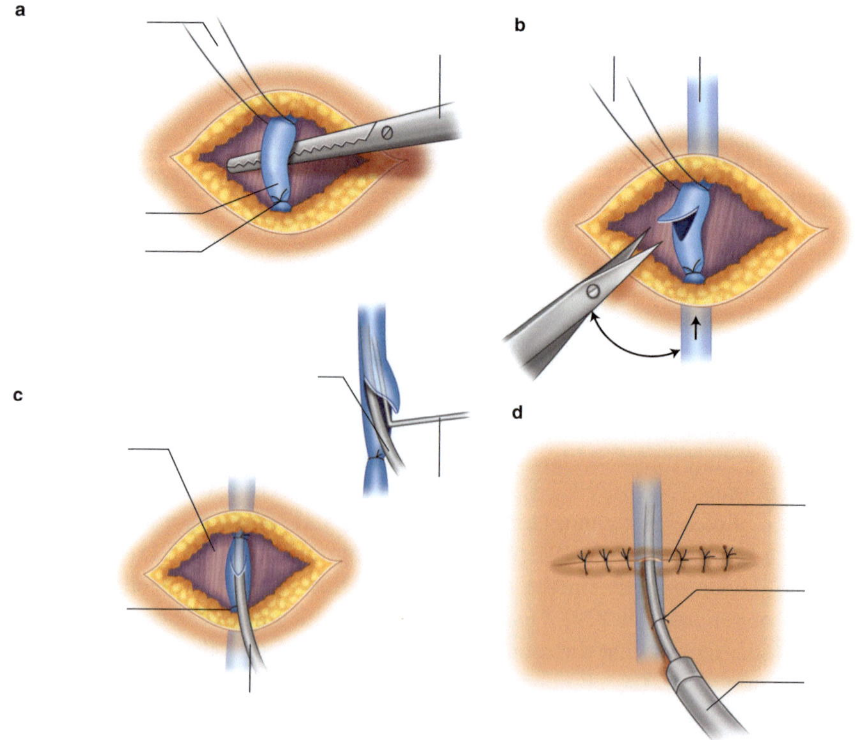

Fig. 10.4 Peripheral venous cutdown technique, including (**a**) identification and isolation of the target vessel, (**b**) venotomy, (**c**) catheter insertion and proximal vessel ligation, and (**d**) repair of skin incision and securement of the catheter

peripheral (e.g., great saphenous) vein is an efficient, though often overlooked, method to secure venous access [35–37]. Venous cutdowns were first described by Keeley and Kirkham in the 1940s, and were employed extensively during the Vietnam War, but in the modern era are typically reserved for critically ill polytrauma patients refractory to ultrasound, intraosseous, and percutaneous central venous intervention [35, 37–42]. This procedure carries a high risk of complications yet remains an effective method of acquiring venous access in patients who are in dire need of life-saving infusions [37, 40, 41].

The technique for venous cutdown is depicted in Fig. 10.4. A tourniquet is applied to the extremity and the cutdown site is sterilized thoroughly. As depicted in Fig. 10.4a, an incision is then made through the skin overlying the vein, and the vein is isolated from the surrounding tissues. During the procedure, two ligatures (e.g., vicryl sutures) are placed around the vein. The distal ligature will be used to tie off the vein, and the proximal ligature will be used to help keep the catheter in the vein. Even after the ligatures are tied off, the ends of the sutures should be kept long until the end of the procedure, as they can be used to elevate the vessel and aid in vessel manipulation. A hemostat can be placed under the vein to further elevate the vessel. The vein is ligated distal to the planned catheter insertion site utilizing the distal suture. As shown in Fig. 10.4b, the vein is then incised with pointed scissors, creating a "V-shaped" incision in the vessel wall. This incision should not be more than half of the vein circumference in length, and scissors are best held at a 45-degree angle relative to the plane of the vessel. The vein must be held gently, especially after it is cut as the vessel may tear with excessive manipulation. A fine-pointed scalpel can be used if small sharp scissors are not available. A catheter introducer is then placed under the venotomy flap, and the catheter is inserted into the vein. The catheter tip should be pointing in the direction of venous flow. As depicted in Fig. 10.4c, the proximal suture is then tied off, wrapping around the catheter while inside the vein, to secure the catheter's position. Once the proximal ligature has been tied off, the extremity tourniquet is released and the venotomy is observed to detect any bleeding. If no bleeding is detected, the suture ends may be cut short, and the skin wound may be closed with interrupted sutures (Fig. 10.4d). The catheter will then be sutured to the skin as well to prevent dislodgement. The catheter insertion site should then be covered with a sterile dressing and tape.

Vein Palpability

Inadequate vein palpability is another common contributor to DVA [1, 2, 8, 9, 13, 43, 44]. Palpability is largely determined by vessel diameter and depth [45]. Tourniquets placed around the extremity of interest are commonly used to overcome this obstacle, as they promote increased venous filling and provide vessel distension during the cannulation attempt. It should be noted that target vein diameter is highly correlated with two important patient characteristics: body habitus and volume status. Obese patients have larger-diameter vessels compared to non-obese patients, and the size of a patient's veins tends to increase with increasing body mass [46–48]. Intravascular blood volume is also important as a predictor of vein distensibility [1]. Hypervolemic patients, with high intravascular blood volume, exhibit distended veins, whereas patients with low intravascular volumes may have vascular collapse [49, 50]. For obvious reasons, a collapsed vein is a harder target. Being thin-walled vessels, veins are especially prone to collapse with external pressure, including the pressure exerted by overly aggressive providers compressing the target insertion site during cannulation attempts. It has been well-established that the appearance of a flat, small-diameter inferior vena cava on echocardiogram, ultrasound, or CT indicates the presence of hypovolemia in trauma and dialysis patients [51–53]. Consequently, venous cannulation is especially difficult in hypotensive, hypovolemic patients. It may be advisable to perform maneuvers known to increase venous distension (e.g., passive leg raise, Trendelenburg positioning) prior to venous cannulation attempts, to increase venous distension prior to cannulation attempts. Blood pressure is also influenced by intravascular volume, and may be increased in hypervolemia and decrease with volume depletion [54, 55]. Not surprisingly, increased vessel diameter is associated with an increased likelihood of successful cannulation [56].

Vein palpability is also predicted by the depth of the target vessel below the surface of the skin [45]. In general, deeper veins are less likely to be palpable, due to increased external pressure exerted by the weight of overlying soft tissues. It has been proposed that high BMI predicts a corresponding increase in vessel depth, due to excessive soft tissue thickness overlying potential target veins [57, 58]. This is a distinct problem for the medical community, as an estimated 160 million Americans are either obese or overweight [59]. Local fluid accumulation – as seen with peripheral edema and hematoma – also increases the distance between skin surface and vessel surface, thereby decreasing vein palpability [60].

Solutions to Enhance Vein Palpability

Topical Treatments

One effective approach to enhancing vein palpability is the application of *heat*. Local warming of the perivascular tissue has been shown to facilitate successful peripheral IV placement due to venous dilatation, engorging the veins to make them more susceptible to needle insertion [61–63]. This can be accomplished via the use of heating devices or warm compresses, with "active warming" proving superior to "passive insulation," regarding both insertion time and cannulation success rates [62]. The application of "dry" heat may be superior to moist heat for the purposes of IV placement – namely, dry towels, compresses, or heating pads in favor of moist towels, compresses, or heating pads [63, 64]. First-attempt IV success rates have been shown to more than double with application of dry heat, when compared to moist heat [63].

Topical application of *nitroglycerin ointment*, usually reserved for patients with cardiovascular syndromes, can also induce local venodilatation [65, 66]. However, transdermal absorption of nitroglycerin ointment also causes a decrease in mean arterial pressure and thoracic fluid content, outcomes that may be undesirable for patients presenting without cardiac complaints or hypotension [67]. Fortunately, the dose required for symptomatic treatment of angina is significantly larger than that required to induce peripheral venodilatation in the skin, cited as 1–2 milligrams, making nitroglycerin application for the purposes of peripheral cannulation a relatively safe endeavor [65].

Eutectic Mixture of Local Anesthetics (EMLA®) cream has been a staple in the management of pediatric patients undergoing painful peripheral needlesticks for decades [68–70]. Children (and adults) often experience significant fear and pain with repeated PIV attempts, activating the sympathetic nervous system and driving peripheral vasoconstriction, a clear obstacle to venous cannulation [62, 71, 72]. Although EMLA® cream has also been shown to induce a transient local cutaneous vasoconstriction, post-EMLA® application of heat or nitroglycerin ointment can counteract this effect [68–70, 73].

Tourniquets

As stated above, tourniquets facilitate venous palpation and allow for easier identification of superficial vessels. Although no consensus exists on a preferred method, the use of either a blood pressure cuff or an elastic tourniquet is commonly used to stimulate venous distension [74–76]. However, increased pressure may not necessarily yield improved results, as the use of two tourniquets (instead of a one) has not been associated with increased PIV cannulation success [77].

Alternative Site Infusion

Volume infusion into a peripheral vein stimulates vessel distension [78]. In patients with inaccessible peripheral veins, clinicians can utilize other modalities to increase intravascular volume and enhance peripheral vein palpability [79]. *Peritoneal* crystalloid infusion is one such method, leveraging capillary absorption within the peritoneal space to provide a steady state of fluid reabsorption into the bloodstream [80]. *Hypodermoclysis*, or subcutaneous saline injection, is another effective means of increasing blood volume without an IV line [81–83]. Neonates (within the first week of life) presenting with small-caliber veins or an excess of subcutaneous fat may also benefit from umbilical vein cannulation [84]. This procedure allows for infusion of medications and fluids directly into the inferior vena cava to improve peripheral venous distension and facilitate subsequent IV attempts [85].

Anatomic Variation of Veins

Although certain common anatomic patterns exist, providers will see great variation in the size, location, and depth of human veins. This inability to predict a patient's vascular anatomy with absolute certainty prior to the vascular access attempt may contribute to difficulties obtaining venous access [86].

For example, the *cubital fossa* of the upper extremity is generally considered the most common site for routine peripheral venipuncture in humans [87–91]. However, this area is also characterized by many highly variable superficial veins, namely, the *cephalic, basilic, median cubital,* and *antebrachial veins* [87, 88, 91]. The most common venous pattern encountered with cannulation of cubital fossa veins is the *"N"-shaped* arrangement. However, a common variation on this pattern is the *"Y"-shape*, in which the median antebrachial vein joins both the basilic and cephalic veins within the cubital fossa. The so-called *"M"-shaped* pattern presents in a minority of patients and looks generally like the more common N-shape, but with diminished or absent cephalic vein contribution [88, 91, 93–95]. A small number of patients also exhibit an *"I"-shaped* configuration of the cubital fossa, in which the cephalic and basilic veins ascend parallel to each other, lacking interconnecting vessels such as the median cubital or median antebrachial veins [88, 91, 93–95]. Still other patients may present with vein arrangements that cannot be classified into any of these categories. Illustrations of these four "named" variants of cubital fossa venous anatomy are provided in Fig. 10.5.

Hazardous Anatomic Structures

In addition to potential variations in the patient's venous anatomy, providers must be aware of specific anatomic structures that can interfere with, or otherwise complicate, venous access attempts. For example, injury to the *brachial artery* during an IV attempt at the cubital fossa will not only risk compromising blood flow to the distal extremity but can lead to hematoma formation due to arterial puncture which may decrease the palpability and visibility of adjacent veins. Prioritizing venous cannulation sites where such "hazardous" structures are less likely to be located will help the provider to prevent iatrogenic injury and likely improve the odds of success. In the cubital fossa, the "safest" venipuncture location (best avoiding potential nerve and arterial damage) is located at the confluence of the *cephalic* and *median cubital veins* [92, 96, 97]. This site is marked with a red "X" in Fig. 10.6, at the apex of a triangle formed by these veins.

The *brachial artery*, a continuation of the *axillary artery* below the lower margin of the *teres major* muscle, is the major blood vessel of the upper arm. This artery travels down the ventral surface of the arm until it reaches the cubital fossa at the elbow, where it divides into the *radial artery* and *ulnar artery*. Thus, injury to the brachial artery can be devastating to the blood supply of the distal upper extremity. The *median nerve*, originating from the brachial plexus in the axilla, initially descends the upper arm *lateral* to the brachial artery but crosses over the brachial artery near the distal attachment of the *coracobrachialis* muscle (at the mid-humerus level) to become situated *medial* to the brachial artery at the level of the cubital fossa. The median nerve is superficial to the elbow joint, just deep to several key venous targets, as illustrated in Fig. 10.7. Providers should be aware of these vital structures and their anatomic position at various levels within the arm and exercise caution with venous cannulation to avoid iatrogenic injury. As the median nerve

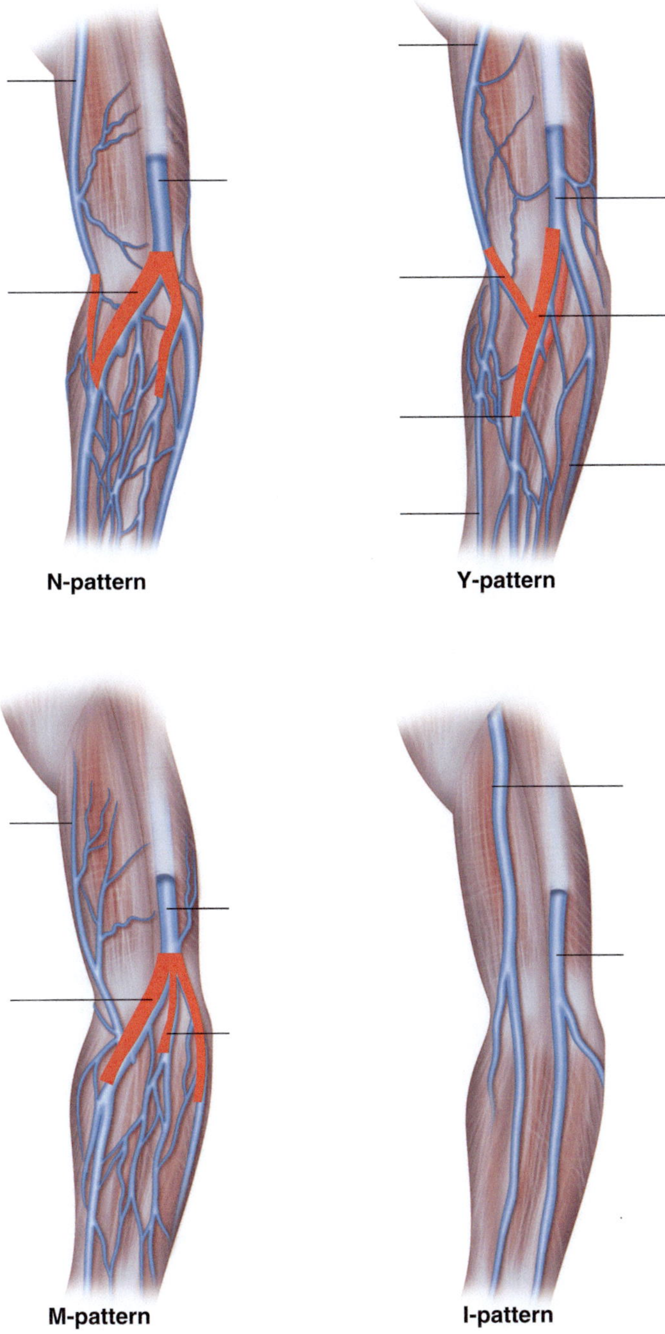

Fig. 10.5 Variations in the superficial venous anatomy of the cubital fossa

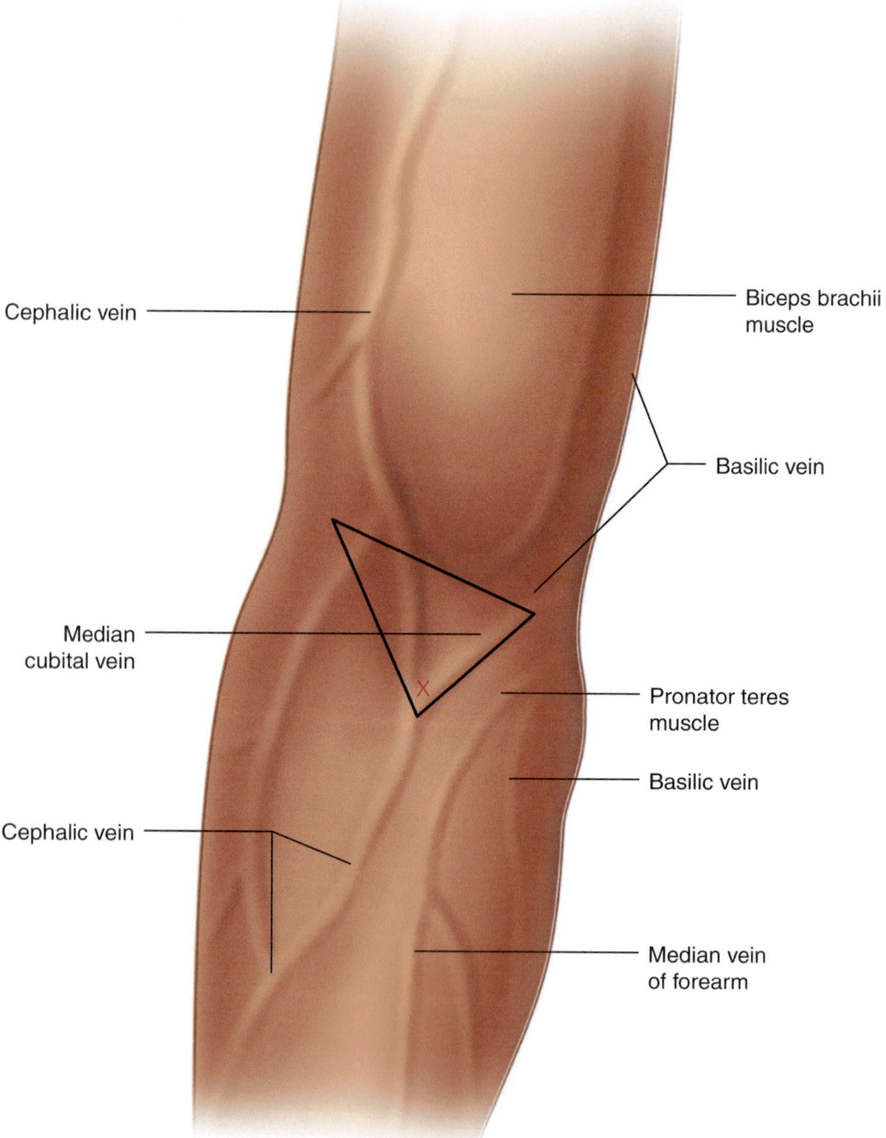

Fig. 10.6 Preferred "safe zone" for venous cannulation within the cubital fossa, at the confluence of the cephalic and median cubital veins

supplies motor function to many of the flexors of the forearm and intrinsic muscles of the hand, injury to the median nerve at the level of the forearm can lead to loss of pronation of the forearm and loss of flexion of the thumb and pointing finger.

Another anatomic feature contributing to DVA is the presence of *venous valves*, which are intraluminal flaps meant to facilitate the proper direction of blood flow returning to the heart [98, 99]. Without valves, venous blood would be more susceptible to the effects of gravity and would tend to accumulate in dependent portions of the body. However, if the tip of an intravenous catheter is situated next to such a valve, the valve can obstruct the lumen of the cannula and prevent the provider from drawing back blood through the catheter. This can confuse the matter of whether the vessel has been successfully cannulated. Although flushing the catheter with saline and confirming the absence of extravasation may alleviate the provider's fears, it is generally best to avoid target sites where valves are commonly encountered, such as venous branching points [9, 89]. Ultrasonography and color Doppler imaging can be used to detect the presence of valves within the superficial veins of the arm and forearm, as can near-infrared vein illumination devices [90, 100, 101]. When considering whether to cannulate the cephalic, basilic, or median cubital vein, it should be recalled that valves are most numerous in the *cephalic vein* [102]. Despite this finding, cephalic vein catheterization

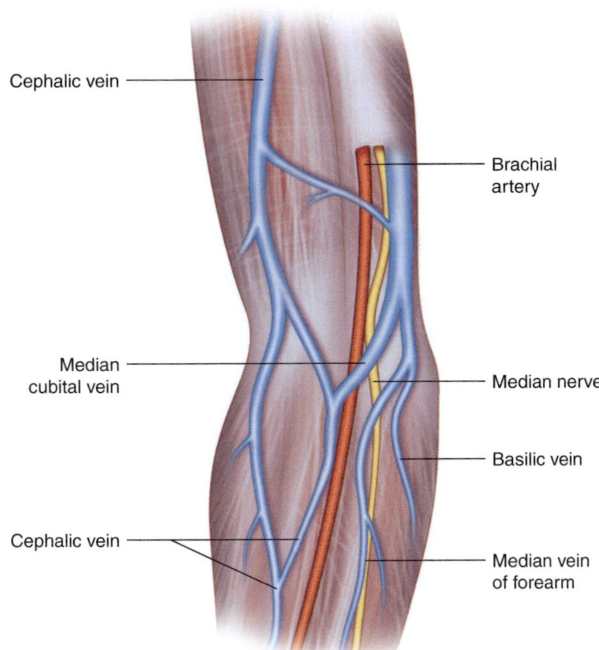

Fig. 10.7 Anatomic relationship between the brachial artery, median nerve, and common peripheral vein targets at the upper extremity

remains preferred over these other candidate veins, due to its relative distance from the subcutaneous nerves and arteries of the forearm [92, 96, 97]. Thus, it is important to consider the "whole picture" of venous anatomy when selecting a target vein or when troubleshooting a failed attempt.

Vessel Size

Vessel palpability is also a function of vessel size, and vein diameter ≤ 2 mm has been shown to be an independent risk factor for DVA [8]. Anticipated vein diameter also guides a clinician's selection of IV catheter gauge. It is recommended that "veins should be larger than twice the diameter of the catheter," to prevent occlusion of the vessel and maintain adequate blood flow around the intravenous catheter [90].

Patient body mass index (BMI) and biological sex can also predict vein diameter [3, 10, 46–48, 58, 90]. Genetic males, on average, possess larger-diameter central and peripheral veins than females, due to the physiologic need for enhanced venous drainage associated with increased muscle mass [47, 58, 90, 103]. Clinicians should target veins that consistently present >2–3 mm in diameter, as these vessels are associated with a high probability of first-attempt IV success [8]. Table 10.1 compares the average cross-sectional size of commonly accessed peripheral veins within the arm, wrist, hand, and foot.

When peripheral IV access cannot be secured, or when multiple attempts at peripheral cannulation could prove detrimental to patient status, providers should consider *central venous catheter (CVC)* placement. Central veins are large-diameter vessels that accommodate high-volume rapid fluid administration [118]. Experienced operators use palpable anatomic landmarks to guide cannulation of these veins in the acute setting, which may be preferred over repeated needlesticks at small-diameter peripheral veins [119]. The ideal CVC site has a low incidence of post-venipuncture complications and a high rate of insertion success [118]. However, available data suggest that there is no one "best" location for central venous access, as each vessel carries its own risks and benefits [120–122]. Table 10.2 highlights the diameters of central veins commonly used as alternatives to peripheral venous access [118, 120].

Table 10.1 Comparison of common peripheral vein diameters [89, 104–117]

Location	Vein	Average Diameter (mm)
Cubital Fossa	Cephalic	2.7
	Basilic	3.0
	Median cubital	3.1
Wrist	Cephalic	2.2
	Basilic	2.1
Hand	Dorsal metacarpals	1.1
Ankle	Great saphenous	2.7
	Lesser saphenous	1.5
Foot	Dorsal metatarsal	1.3

Table 10.2 Comparison of central vein diameters [103, 123–126]

Vessel	Average diameter (mm)
Internal jugular vein	16.5 (right)
	11.8 (left)
Subclavian vein	11.6
Femoral vein	10.3

Skin Characteristics

Skin toughness is an independent variable associated with the likelihood of failed peripheral venous cannulation [14, 15]. Tattoos and scarring both contribute to increased skin resistance to needle puncture, in addition to decreasing vein visibility [14]. Comorbidities or localized soft tissue conditions that affect skin thickness, such as scleroderma, cellulitis, and peripheral edema, should also be considered when deciding upon a site for peripheral venous cannulation.

The *modified Rodnan skin score (mRSS)* is used to evaluate skin thickness at different areas of the body [127]. Determination of skin thickness with this scale is accomplished by using the provider's thumb and index finger to gently pinch an area of the skin and look for the presence of wrinkles or skin folds [127]. An mRSS of zero indicates "normal" skin thickness with the presence of fine wrinkles, while an mRSS of one describes "mild" thickness with the presence of wrinkles and/or skin folds, an mRSS of two indicates "moderate" thickness with no wrinkles and difficulty in making skin folds, and an mRSS of three indicates "severe" skin thickness with an inability to make folds [127]. We propose that areas of skin with an mRSS ≥ 2 should be avoided during initial cannulation attempts, as this may be associated with a decreased likelihood of venipuncture success. Unfortunately, a useful clinical algorithm for predicting skin toughness has not been established.

Patient Compliance

Patient behavior and compliance with the venous access attempt is another important consideration. Needle puncture may cause significant psychological stress for patients, especially within the pediatric population [128, 129]. Refusal of venous attempts and even physiological events (e.g., vasovagal syncope) can result from the psychological stress induced by venous puncture attempts [129]. For this reason, we recommend that providers seek out patient preferences regarding the site of venous puncture or cannulation, when feasible. Patient compliance (and willingness to permit future IV attempts) may be enhanced by enlisting the patient to assist in selecting a target vein for cannulation [130].

Patients believed to be under the influence of drugs or alcohol exhibit an increased risk of violent behavior [131, 132]. In addition, substance abuse can aggravate pre-existing psychiatric conditions or heighten aggression toward providers, which may further limit opportunities for safe venous cannulation. Unfortunately, 40–50% of trauma patients present with signs and symptoms of alcohol use, and they may require rapid venous cannulation despite combative behavior [132, 133]. Involuntary noncompliance with venous cannulation may also be encountered, as in *status epilepticus*, presenting a real danger to both patient and provider during the IV attempt [134]. Alternate routes of access may need to be considered for the administration of anti-epileptic medications in seizure patients, especially when patients are unable to comply with provider requests to limit spontaneous movement during the attempt.

Intramuscular (IM) injection of ketamine, fentanyl, or other measures to control agitation and/or moderately sedate patients may help to ensure clinician safety during venous access attempts in agitated patients [135]. Moderate sedation should be considered to allow providers to establish medical control over the behavior of voluntarily- or involuntarily-violent patients, optimizing appropriate venous access attempts [135]. Intramuscular drug administration is also recommended with benzodiazepine therapy for patients who are actively seizing, although intranasal (IN) and buccal routes of application may suffice [133]. Patient sedation is often critical in emergent settings to avoid procedural complications, patient deterioration, and harm to emergency care providers during vascular access attempts [133, 135].

Provider Causes of DVA

Although often overlooked, clinician and provider characteristics appear to be major contributors to DVA in emergent settings. High-stress situations, lack of procedural knowledge, fatigue, and distractions can impair any member of the healthcare team and may prove detrimental to catheter insertion. Physician attitude and bias toward procedural outcomes also play an important role in cannulation success [136]. Management of these preventable factors should be a priority for emergency care providers. Even in patients with no identifiable DVA risk factors, provider influences can quickly undermine venous access attempts.

Distractibility

Physician distractibility is a leading cause of procedural error [137]. Especially in emergency departments, where high workload and patient complexity are commonplace, clinicians can find themselves juggling multiple tasks at once [7, 138, 139]. This results in increased cognitive demand, including distraction by both internal and external sources [137]. Internal distractions may manifest when a provider is responsible for many patients at once, physically performing one task while mentally preoccupied with other tasks. This compromises the provider's ability to focus on the task at hand, which can lead to preventable procedural complications [137]. External distractions, whether provided by patients or other members of the healthcare team, interrupt provider concentration [137]. Distracted providers may repeat cannulation attempts at inaccessible veins, disregard appropriate sterile techniques, or utilize ineffective strategies to improve vein visibility or palpability [89]. Solutions to decrease a provider's "cognitive load," by minimizing external distractions, may help to optimize efficiency in obtaining vascular access [137, 140]. As much as feasible, providers should seek assistance from other staff to minimize external distractions and mentally prepare prior to the venous access attempt, by focusing their attention solely on the job at hand. Cognitive offloading may be facilitated by maintaining a task checklist [137, 138]. Other simple solutions, such as avoiding small talk with other providers or closing doors upon entering a patient's room, have also been suggested to help clinicians focus on individual assignments [137]. Department-wide reform may even be necessary to improve DVA outcomes, with implementation of training or educational courses aimed at identifying distraction-prone tasks, including venous access [137]. Simulated venous access attempts may also be helpful in recognizing the degree to which internal and external distractions impair provider performance, and these lessons may then be translated to clinical practice [137, 139].

Fatigue

Adequate sleep is paramount to physician performance [139, 141]. Providers who receive less than the recommended 7–9 hours of sleep per night suffer from impaired alertness, altered cognition, and decreased fine motor function [139, 141–143]. These provider traits are associated with poor patient outcomes and increased incidence of procedural errors [139, 142]. Fatigued providers may be especially affected, as sleep deprivation has been shown to be associated with an increased incidence of self-needlestick injuries [142]. Provider adherence to proper sleep habits is of paramount importance in minimizing fatigue. Such measures include avoiding caffeine, nicotine, bright light exposure, and exercise immediately prior to bedtime, to optimize sleep initiation and quality [143].

High-Pressure Situations

High-stakes circumstances are known to place significant stress on healthcare personnel [140, 144, 145]. Such scenarios are complicated by the need for emergent medical intervention, with patient outcomes often dependent upon clinician performance under pressure [140]. This stress can impair providers' ability to make important decisions, potentially exacerbating DVA and increasing the risk of avoidable patient deterioration [7, 140, 145]. Provider manuals outlining the proper management of critically ill patients may aid decision-making under stressful conditions [140, 144]. Making such resources readily accessible within environments that are prone to critical events, such as the ED or ICU, could serve clinicians and patients well during high-stakes scenarios [140, 144].

Experience and Bias

Lack of previous formal training and adequate previous experience in vascular access have been shown to be associated with decreased competence in establishing venous access [146, 147]. This effect is likely due to a combination of inexperience and lack of confidence. Decreased confidence due to provider inexperience has been shown to predict the likelihood of failed cannulation attempts [147]. Although increased operator experience is beneficial to vascular access success rates, it may also impair clinician judgment with DVA patients. If a provider anticipates DVA prior to IV placement, there is a greater likelihood of first-attempt cannulation failure [136]. In some cases, this may be a "self-fulfilling prophecy," in which the provider dooms the access attempt before even starting it. Ideally, a determination of DVA should be based upon all the available evidence, not just the patient's DVA risk factors. However, the provider may be biased from past experiences with peripheral IV attempts on other patients or even failed previous attempts on the same patient during a previous care episode. Providers with experience in managing DVA patients may be more inclined to assume the presence of DVA, resulting in earlier declaration of failure or immediate utilization of alternate access techniques. Thus, an appreciation of DVA concepts is a two-edged sword, which can be used to help, or hinder, the venous access attempt. Providers should be encouraged to approach each patient with a fresh and objective assessment of their risk for DVA and make whatever attempts at venous access that may be considered reasonable in the setting of the patient's presenting condition. While early recognition of DVA is essential in streamlining venous access attempts, providers must remain vigilant to not assume DVA when the condition may not exist.

One method of reducing the inappropriate declaration of DVA is the practice of pairing potential DVA patients with experienced IV operators. This practice has been associated with a higher likelihood of first-attempt IV success [11, 43, 148]. This may be especially helpful in emergent settings, when critically ill patients are most likely to benefit from expeditious venous access. The importance of availing the clinical team with experienced DVA providers cannot be overstated. Previous studies have shown that exposing inexperienced vascular access providers to instructional books or videos on IV insertion is not associated with increased cannulation success rates [146]. Based on the available evidence, it appears that a skilled provider's experience with DVA seems to be the best predictor of appropriate DVA management. Providers with an inadequate understanding of the risk factors for DVA may benefit from review of current DVA guidelines regarding presentation and treatment modalities, thereby refining individual perceptions of how DVA appears in the emergent clinical setting. However, DVA management appears to be best handled by experienced IV operators who already understand the intricacies of IV placement in DVA patients.

Environment Causes of DVA

Environmental risk factors can impair both patients and providers. Unfortunately, identifying specific environmental risk factors for DVA can be a difficult task. Healthcare providers and institutions should be aware of the potential pitfalls encountered with short-staffing, resource unavailability, and chaotic settings and how these circumstances contribute to the presence of DVA.

Venous catheterization requires a wide array of equipment, which may not always be available to the emergency care provider [89]. The relative unavailability of VADs/VASDs, sterilizing accessories, tubing, and personal protective gear can impair provider function and delay appropriate intervention [149, 150]. Stocking DVA-specific "crash carts" or toolkits with devices and adjuncts needed to facilitate emergent cannulation can reduce delays in cannulating patients with difficult vascular access [151, 152]. However, daily organization and maintenance of these toolkits are essential [151, 153].

Staffing shortages are associated with increased adverse patient events [150, 154]. In hospitals with inadequate staffing ratios, specialized personnel may not be available to assist with more complex, occupation-specific tasks. DVA patients can be particularly affected by such environmental factors, especially in the absence of experienced vascular access specialists. Providers for DVA patients must be given adequate assistance from others with patient positioning, minimizing patient stress and otherwise facilitating the venous access attempt [89].

Providers should optimize their physical environment as much as possible when preparing to establish venous access. Noise and light conditions can have a significant impact upon physician performance [7, 138]. Poor overhead lighting negatively effects vein visibility [4], and high levels of noise may worsen provider distractibility [137]. The presence of stressed patient family members, especially in high-stakes circumstances, can further compromise provider focus [137, 138]. These added distractions interfere with the execution of careful, rehearsed treatment steps and can place the patient at risk of complications [137, 155]. Providers and institutions should consider the implementation of policies limiting the presence of nonessential personnel within treatment rooms during venous access attempts [156]. This will decrease distraction and avoid crowding, thereby freeing up additional space for procedures or resuscitative measures [156].

Additional DVA Risk Factors

Comorbid Conditions

Certain sequelae of previous comorbid conditions may also limit the potential target sites for venous access. Patients presenting with limb amputations or contractures provide fewer options for peripheral vein cannulation, potentially forcing clinicians to consider CVC or IO techniques early in the management algorithm. The existence of an arteriovenous fistula (AVF) or graft (AVG) for the purposes of hemodialysis can present an obstacle to venous catheter placement, as venous access is generally contraindicated in limbs containing preexisting fistulae [157]. Patients engaged in routine hemodialysis due to advanced renal failure may require conservation of their dialysis site for life-sustaining hemodialysis treatments. These extremities may be tempting sites for venous cannulation, as they are prominent and appear to be readily accessible for purposes of emergent infusion. However, the provider should be aware of the potential risks of cannulating such hemodialysis sites for emergent infusion of medications and fluids. Cannulation of a hemodialysis site for emergent infusion does introduce the risk of disruption or destruction of the site for future hemodialysis, due to clot formation or injury to the AV fistula site, which could cause thrombosis of the site and render this access point unusable for future dialysis treatments. This is a major risk, as many hemodialysis patients may not be able to be dialyzed at this site due to thrombosis or other injuries to the fistula site resulting from emergent cannulation. Furthermore, medications or fluids administered via an AV fistula site may not be delivered efficiently to the venous system, since the AV fistula is, by definition, connected to both the arterial and the venous circulation. We suggest that extremities possessing an AV fistula or graft not be utilized for emergent venous cannulation unless adequate efforts have been made to establish alternative venous access in other extremities first. In general, AV fistulas or grafts should not be utilized for emergent vascular access until attempts at venous access at other extremities have been exhausted and the provider feels that no other venous access is possible.

When patients with AV grafts or fistulas present in emergent settings, we suggest that the extremity containing the AV graft or fistula not be utilized for venous access. In such patients, providers should immediately look to alternate extremities (or consider central venous access) for cannulation [34]. If the patient has already received AV fistulas or grafts to both upper extremities, providers may need to utilize more rarely cannulated peripheral veins, such as lower extremity vessels of the ankle and foot.

Vascular Trauma and Vein Disease

A history of vascular trauma, such as that seen in IV drug abusers or patients with chronic medical conditions requiring frequent needlesticks, increases the likelihood of PIV placement failure. In one study, diabetes mellitus and sickle cell disease appear to be positively correlated with an increased risk of DVA [1]. In response to vascular trauma from repetitive needle insertion, inflammatory markers within the venous endothelium stimulate formation of fibrous tissue [158]. This results in intimal hyperplasia and vessel wall thickening, which can permanently hinder attempts at cannulation due to scarring and stenosis of the venous lumen [158, 159]. Patients with chronic venous disease, such as those with a history of deep vein thrombosis (DVT) or varicose veins, suffer from a similar mechanism of venous scar formation [3].

Coagulopathies

Coagulation disorders are also a significant predictor of difficult venous cannulation [3]. Patients with coagulopathies (e.g., hemophilia, von Willebrand's disease, therapeutic anticoagulation, or antiplatelet therapy) undergoing any procedure that breaks the skin (no matter how minimally invasive) are more likely to form a hematoma at an IV site than patients without coagulopathy. This underscores the importance of a successful first IV attempt, as failed attempts diminish the likelihood of future success in the immediate area [3].

History of Chemotherapy

Traditionally, infusion of chemotherapy drugs has been linked to the presence of DVA in cancer patients [2, 160]. Vesicant chemotherapeutic agents, such as the anthracyclines and *vinca* alkaloids, are known to cause significant endothelial vascular dysfunction and tissue necrosis [161, 162]. This damage to the vessel intima increases the difficulty of subsequent cannulation [17]. However, such adverse phenomena are exclusive to peripheral vasculature and do not occur with chemotherapeutic infusion through the central veins [163]. The advent of implantable central venous catheters for use in cancer patients did not occur until the 1980s, which may explain the historical association between chemotherapy and peripheral vein DVA [164]. Modern-day criteria for the administration of vesicant chemotherapeutic drugs continue to recommend the use of central venous access devices, such as PICC lines or Mediports, to avoid vascular remodeling and DVA development in cancer patients [34, 165, 166]. Exhaustion of physiologic venous supply is an extremely common phenomenon in patients with end-stage renal disease (ESRD) [167, 168]. Arteriovenous fistulas and grafts represent a relatively high-pressure vascular region, which is not ideal for the infusion of fluids or medications, due to the increased intrinsic vascular resistance to infusion caused by fistulization of the venous and arterial systems. The long-term complications from emergent cannulation will usually far outweigh any immediate benefits.

The Effects of Aging

Elastic fibers located within the perivascular connective tissue allow veins to deform under stress and to subsequently recoil against pressure [169]. Loss of these elastic fibers with the aging process may increase the risk of a "blown" vein (i.e., vascular rupture upon introduction of a needle) or venous collapse with early infusion [170]. Aging is also associated with increased venous and arterial calcification, which causes hardening or stiffening of vessels, making them more resistant to needle puncture [171–177]. These calcifications may prevent full occlusion of the vessel with pressure, following needle retraction [174]. This leads to an increased risk of bleeding and hematoma formation [174]. Providers should be aware that advanced age may increase the risk of DVA and should plan accordingly.

Certain patients already possess established venous access sites associated with chronic medical conditions. For example, indwelling catheters and subcutaneous ports are commonly available in chemotherapy patients, as they are used for repeated and prolonged infusions of chemotherapy drugs as a means of avoiding recurrent needle sticks. Such devices can accommodate high-volume flow [178]. This makes them ideal for use under emergent conditions, especially when peripheral cannulation is either delayed or impossible. However, indwelling devices are susceptible to both blood clots (the rationale for periodic flushing of the device with dilute heparin to maintain patency) and bacterial colonization, which may increase patient mortality [178, 179].

Pathways for DVA Management

Because of the rising incidence of DVA within the general population, the medical community must make a concerted effort to change the way in which healthcare providers approach this problem. Difficult venous access is a dynamic issue that depends upon many factors, and providers should recognize both provider-specific and institutional limitations that impact their ability to provide adequate and efficient vascular access. When confronted with seemingly inaccessible peripheral veins, providers should have already adopted a clearly outlined algorithm for intervention, complete with multiple solutions to augment first-attempt IV success. This must be supplemented with a checklist of possible auxiliary solutions, in the event of standard landmark-based IV failure. Equipping healthcare teams with these tools and tactics can help emergent responders define a path toward consistent vascular access success [180].

The initial survey of any DVA patient should account for the patient's complete medical status. The acuity of a patient's need for venous access will direct treatment steps and should guide the provider's choice of VAD [40]. Providers should select VADs based upon the presence or absence of critical illness and the proposed duration of IV therapy, according to Centers for Disease Control and Prevention (CDC) and Michigan Appropriateness Guide for Intravenous Catheters (MAGIC) guidelines [34, 122]. Peripheral IV catheterization (with or without ultrasound guidance) is indicated in stable DVA patients with a projected length of therapy ≤14 days [34]. Providers should consider PICC placement after 6 days of therapy in DVA patients, in order to decrease the risk of thrombophlebitis associated with repetitive needlesticks [34].

If the provider has decided that their patient is stable enough to tolerate peripheral vein cannulation, a limited number of attempts at PIV access should be allowed, even in patients experiencing DVA [40, 181]. However, the acceptable number of failed PIV cannulation attempts should be established prior to the first attempt, ideally informed by prior consultation with the patient. Failure of these initial PIV attempts should be followed by adjunct topical treatments and/or the use of VASDs (including ultrasound guidance) [40]. Sou et al. incorporated US-guided PIV into their own "DiVA pathway," and this protocol was found to significantly reduce the need for CVC placement in patients experiencing DVA [2]. For those vascular access teams unable to achieve PIV placement within a short predetermined window of time (e.g., 2 minutes), we suggest that ultrasound should be the "go-to" solution for appropriate patients. Unstable patients who remain refractory to peripheral IV access after adequate attempts should be considered candidates for immediate CVC or IO line placement [40, 181].

Published DVA algorithms suggest that at least two attempts at peripheral IV access should be tolerated in critically ill patients before resorting to CVC or IO line placement [40, 181]. However, providers should be prepared to override these recommendations under emergent conditions. The MAGIC recommendations suggest that CVCs be used in critically ill DVA patients – with a projected duration of IV therapy lasting ≤ 14 days – at the onset of treatment [34]. Clinicians should utilize this option if rapid fluid and drug administration, cardiac pacing, or monitoring of central venous pressure is anticipated [6]. The provider must keep in mind, however, that CVC cannulation carries a high risk of complications that could potentially worsen a patient's condition [6, 182]. In patients that cannot tolerate these risks, IO cannulation may be a superior option. Intraosseous vascular access can be accomplished without interrupting chest compressions (if necessary) and can be completed more quickly than CVC placement [6, 182, 183]. Since IO catheters are only currently recommended for dwell times ≤ 2 days, providers should use IO catheters as part of a "bridging" strategy to temporarily infuse fluids and medications while planning for more definitive venous access [6, 79].

Conclusions

Difficult vascular access is a multifaceted problem that all emergency care providers should understand. Rather than a feature or comorbidity of at-risk patients, DVA exists as a condition influenced by time constraints, as well as many patient-specific, provider-specific, and environmental factors. These factors must all be considered when managing difficult vascular access under emergent conditions. Due to recent advances in healthcare, patients are living longer with chronic conditions than ever before. Consequently, patient-specific factors contributing to the presence of DVA will likely represent an increasing challenge to providers in the future. Individual providers and institutions should seek to optimize the conditions under which venous access occurs for all our patients, not just those deemed to be at risk for DVA. Considering the importance of timing in the management of acutely ill patients, providers should seek out ways to provide venous access more efficiently and effectively. This necessitates an understanding and appreciation of alternative methods of gaining venous access under DVA conditions, including the use of adjunct devices and indirect venous access methods.

Key Concepts

- Rather than simply a comorbidity or feature of at-risk patients, DVA should be considered a *condition* influenced by time constraints, as well as patient-specific, provider-specific, and environmental factors.
- Solutions aimed at reducing the clinical burden of DVA must address each of these factors and may require significant provider-specific and institutional changes.
- Patient-specific factors, such as inadequate vein visibility and palpability, are important obstacles to successful venous cannulation. Vascular access support devices and other adjuncts may help to overcome these obstacles.
- Providers should be aware of alternative methods of gaining direct or indirect venous access and have adequate prior training and confidence in their use.
- Providers should prepare for instances of DVA in advance, by developing management plans that incorporate specific triggers (e.g., timing, number of failed attempts) to guide venous access attempts under stressful or chaotic conditions.
- Algorithms for the management of DVA can equip healthcare providers with stepwise solutions for DVA. Providers should become familiar with evidence-based algorithms for DVA and consider their use.

References

1. Fields JM, Piela NE, Au AK, Bon S. Risk factors associated with difficult venous access in adult ED patients. Am J Emerg Med. 2014;32(10):1179–82.
2. Sou V, McManus C, Mifflin N, et al. A clinical pathway for the management of difficult venous access. BMC Nurs. 2017;16(1):1–7.
3. Civetta G, Cortesi S, Mancardi M, et al. EA-DIVA score (enhanced adult DIVA score): a new scale to predict difficult preoperative venous cannulation in adult surgical patients. J Vasc Access. 2019;20(3):281–9.
4. Kuensting LL, DeBoer S, Holleran R, et al. Difficult venous access in children: taking control. J Emerg Nurs. 2009;35(5):419–24.
5. Keleekai NL, Schuster CA, Murray CL, et al. Improving nurses' peripheral intravenous catheter insertion knowledge, confidence, and skills using a simulation-based blended learning program. Simul Healthc. 2016;11(6):376–84.
6. Leidel BA, Kirchhoff C, Bogner V, et al. Comparison of intraosseous versus central venous vascular access in adults under resuscitation in the emergency department with inaccessible peripheral veins. Resuscitation. 2012;83(1):40–5.
7. Zavala AM, Day GE, Plummer D, et al. Decision-making under pressure: medical errors in uncertain and dynamic environments. Aust Health Rev. 2018;42(4):395–402.
8. van Loon FHJ, Puijn LAPM, Houterman S, et al. Development of the A-DIVA scale: a clinical predictive scale to identify difficult intravenous access in adult patients based on clinical observations. Medicine (Baltimore). 2016;95(16):e3428.
9. Piredda M, Biagioli V, Barella B, et al. Factors affecting difficult peripheral intravenous cannulation in adults: a prospective observational study. J Clin Nurs. 2017;26(7–8):1074–84.

10. Sebbane M, Claret P-G, Lefebvre S, et al. Predicting peripheral venous access difficulty in the emergency department using body mass index and a clinical evaluation of venous accessibility. J Emerg Med. 2013;44(2):299–305.

11. Carr PJ, Rippey JC, Budgeon CA, et al. Insertion of peripheral intravenous cannulae in the emergency department: factors associated with first-time insertion success. J Vasc Access. 2016;17(2):182–90.

12. Rodríguez-Calero MA, Blanco-Mavillard I, Morales-Asencio JM, et al. Defining risk factors associated with difficult peripheral venous cannulation: a systematic review and meta-analysis. Heart Lung. 2020;49(3):273–86.

13. Riker MW, Kennedy C, Winfrey BS, et al. Validation and refinement of the difficult intravenous access score: a clinical prediction rule for identifying children with difficult intravenous access. Acad Emerg Med. 2011;18(11):1129–34.

14. Ehrhardt BS, Givens KE, Lee RC. Making it stick: developing and testing the Difficult Intravenous Access (DIVA) tool. Am J Nurs. 2018;118(7):56–62.

15. Jacobson AF, Winslow EH. Variables influencing intravenous catheter insertion difficulty and failure: an analysis of 339 intravenous catheter insertions. Heart Lung. 2005;34(5):345–59.

16. Chiao FB, Resta-Flarer F, Lesser J, et al. Vein visualization: patient characteristic factors and efficacy of a new infrared vein finder technology. Br J Anaesth. 2013;110(6):966–71.

17. Lamperti M, Pittiruti M. Difficult peripheral veins: turn on the lights. Br J Anaesth. 2013;110(6):888–91.

18. Curtis SJ, Craig WR, Logue E, et al. Ultrasound or near-infrared vascular imaging to guide peripheral intravenous catheterization in children: a pragmatic randomized controlled trial. CMAJ. 2015;187(8):563–70.

19. Demir D, Inal S. Does the use of a vein visualization device for peripheral venous catheter placement increase success rate in pediatric patients? Pediatr Emerg Care. 2019;35(7):474–9.

20. Basadonna G. AccuVein vein illumination device (AV400) improves first attempt success rate for IV placement in obese patients. AccuVein [Internet]. 2016. Cited 2020 June 9. Available from: https://www.accuvein.com/assets/Clinical-Studies-Umass-Obese.pdf.

21. Gümüş M, Başbakkal Z. Efficacy of Veinlite PEDI in pediatric peripheral intravenous access: a randomized controlled trial. Pediatr Emerg Care. 2018;37:145.

22. McNeely HL, Ream TL, Thrasher JM, et al. Utilization of a biomedical device (VeinViewer®) to assist with peripheral intravenous catheter (PIV) insertion for pediatric nurses. J Spec Pediatr Nurs. 2018;23(2):e12208.

23. Perry AM, Caviness AC, Hsu DC. Efficacy of a near-infrared light device in pediatric intravenous cannulation: a randomized controlled trial. Pediatr Emerg Care. 2011;27(1):5–10.

24. Rothbart A, Yu P, Müller-Lobeck L, et al. Peripheral intravenous cannulation with support of infrared laser vein viewing system in a pre-operation setting in pediatric patients. BMC Res Notes. 2015;8(1):463.

25. Kim MJ, Park JM, Rhee N, et al. Efficacy of VeinViewer in pediatric peripheral intravenous access: a randomized controlled trial. Eur J Pediatr. 2012;171(7):1121–5.

26. Katsogridakis YL, Seshadri R, Sullivan C, Waltzman ML. Veinlite transillumination in the pediatric emergency department: a therapeutic interventional trial. Pediatr Emerg Care. 2008;24(2):83–8.

27. Cantor-Peled G, Halak M, Ovadia-Blechman Z. Peripheral vein locating techniques. Imaging Med. 2016;8(3):83–8.

28. García AM, Horche PR. Light source optimizing in a biphotonic vein finder device: experimental and theoretical analysis. Results Phys. 2018;11:975–83.

29. Translite LLC. Veinlite quick guide. Veinlite [Internet]. Cited 2020 June 9. Available from: https://www.theemsstore.com/download.aspx?fileId=341.

30. van Loon FH, Buise MP, Claassen JJ, et al. Comparison of ultrasound guidance with palpation and direct visualisation for peripheral vein cannulation in adult patients: a systematic review and meta-analysis. Br J Anaesth. 2018;121(2):358–66.

31. Egan G, Healy D, O'Neill H, et al. Ultrasound guidance for difficult peripheral venous access: systematic review and meta-analysis. Emerg Med J. 2013;30(7):521–6.

32. Currie M, Zhu B, Huecker MR. Ultrasound intravascular access. StatPearls [Internet]. 2019 Jul 3. Cited 2020 June 9. Available from: https://www.ncbi.nlm.nih.gov/books/NBK448093/.
33. Saugel B, Scheeren TW, Teboul JL. Ultrasound-guided central venous catheter placement: a structured review and recommendations for clinical practice. Crit Care. 2017;21(1):225.
34. Chopra V, Flanders SA, Saint S, et al. The Michigan Appropriateness Guide for Intravenous Catheters (MAGIC): results from a multispecialty panel using the RAND/UCLA appropriateness method. Ann Intern Med. 2015;163(6_Supplement):S1–40.
35. Yin J, Zhang X, Cheng G. IP267 external jugular vein cutdown approach vs percutaneous approach for totally implantable venous access device placement: a safe, fast, and cheap method. J Vasc Surg. 2017;65(6):S126.
36. Cavallaro G, Iorio O, Iossa A, et al. A prospective evaluation on external jugular vein cutdown approach for TIVAD implantation. World J Surg Oncol. 2015;13(1):243.
37. Lee MM, Loyd JW. Saphenous vein cutdown. StatPearls [Internet]. 2019. Cited 2020 June 9. Available from: https://pubmed.ncbi.nlm.nih.gov/30422475/.
38. Keeley JL. Intravenous injections and infusions. Am J Surg. 1940;50(3):485–90.
39. Kirkham JH. Infusion into the internal saphenous vein at the ankle. Lancet. 1945;246(6382):815–7.
40. Mbamalu D, Banerjee A. Methods of obtaining peripheral venous access in difficult situations. Postgrad Med J. 1999;75(886):459–62.
41. Chappell S, Vilke GM, Chan TC, et al. Peripheral venous cutdown. J Emerg Med. 2006;31(4):411–6.
42. Roberts JR. Roberts and Hedges' clinical procedures in emergency medicine and acute care e-book. Elsevier Health Sciences; 2017.
43. Carr PJ, Rippey JC, Cooke ML, et al. Factors associated with peripheral intravenous cannulation first-time insertion success in the emergency department. A multicentre prospective cohort analysis of patient, clinician and product characteristics. BMJ Open. 2019;9(4):e022278.
44. Yalçınlı S, Akarca FK, Can Ö, et al. Factors affecting the first-attempt success rate of intravenous cannulation in older people. J Clin Nurs. 2019;28(11–12):2206–13.
45. Ichimura M, Matsumura Y, Sasaki S, et al. The characteristics of healthy adults with hardly palpable vein—relations between easy venous palpation and physical factors. Int J Nurs Pract. 2015;21(6):805–12.
46. Twardowski ZJ, Seger RM. Measuring central venous structures in humans: implications for central-vein catheter dimensions. J Vasc Access. 2002;3(1):21–37.
47. Keiler J, Seidel R, Wree A. The femoral vein diameter and its correlation with sex, age and body mass index–an anatomical parameter with clinical relevance. Phlebology. 2019;34(1):58–69.
48. Mortensen JD, Talbot S, Burkart JA. Cross-sectional internal diameters of human cervical and femoral blood vessels: relationship to subject's sex, age, body size. Anat Rec. 1990;226(1):115–24.
49. Stawicki SP, Adkins EJ, Eiferman DS, et al. Prospective evaluation of intravascular volume status in critically ill patients: does inferior vena cava collapsibility correlate with central venous pressure? J Trauma Acute Care Surg. 2014;76(4):956–64.
50. Zhang X, Luan H, Zhu P, et al. Does ultrasonographic measurement of the inferior vena cava diameter correlate with central venous pressure in the assessment of intravascular volume in patients undergoing gastrointestinal surgery? J Surg Res. 2014;191(2):339–43.
51. Prencipe M, Granata A, D'Amelio A, et al. Usefulness of US imaging in overhydrated nephropathic patients. J Ultrasound. 2016;19(1):7–13.
52. Ferrada P, Vanguri P, Anand RJ, et al. Flat inferior vena cava: indicator of poor prognosis in trauma and acute care surgery patients. Am Surgeon. 2012;78(12):1396–8.
53. Liao YY, Lin HJ, Lu YH, et al. Does CT evidence of a flat inferior vena cava indicate hypovolemia in blunt trauma patients with solid organ injuries? J Trauma. 2011;70(6):1358–61.
54. Kreimeier U. Pathophysiology of fluid imbalance. Crit Care. 2000;4(2):S3–7.
55. Hür E, Özişik M, Ural C, et al. Hypervolemia for hypertension pathophysiology: a population-based study. Biomed Res Int. 2014;2014:895401.

56. Panebianco NL, Fredette JM, Szyld D, et al. What you see (sonographically) is what you get: vein and patient characteristics associated with successful ultrasound-guided peripheral intravenous placement in patients with difficult access. Acad Emerg Med. 2009;16(12):1298–303.
57. Seyahi N, Kahveci A, Altiparmak MR, et al. Ultrasound imaging findings of femoral veins in patients with renal failure and its impact on vascular access. Nephrol Dial Transpl. 2005;20(9):1864–7.
58. Kim IS, Kang SS, Park JH, et al. Impact of sex, age and BMI on depth and diameter of the infraclavicular axillary vein when measured by ultrasonography. Eur J Anaesthesiol. 2011;28(5):346–50.
59. Murray C, Ng M, Mokdad A. The vast majority of American adults are overweight or obese, and weight is a growing problem among US children. IHME [Internet]. 2014 May 28. Cited 2020 June 9. Available from: http://www.healthdata.org/news-release/vast-majority-american-adults-are-overweight-or-obese-and-weight-growing-problem-among.
60. Gregg SC, Murthi SB, Sisley AC, et al. Ultrasound-guided peripheral intravenous access in the intensive care unit. J Crit Care. 2010;25(3):514–9.
61. Homayouni A, Tabari-Khomeiran R, Asadi-Louyeh A. Investigating the effect of local warming on vein diameter in the antecubital area in adults aged 20-40 years. Br J Nurs. 2019;28(8):S20–6.
62. Lenhardt R, Seybold T, Kimberger O, et al. Local warming and insertion of peripheral venous cannulas: single blinded prospective randomised controlled trial and single blinded randomised crossover trial. BMJ. 2002;325(7361):409.
63. Fink RM, Hjort E, Wenger B, et al. The impact of dry versus moist heat on peripheral IV catheter insertion in a hematology-oncology outpatient population. Oncol Nurs Forum. 2009;36(4):E198–204.
64. Biyik Bayram S, Caliskan N. Effects of local heat application before intravenous catheter insertion in chemotherapy patients. J Clin Nurs. 2016;25(11–12):1740–7.
65. Hecker JF, Lewis GB, Stanley H, Smith RM. Nitroglycerine ointment as an aid to venepuncture. Survey Anesthesiol. 1983;27(5):279.
66. Roberge RJ, Kelly M, Evans TC, et al. Facilitated intravenous access through local application of nitroglycerin ointment. Ann Emerg Med. 1987;16(5):546–9.
67. Mumma BE, Dhingra KR, Kurlinkus C, Diercks DB. Hemodynamic effects of nitroglycerin ointment in emergency department patients. J Emerg Med. 2014;47(2):192–7.
68. Huff L, Hamlin A, Wolski D, et al. Atraumatic care: EMLA cream and application of heat to facilitate peripheral venous cannulation in children. Issues Compr Pediatr Nurs. 2009;32(2):65–76.
69. Schreiber S, Ronfani L, Chiaffoni GP, et al. Does EMLA cream application interfere with the success of venipuncture or venous cannulation? A prospective multicenter observational study. Eur J Pediatr. 2013;172(2):265–8.
70. Egekvist H, Bjerring P. Effect of EMLA cream on skin thickness and subcutaneous venous diameter. A randomized, placebo-controlled study in children. Acta Derm Venereol. 2000;80(5):340–3.
71. Chalacheva P, Khaleel M, Sunwoo J, et al. Biophysical markers of the peripheral vasoconstriction response to pain in sickle cell disease. PLoS One. 2017;12(5):e0178353.
72. Hayashi N, Someya N, Maruyama T, et al. Vascular responses to fear-induced stress in humans. Physiol Behav. 2009;98(4):441–6.
73. Andrew M, Barker D, Laing R. The use of glyceryl trinitrate ointment with EMLA cream for iv cannulation in children undergoing routine surgery. Anaesth Intensive Care. 2002;30(3):321–5.
74. Kule A, Hang B, Bahl A. Preventing the collapse of a peripheral vein during cannulation: an evaluation of various tourniquet techniques on vein compressibility. J Emerg Med. 2014;46(5):659–66.
75. Nelson D, Jeanmonod R, Jeanmonod D. Randomized trial of tourniquet vs blood pressure cuff for target vein dilation in ultrasound-guided peripheral intravenous access. Am J Emerg Med. 2014;32(7):761–4.

76. Tran T, Lund SB, Nichols MD, Kummer T. Effect of two tourniquet techniques on peripheral intravenous cannulation success: a randomized controlled trial. Am J Emerg Med. 2019;37(12):2209–14.

77. Price J, Xiao J, Tausch K, et al. Single versus double tourniquet technique for ultrasound-guided venous catheter placement. West J Emerg Med. 2019;20(5):719–25.

78. Cui J, Leuenberger UA, Gao Z, Sinoway LI. Sympathetic and cardiovascular responses to venous distension in an occluded limb. Am J Phys. 2011;301(6):R1831–7.

79. Rudland S. A further communication from the front. J Roy Nav Med Serv. 1991;77(3):235–6.

80. Åsheim P, Uggen PE, Aasarød K, Aadahl P. Intraperitoneal fluid therapy: an alternative to intravenous treatment in a patient with limited vascular access. Anaesthesia. 2006;61(5):502–4.

81. Sasson M, Shvartzman P. Hypodermoclysis: an alternate infusion technique. Am Fam Physician. 2001;64(9):1575.

82. Remington R, Hultman T. Hypodermoclysis to treat dehydration: a review of the evidence. J Am Geriatr Soc. 2007;55(12):2051–5.

83. Humphrey P. Hypodermoclysis: an alternative to IV infusion therapy. Nursing. 2011;41(11):16–7.

84. Scott-Warren VL, Morley RB. Paediatric vascular access. BJA Educ. 2015;15(4):199–206.

85. Lewis K, Spirnak PW. Umbilical vein catheterization. StatPearls [Internet]. 2020 Feb 21. Cited 2020 June 9. Available from: https://pubmed.ncbi.nlm.nih.gov/31751059/.

86. Kusztal M, Weyde W, Letachowicz K, et al. Anatomical vascular variations and practical implications for access creation on the upper limb. J Vasc Access. 2014;15(7_suppl):70–5.

87. Pires L, Ráfare AL, Peixoto BU, et al. The venous patterns of the cubital fossa in subjects from Brazil. Morphologie. 2018;102(337):78–82.

88. Ukoha UU, Oranusi CK, Okafor JI, et al. Patterns of superficial venous arrangement in the cubital fossa of adult Nigerians. Niger J Clin Pract. 2013;16(1):104–9.

89. Beecham GB, Tackling G. Peripheral line placement. StatPearls [Internet]. 2019 Oct 14. Cited 2020 June 9. Available from: https://www.ncbi.nlm.nih.gov/books/NBK539795/.

90. Gagne P, Sharma K. Relationship of common vascular anatomy to cannulated catheters. Int J Vasc Med. 2017;19:2017.

91. Lee H, Lee SH, Kim SJ, et al. Variations of the cubital superficial vein investigated by using the intravenous illuminator. Anat Cell Biol. 2015;48(1):62–5.

92. Yamada K, Yamada K, Katsuda I, Hida T. Cubital fossa venipuncture sites based on anatomical variations and relationships of cutaneous veins and nerves. Clin Anat. 2008;21(4):307–13.

93. Bains KN, Lappin SL. Anatomy, shoulder and upper limb, elbow cubital fossa. StatPearls [Internet]. 2019 Feb 8. Cited 2020 June 9. Available from: https://www.ncbi.nlm.nih.gov/books/NBK459250/.

94. Yammine K, Erić M. Patterns of the superficial veins of the cubital fossa: a meta-analysis. Phlebology. 2017;32(6):403–14.

95. Simundic AM, Bölenius K, Cadamuro J, et al. Joint EFLM-COLABIOCLI recommendation for venous blood sampling. Clin Chem Lab Med. 2018;56(12):2015–38.

96. Mikuni Y, Chiba S, Tonosaki Y. Topographical anatomy of superficial veins, cutaneous nerves, and arteries at venipuncture sites in the cubital fossa. Anat Sci Int. 2013;88(1):46–57.

97. Mukai K, Nakajima Y, Nakano T, et al. Safety of venipuncture sites at the cubital fossa as assessed by ultrasonography. J Patient Saf. 2020;16(1):98.

98. Gottlob R, May R. Venous valves. Springer; 1986.

99. Center for Vein Restoration [Internet]. What are venous valves and why are they so important? 2018 Mar 16. Cited 2020 June 9. Available from: https://www.centerforvein.com/blog/venous-valves.

100. Necas M. Duplex ultrasound in the assessment of lower extremity venous insufficiency. AJUM. 2010;13(4):37–45.

101. Emergency Medicine News [Internet]. Vein visualization aids providers; 2017 Apr. Cited 2020 June 9. Available from: https://journals.lww.com/em-news/fulltext/2017/04181/technology___inventions__vein_visualization_aids.2.aspx.

102. Shima H, Ohno K, Shimizu T, et al. Anatomical study of the valves of the superficial veins of the forearm. J Cranio Maxill Surg. 1992;20(7):305–9.
103. Fronek A, Criqui MH, Denenberg J, Langer RD. Common femoral vein dimensions and hemodynamics including Valsalva response as a function of sex, age, and ethnicity in a population study. J Vasc Surg. 2001;33(5):1050–6.
104. Chang TS. Principles, techniques and applications in microsurgery. World Scientific; 1986.
105. Johnston WF, West JK, LaPar DJ, et al. Greater saphenous vein evaluation from computed tomography angiography as a potential alternative to conventional ultrasonography. J Vasc Surg. 2012;56(5):1331–7.
106. Rumack CM, Levine D. Diagnostic ultrasound e-book. Elsevier Health Sciences; 2017.
107. Seidel AC, Miranda F Jr, Juliano Y, Novo NF. Relationship between the diameter of great saphenous vein and body mass index. J Vasc Bras. 2005;4(3):265–9.
108. Zhang SX, Schmidt HM. Clinical anatomy of the subcutaneous veins in the dorsum of the hand. Ann Anat. 1993;175(4):381–4.
109. Pirozzi N, Apponi F, Napoletano AM, et al. Microsurgery and preventive haemostasis for autogenous radial–cephalic direct wrist access in adult patients with radial artery internal diameter below 1.6 mm. Nephrol Dial Transpl. 2010;25(2):520–5.
110. van Bemmelen PS, Kelly P, Blebea J. Improvement in the visualization of superficial arm veins being evaluated for access and bypass. J Vasc Surg. 2005;42(5):957–62.
111. Intravenous Therapy Skills [Internet]. Veins used for IV therapy; 2017 Apr. Cited 2020 June 9. Available from: learningcentral.health.unm.edu/learning/user/onlineaccess/CE/CE1001/anatomy/veins.html.
112. Shima H, Ohno K, Michi KI, et al. An anatomical study on the forearm vascular system. J Cranio Maxill Surg. 1996;24(5):293–9.
113. Ishaque B, Zayed MA, Miller J, et al. Ethnic differences in arm vein diameter and arteriovenous fistula creation rates in men undergoing hemodialysis access. J Vasc Surg. 2012;56(2):424–32.
114. Spivack DE, Kelly P, Gaughan JP, van Bemmelen PS. Mapping of superficial extremity veins: normal diameters and trends in a vascular patient-population. Ultrasound Med Biol. 2012;38(2):190–4.
115. Kiray A, Ergür I, Tayefi H, et al. Anatomical evaluation of the superficial veins of the upper extremity as graft donor source in microvascular reconstructions: a cadaveric study. Acta Orthop Traumato. 2013;47(6):405–10.
116. Lynn Hadaway Associates [Internet]. Peripheral veins – size matters; 2018 July 5. Cited 2020 June 9. Available from: http://hadawayassociates.com/lynns-blog/peripheral-veins-size-matters.
117. Sharp R, Childs J, Bulmer AC, Esterman A. The effect of oral hydration and localised heat on peripheral vein diameter and depth: a randomised controlled trial. Appl Nurs Res. 2018;42:83–8.
118. Akaraborworn O. A review in emergency central venous catheterization. Chin J Traumatol. 2017;20(3):137–40.
119. Bannon MP, Heller SF, Rivera M. Anatomic considerations for central venous cannulation. Risk Manag Healthc Policy. 2011;4:27–39.
120. Parienti JJ, Mongardon N, Mégarbane B, et al. Intravascular complications of central venous catheterization by insertion site. N Engl J Med. 2015;373(13):1220–9.
121. Ikusika O, Waxman M, Asher S, Cohen J. 1090: recommended site for central venous catheter placement: a review of current practice guidelines. Crit Care Med. 2013;41(12):A275.
122. Allen G. 2011 CDC guidelines for the prevention of intravascular catheter-associated infections: strategies to reduce intravascular catheter-associated infections. Ethicon, Inc; 2011.
123. Tartière D, Seguin P, Juhel C, et al. Estimation of the diameter and cross-sectional area of the internal jugular veins in adult patients. Crit Care. 2009;13(6):1–4.
124. Asouhidou I, Natsis K, Asteri T, et al. Anatomical variation of left internal jugular vein: clinical significance for an anaesthesiologist. Eur J Anaesthesiol. 2008;25(4):314–8.

125. Zhu P, Zhang X, Luan H, et al. Ultrasonographic measurement of the subclavian vein diameter for assessment of intravascular volume status in patients undergoing gastrointestinal surgery: comparison with central venous pressure. J Surg Res. 2015;196(1):102–6.
126. Sharifian H, Gharekhanloo F. Evaluation of average diameter of lower extremity veins in acute and chronic thrombosis and comparison with normal persons by doppler sonography. Acta Med Iran. 2003;41(3):180–2.
127. Khanna D, Furst DE, Clements PJ, et al. Standardization of the modified Rodnan skin score for use in clinical trials of systemic sclerosis. J Scleroderma Relat Disord. 2017;2(1):11–8.
128. Stoltz P, Manworren RC. Comparison of children's venipuncture fear and pain: randomized controlled trial of EMLA® and J-Tip Needleless Injection System®. J Pediatr Nurs. 2017;37:91–6.
129. Deacon B, Abramowitz J. Fear of needles and vasovagal reactions among phlebotomy patients. J Anxiety Disord. 2006;20(7):946–60.
130. Cooke M, Ullman AJ, Ray-Barruel G, et al. Not" just" an intravenous line: consumer perspectives on peripheral intravenous cannulation (PIVC). An international cross-sectional survey of 25 countries. PLoS One. 2018;13(2):e0193436.
131. Volavka J, Swanson J. Violent behavior in mental illness: the role of substance abuse. JAMA. 2010;304(5):563–4.
132. Hadjizacharia P, O'Keeffe T, Plurad DS, et al. Alcohol exposure and outcomes in trauma patients. Eur J Trauma Emerg S. 2011;37(2):169–75.
133. NIH [Internet]. Alcohol and trauma; 1989. Cited 2020 June 9. Available from: pubs.niaaa.nih.gov/publications/aa03.html.
134. Silverman EC, Sporer KA, Lemieux JM, et al. Prehospital care for the adult and pediatric seizure patient: current evidence-based recommendations. West J Emerg Med. 2017;18(3):419–36.
135. Scheppke KA, Braghiroli J, Shalaby M, Chait R. Prehospital use of IM ketamine for sedation of violent and agitated patients. West J Emerg Med. 2014;15(7):736–41.
136. van Loon FH, van Hooff LW, de Boer HD, et al. The modified A-DIVA scale as a predictive tool for prospective identification of adult patients at risk of a difficult intravenous access: a multicenter validation study. J Clin Med. 2019;8(2):144.
137. Feil M. Distractions and their impact on patient safety. PA PSRS Patient Saf Advis. 2013;10(1):1–0.
138. Rivera-Rodriguez AJ, Karsh BT. Interruptions and distractions in healthcare: review and reappraisal. Qual Saf Health Care. 2010;19(4):304–12.
139. Westbrook JI, Raban MZ, Walter SR, Douglas H. Task errors by emergency physicians are associated with interruptions, multitasking, fatigue and working memory capacity: a prospective, direct observation study. BMJ Qual Saf. 2018;27(8):655–63.
140. Kazior MR, Wang J, Stiegler MP, et al. Emergency manuals improved novice physician performance during simulated ICU emergencies. J Educ Perioper Med. 2017;19(3):E608.
141. Parker JB. The effects of fatigue on physician performance-an underestimated cause of physician impairment and increased patient risk. Can J Anaesth. 1987;34(5):489–95.
142. Comondore VR, Wenner JB, Ayas NT. The impact of sleep deprivation in resident physicians on physician and patient safety: is it time for a wake-up call? BCMJ. 2008;50(10):560–4.
143. Howard SK. Sleep deprivation and physician performance: why should I care? Proc (Bayl Univ Med Cent). 2005;18(2):108–12.
144. Ali S, Thomson D, Graham TA, et al. High stakes and high emotions: providing safe care in Canadian emergency departments. Open Access Emerg Med. 2017;9:23–6.
145. Kent J, Thornton M, Fong A, et al. Acute provider stress in high stakes medical care: implications for trauma surgeons. J Trauma Acute Care Surg. 2020;88(3):440–5.
146. Woelfel IA, Takabe K. Successful intravenous catheterization by medical students. J Surg Res. 2016;204(2):351–60.

147. Dehmer JJ, Amos KD, Farrell TM, et al. Competence and confidence with basic procedural skills: the experience and opinions of fourth-year medical students at a single institution. Acad Med. 2013;88(5):682–7.
148. Lapostolle F, Catineau J, Garrigue B, et al. Prospective evaluation of peripheral venous access difficulty in emergency care. Intensive Care Med. 2007;33(8):1452–7.
149. Moyimane MB, Matlala SF, Kekana MP. Experiences of nurses on the critical shortage of medical equipment at a rural district hospital in South Africa: a qualitative study. Pan Afr Med J. 2017;28(1):157.
150. Bradley S, Kamwendo F, Chipeta E, et al. Too few staff, too many patients: a qualitative study of the impact on obstetric care providers and on quality of care in Malawi. BMC Pregnancy Childbirth. 2015;15(1):65.
151. Pennsylvania Patient Safety Advisory [Internet]. Clinical emergency: are you ready in any setting? 2010 June. Cited 2020 June 9. Available from: http://patientsafety.pa.gov/ADVISORIES/Documents/201006_52.pdf.
152. Singh MM, Saini RS, Raj A. Evaluation of availability and effectiveness of crash cart in public and pvt hospitals. PIJR. 2019;8(2):20–24.
153. Verhoeff K, Saybel R, Mathura P, et al. Ensuring adequate vascular access in patients with major trauma: a quality improvement initiative. BMJ Open Qual. 2018;7(1):e000090.
154. Hughes R, editor. Patient safety and quality: an evidence-based handbook for nurses. Rockville: Agency for Healthcare Research and Quality; 2008.
155. Brasel KJ, Entwistle JW, Sade RM. Should family presence be allowed during cardiopulmonary resuscitation? Ann Thorac Surg. 2016;102(5):1438–43.
156. Traylor M. Should family be permitted in a trauma bay? AMA J Ethics. 2018;20(5):455–63.
157. Texas Heart Institute [Internet]. Vascular access for hemodialysis; 2020. Cited 2020 June 9. Available from: https://www.texasheart.org/heart-health/heart-information-center/topics/vascular-access-for-hemodialysis/.
158. Skandalou EI, Apostolidou-Kiouti FD, Minasidis ID, Skandalos IK. Left brachiocephalic vein stenosis due to the insertion of a temporal right subclavian hemodialysis catheter. Case Rep Vasc Med. 2017;22:2017.
159. UPMC [Internet]. Vascular trauma; 2019. Cited 2020 June 9. Available from: https://www.upmc.com/services/heart-vascular/conditions-treatments/vascular-trauma.
160. Kaur P, Rickard C, Domer GS, Glover KR. Dangers of peripheral intravenous catheterization: the forgotten tourniquet and other patient safety considerations. In: Stawicki SP, Firstenberg MS, editors. Vignettes in patient safety, vol. 4. IntechOpen; 2019.
161. Cameron AC, Touyz RM, Lang NN. Vascular complications of cancer chemotherapy. Can J Cardiol. 2016;32(7):852–62.
162. Kreidieh FY, Moukadem HA, El Saghir NS. Overview, prevention and management of chemotherapy extravasation. World J Clin Oncol. 2016;7(1):87.
163. Schulmeister L. Safe management of chemotherapy: infusion-related complications. Clin J Oncol Nurs. 2014;18(3):283.
164. Zerati AE, Wolosker N, de Luccia N, Puech-Leão P. Totally implantable venous catheters: history, implantation technique and complications. J Vasc Bras. 2017;16(2):128–39. https://doi.org/10.1590/1677-5449.008216.
165. Boschi R, Rostagno E. Extravasation of antineoplastic agents: prevention and treatments. Pediatr Rep. 2012;4(3):e28.
166. Gallieni M, Pittiruti M, Biffi R. Vascular access in oncology patients. CA-Cancer J Clin. 2008;58(6):323–46.
167. Vachharajani TJ, Agarwal AK, Asif A. Vascular access of last resort. Kidney Int. 2018;93(4):797–802.
168. Hajji M, Harzallah A, Kaaroud H, et al. Exhaustion of vascular capital in patients on hemodialysis: what will be the outcome? Pan Afr Med J. 2016;25:237.
169. Sherratt MJ. Tissue elasticity and the ageing elastic fibre. Age. 2009;31(4):305–25.

170. Healthline [Internet]. What can cause a blown vein and how to treat it. 2019 Nov. Cited 2020 June 9. Available from: www.healthline.com/health/blown-vein.

171. Pedigo SL, Guth CM, Hocking KM, et al. Calcification of human saphenous vein associated with endothelial dysfunction: a pilot histopathophysiological and demographical study. Front Surg. 2017;4:6.

172. Demer LL, Tintut Y. Vascular calcification: pathobiology of a multifaceted disease. Circulation. 2008;117(22):2938–48.

173. Schmidli J, Widmer MK, Basile C, et al. Editor's choice–vascular access: 2018 clinical practice guidelines of the European Society for Vascular Surgery (ESVS). Eur J Vasc Endovasc Surg. 2018;55(6):757–818.

174. Bodenham A. Vascular access. Rev Méd Clin Las Condes. 2017;28(5):701–12.

175. Rocha-Singh KJ, Zeller T, Jaff MR. Peripheral arterial calcification: prevalence, mechanism, detection, and clinical implications. Catheter Cardiovasc Interv. 2014;83(6):E212–20.

176. Nemcsik J, Kiss I, Tislér A. Arterial stiffness, vascular calcification and bone metabolism in chronic kidney disease. World J Nephrol. 2012;1(1):25.

177. Giachelli CM. Vascular calcification mechanisms. Clin J Am Soc Nephrol. 2004;15(12):2959–64.

178. Teichgräber UK, Pfitzmann R, Hofmann HA. Central venous port systems as an integral part of chemotherapy. Dtsch Arztebl Int. 2011;108(9):147.

179. Cridlig J, Kessler M, Cao-Huu T. Arteriovenous fistula or catheter: creating an optimal vascular access for hemodialysis. In: Hemodialysis. IntechOpen; 2013.

180. Carr PJ, Higgins NS, Rippey J, et al. Tools, clinical prediction rules, and algorithms for the insertion of peripheral intravenous catheters in adult hospitalized patients: a systematic scoping review of literature. J Hosp Med. 2017;12:851.

181. Gazin N, Auger H, Jabre P, et al. Efficacy and safety of the EZ-IO™ intraosseous device: out-of-hospital implementation of a management algorithm for difficult vascular access. Resuscitation. 2011;82(1):126–9.

182. Bloch SA, Bloch AJ, Silva P. Adult intraosseous use in academic EDs and simulated comparison of emergent vascular access techniques. Am J Emerg Med. 2013;31(3):622–4.

183. Anson JA. Vascular access in resuscitation: is there a role for the intraosseous route? Anesthesiology. 2014;120(4):1015–31.

Decision-Making for Emergent Vascular Access

James H. Paxton and Alexandra Lemieux

Introduction

Decision-making on emergent vascular access can be challenging, even for the most experienced provider. As mentioned in previous chapters, many factors must be considered when deciding upon which type of vascular access device (VAD) to use, including patient-specific, provider-specific, environmental, and time-related factors. Despite these challenges, it is still possible for providers to develop *a structured, systematic approach to their own decision-making* regarding establishing vascular access under emergent conditions. This chapter will outline some of the existing evidence on how to select the right VAD for a specific patient, operating under the assumption that providing vascular access in an emergency differs from providing access under other clinical circumstances.

The first and most crucial step in deciding upon the proper VAD for use under emergent circumstances is making an *accurate and rapid assessment of the circumstances* surrounding that decision. The ability to make such assessments constitutes a unique skill set that emergency care providers will develop over time and with proper training. While it is possible to establish guidelines and policies relating to the use of VADs for specific patient populations and circumstances, even the most comprehensive clinical guidelines cannot account for all possible situations. Consequently, decision-making in emergent vascular access is as much an "art" as a "science." Like all artists, providers of emergent vascular access will bring their own unique talents, perspectives, and understanding of the patient's clinical

J. H. Paxton (✉)
Department of Emergency Medicine, Wayne State University School of Medicine, Detroit, MI, USA
e-mail: james.paxton@wayne.edu

A. Lemieux
Wayne State University School of Medicine, Detroit, MI, USA
e-mail: fh1310@wayne.edu

© Springer Nature Switzerland AG 2021
J. H. Paxton (ed.), *Emergent Vascular Access*,
https://doi.org/10.1007/978-3-030-77177-5_11

condition and circumstances to the task. In this chapter, we will provide some of the tools needed to make the "right" decisions for patients, although the final solution will always be dependent on providers' ability to recognize when and how to use those tools.

Have a Game Plan

Providers should *develop a vascular access "game plan"* before starting the first vascular access attempt. This might be a simple mental algorithm that the provider has used on innumerable previous patients, but should include next steps that the provider will take if preceding approaches are unsuccessful, and must be able to be quickly adapted to changing circumstances. Under stressful and time-limited conditions, providers should have at least a rough sketch of this game plan going into the encounter, with the understanding that the plan will be modified as conditions change. This may help to prevent bad decision-making "in the heat of the moment" and should enable providers to gather the anticipated resources prior to needing them.

One example of such a game plan might be: "Try for a visualized/palpable vein large-bore peripheral IV in the upper extremity. If no PIV is established after two attempts and the patient is stable, consider US-PIV. If the patient is unstable, establish a proximal humerus IO or EJ PIV." Establishing such a vascular access plan *a priori* provides a cognitive framework for the provider that will facilitate rapid transition from one failed effort to the next sequential step, without requiring a cognitive pause on the part of the provider. This type of cognitive unloading should help the provider to focus upon the task at hand, rather than subconsciously (or consciously) worrying about what the next step should be. Most providers who are involved in establishing emergent vascular access on a regular basis already have a mental algorithm that they use regularly, even if they don't recognize it. For those who do not yet have one, efforts to develop such a mental algorithm should help to enhance efficiency and increase the likelihood of successful line placement.

Environmental Limitations

Before considering patient- or provider-specific circumstances, it is important for providers to *accurately assess the environment that they are working in*. Importantly, a provider's environment is not only the *physical space* in which the provider is working, although this is an important aspect. Providers must also consider what local tools and resources are available to them to assist in performing their task. Austere environments (e.g., the prehospital environ) are characterized by limited access to technologies and assistance in establishing vascular access. For providers who are accustomed to working in a specific clinical environment, these limitations will be intuitively incorporated into the provider's decision-making. But individuals who are working in a new or unfamiliar environment should assess their environment carefully before establishing a plan for meeting the patient's vascular access needs. Providers must know what VADs are available to them, including which adjunct and assistive technologies (e.g., ultrasound, vein-finding devices, etc.) may be available when needed. This includes not just knowing what tools are generally available but being aware of any shortages in stocking supplies, where supplies are kept in one's clinical space, and proactively arranging supplies in one's space (within the realm of possibility) to accommodate anticipated needs during the acute care episode. Providers should try to learn from their difficulties with prior attempts and modify future approaches to prevent those difficulties in the future. One should always hope for the best conditions but plan (and prepare) for the worst.

An accurate assessment of one's environment will help to rule in or rule out the ability to use specific types of vascular access devices or useful adjuncts. A few key questions that providers should ask themselves when assessing their environment include:

- *Where am I?* Providers who are treating a patient in a dark hallway or abandoned building should expect more austere conditions than providers working in a well-lit emergency department or inpatient hospital room. Access to adequate lighting, a crash cart, a stash of medical supplies, or other needed resources will always be dictated by the location of the intervention effort.
- *What did I bring with me?* This may be the easiest thing for a seasoned vascular access specialist to assess. Rapid response teams and prehospital providers will know exactly what is in their "pack," although those new to the emergency department or inpatient setting may not know what they have available at their fingertips, especially if they did not bring it themselves. Providers should also consider what specialized knowledge and training they bring to the patient's care. Sometimes the most valuable tool that a provider can offer to the patient is their own skill set.
- *What resources are summonable?* In any environment, it is important for providers to consider what additional resources can be quickly recruited to the vascular access attempt. Providers must know how to find what they need and which devices and adjuncts may be quickly obtained in their care environment.
- *Is assistance available?* Providers who are working alone will have fewer options, especially if the patient is unstable and requires simultaneous completion of other (i.e., non-vascular access) tasks. Optimally, the vascular access specialist should be focused on establishing vascular access, *not* providing chest compressions, transporting the patient, intubating the patient, etc. Providers must know their limits, including when to ask for help.

Clearly, many such questions about the environment are best asked and answered well before the immediate need for emergent vascular access occurs. For those who are new to the world of emergent vascular access, this educational process will be revealing. Providers should not wait until their patient is crashing to ask these questions. For those who have a long track record of providing emergent vascular access, the answers may be familiar but should bear occasional reassessment. After all, circumstances can change.

Patient Assessment

Once the provider has assessed where they are, and what resources they can quickly access, they must focus on the characteristics unique to the patient and their emergent medical condition. More than likely, these patient characteristics will not already be well-known to the provider. Unfortunately, critically ill or unstable patients may not have the time or ability to educate the provider about their medical history or previous vascular access attempts. Family members or others familiar with the patient may not be available, and medical records may be scarce or unavailable. Emergency care providers are accustomed to this dearth of information on their patients, but it may be unsettling to those less familiar with such circumstances. It is imperative that providers approach each encounter requiring emergent vascular access as objectively as possible, understanding that limited information about the patient's medical condition and past medical history are the rule, rather than the exception. Providers must be able to assess the patient rapidly, with limited information and a critical eye toward how they can achieve your primary objective – to establish vascular access quickly and with a minimum of risk to the patient.

Although each patient's needs are different, providers can still employ a systematic method of patient assessment when establishing emergent vascular access. The experienced provider will begin their assessment even before they have examined the patient. The patient's *ability to assist and comply* with vascular access attempts should be evident within seconds of meeting them, including behavior or exam findings that suggest limiting circumstances such as intoxication, agitation, diminished mental capacity, cardiac arrest, and uncontrollable movement. Such global patient factors will dramatically change the provider's approach, and providers should have a "go-to" approach for managing uncooperative patients that will likely differ from the approach taken with a cooperative patient.

If the patient is awake and able to communicate, important information may be obtained very rapidly from the patient within seconds. When feasible, patients should be *asked about their own vascular access preferences* as well as their self-reported contraindications to considering specific insertion sites and/or modalities. Compliance with vascular access attempts among alert patients may be enhanced by consulting the patient on their VAD preferences. The discovery of relevant physical exam findings (e.g., hemodialysis fistulas, venous scarring, small-caliber veins, etc.) may also be accelerated by simply asking the patient about the success or failure of previous vascular access attempts or access sites that they believe to be "off-limits" to providers.

Unfortunately, hemodynamically unstable patients may be uncooperative and/or unreliable historians. Even stable patients have myriad reasons for not complying with vascular access attempts, including the presence of alcohol or other intoxicants, acute psychiatric illness, dementia, or agitation due to pain and anxiety (just to name a few). When assessing an unstable patient, providers should be prepared for the likelihood that the patient will not be able to provide any helpful information during the assessment, and they may even fight one's efforts to establish adequate vascular access. Any other baseline assumption is counterproductive. Understanding this, *providers should approach the patient encounter expecting to intuit their way through the process, including a strong reliance on physical exam findings and circumstantial evidence.* Input from the patient, though valuable and worth seeking, may not be forthcoming.

Before anchoring upon a specific VAD insertion site or device, the provider should perform a brief but adequate physical examination of the patient. The purpose of this examination is to *identify the presence of physical characteristics that could influence the provider's choice of site and device* in forthcoming vascular access attempts. A systematic approach is of value here. The provider should expose the patient by removing clothing and other obstacles to full evaluation of their upper extremities, chest, and neck. The patient should be examined for surgical scars or evidence of repeated venous access attempts, as well as extremity swelling or soft tissue patterns that could make cannulation unlikely. The presence of an active hemodialysis fistula or graft will alert the provider to this important limitation, as venous access should not be performed on the same extremity, to preserve dialysis access. Although nonfunctional (e.g., clotted and unsalvageable) hemodialysis sites may be considered for venous cannulation under austere circumstances, it is always preferred to avoid cannulating an extremity with altered anatomy, and the contralateral extremity should be considered first. If the salvageability of the hemodialysis site is unknown to the provider (as is often the case), providers should assume that the extremity is off-limits. For cardiac arrest patients, especially when IO access may be required, it is important to examine both the shoulder and knee joints for surgical scars as joint surgery is a relative contraindication to placement of an IO catheter at that location. Providers should look for long-bone fractures or joint dislocations, to avoid placing an IV or IO on the same extremity as an acute orthopedic injury or disruption of the bony cortex. Acute orthopedic injuries may compromise venous/lymphatic drainage from the extremity. Mastectomy scars may suggest that IV or IO placement should be avoided on the ipsilateral upper extremity due to potentially impaired lymphatic drainage following previous lymph node dissection. These and other contraindications to specific insertion sites can help the provider to immediately rule out certain access points, allowing the provider to prioritize available appropriate insertion sites in their placement algorithm.

An *"anatomic inventory"* (Table 11.1) can provide one means of rapidly assessing the emergent patient's physical state as it relates to potential vascular access sites. This type of approach will quickly identify key anatomic considerations that may compromise the patient's ability to receive specific device types or vascular access sites.

The key component of such an anatomic assessment is the provider's ability to rapidly evaluate the patient and identify key physical examination findings suggesting which vascular access sites and devices may be compromised for the patient.

When assessing a patient's vascular access needs, providers should also attempt to predict how the VAD will be used during the patient's subsequent care. In the acute setting, it may be necessary to establish "bridging" access to stabilize the patient's condition while appropriate definitive vascular access is being attempted.

Table 11.1 Anatomic inventory for rapid assessment of vascular access obstacles

Anatomic finding	Key obstacles	Types of VAD compromised
Altered mental status	Inability to follow commands or comply with assessment and VAD insertion effort	PIV, CVC, IO
Unstable vital signs	Venous collapse, reduced pulse perception	PIV, CVC
Cardiac arrest	Venous collapse, impaired circulation, extremity movement, chest compressions	
Neck scarring	Central venous collapse, venous obstruction	CVC
Extremity scarring	Peripheral venous collapse, venous fragility	PIV
Surgical scarring at joints (e.g., shoulder, knee)	Distorted bony landmarks, disrupted drainage from intraosseous space	IO
Traumatic orthopedic deformity	Soft tissue swelling, disrupted bony cortex, distorted anatomy, impaired venous drainage	PIV, IO
AV graft or fistula	Need for dialysis site preservation, distorted anatomy, impaired blood flow	PIV
Rash or cellulitis	Risk of infectious complications	PIV, IO
Extremity edema	Obscured anatomy, impaired venous drainage	PIV, IO
Pre-existing access (e.g., PICC line, PIV line, etc.)	Need to preserve long-term vascular access, questionable functioning of existing device	PIV, IO, CVC
Isolated diminished extremity pulse	Impaired blood flow, increased risk of extremity malperfusion	PIV, IO

Table 11.2 Examples of patient needs to consider with the initial vascular access attempt

Immediate needs (stabilization)	Short-term needs (hospitalization)	Long-term needs (post-hospitalization)
Intubation (RSI)	Continuous infusions	Central vein preservation
Vasopressors	Vasopressors	Minimal risk of CRBSI
Fluids (bolus)	Fluids (maintenance)	Minimal risk of CRT
Antibiotics	Antibiotics (inpatient)	Antibiotics (long-term)
Hyperosmolar agents	"As-needed" medications	
Anticoagulation	Anticoagulation	
ACLS medications/CPR	Parenteral nutrition	
Blood sampling	Blood sampling	
Hemodynamic monitoring	Hemodynamic monitoring	
Intravenous contrast	Intravenous contrast	
Patient preference	Patient comfort	
Interventional procedures	Low risk of line failure	
Low risk of complications	Low risk of complications	

Note: *RSI* rapid sequence induction, *CRBSI* catheter-related bloodstream infection, *CRT* catheter-related thrombosis, *ACLS* advanced cardiac life support, *CPR* cardiopulmonary resuscitation

However, *providers should always seek to establish definitive vascular access that satisfies all the patient's anticipated needs on the first vascular access attempt*. This might prevent additional VAD placement from being necessary and may ultimately improve the quality of care afforded to the patient. Examples of important considerations when assessing a patient's needs for immediate vascular access are provided in Table 11.2. Each of these considerations should be assessed for the patient prior to making first attempts at establishing access.

Presenting Medical Conditions

The patient's presenting condition is an important consideration when assessing vascular access needs. Some patients may not require immediate access, although the underlying assumption in this chapter is that emergent vascular access is required. Other patients (e.g., cardiac arrest) may require immediate intervention that is only possible through a VAD. Many patients will fall somewhere in between these two extremes. The primary distinction here is the *time-sensitive need for an intervention that requires a vascular access device.* This determination should be made by the medical provider who is treating the patient's medical condition, and this person may not always be the same person who is providing vascular access. In such cases, communication between the medical provider and the vascular access provider is paramount to appropriate and successful line placement. As discussed previously in Chap. 10, time constraints are an important contributor to difficult vascular access. Consequently, providers should give themselves as much time as possible to plan and execute VAD placement but must also avoid delays. Thus, the provider must strike a balance between the needs of the patient for immediate therapy and the needs of the provider.

The *presence of specific medical conditions* may also guide the selection of an appropriate VAD. For example, patients presenting with suspected septic shock may reasonably be expected to require large volumes of bolus crystalloid infusion and vasopressors. Although fluids may be delivered by various routes, vasopressor infusion should be delivered by central venous access. In this case, the provider should anticipate that central venous access may be required, although a bridging device (e.g., large-bore peripheral IV) may be established to initiate fluid infusion. This will allow the patient to receive required antibiotics and fluids early, which may improve the patient's intravascular volume and enhance the likelihood of a successful subsequent central line attempt by enlarging the central vein targets. In some cases, "fluid-responsive" patients suspected of septic shock may improve hemodynamically after receiving fluids alone, thereby postponing or eliminating the need for central venous access. An awareness of the patient's suspected medical condition, as well as the appropriate interventions planned to treat this condition, may allow such a staged approach to vascular access. This example highlights the need to predict a patient's future vascular access needs, as well as the importance of modifying or adapting the vascular access plan in response to subsequent events.

The need for *infusion of crystalloid* (e.g., normal saline, lactated Ringer's solution) or colloid (e.g., hetastarch, albumin) solutions is a common indication for vascular access device placement. In the acute setting, providers often think of fluid infusion in terms of "bolus" aliquots of large volumes infused over a short period of time. As discussed in Chap. 2, fluid flow rates are dependent on a variety of factors, including internal catheter diameter, catheter length, fluid viscosity, and infusion pressure gradients. Longer, thinner catheters typically have lower maximal flow rates than shorter, wider catheters. Larger veins typically have lower resistance to flow than smaller veins. Higher viscosity fluids may infuse more slowly than less viscous fluids. Understanding these concepts will inform the provider's choice of vascular access device and decisions on whether to use devices that enhance the infusion pressure gradient (e.g., pressure bags, infusion pumps). Blood products are more viscous than crystalloid fluids, and fluids containing red blood cells (e.g., whole blood, packed red blood cells) introduce the additional concern of red blood cell (RBC) lysis, which can cause or worsen hyperkalemia and reduce the effectiveness of the RBCs infused. It is important to predict the patient's need for immediate bolus fluid infusion when planning VAD placement. In many cases, multiple VADs may be indicated to accommodate the patient's need for immediate bolus infusion, especially when other medications (e.g., antibiotics, electrolyte replacement) may be competing for infusion space at the same time.

Many sources recommend selection of the proper gauge catheter based upon the patient's presentation and the indications for VAD placement. Commonly recommended indications for different gauges of peripheral IV insertion are illustrated in Fig. 11.1.

The Advanced Trauma Life Support (ATLS) guidelines recommend the immediate establishment of two large-bore (i.e., 18-gauge or larger) peripheral IV lines at the forearm or antecubital fossae for adult major trauma victims [1]. These patients often require large volumes of crystalloid fluid and blood products; both indications suggest the need for large-bore catheters.

The American Heart Association (AHA) Advanced Cardiac Life Support (ACLS) guidelines recommend attempting PIV insertion prior to the use of other vascular access techniques for victims of cardiac arrest, although no specific guidance is offered regarding the gauge or location of PIV insertion [2]. The only caveat to this is that *PIV insertion is recommended to be above the diaphragm for pregnant patients*, although common practice for all cardiac arrest victims is to seek PIV

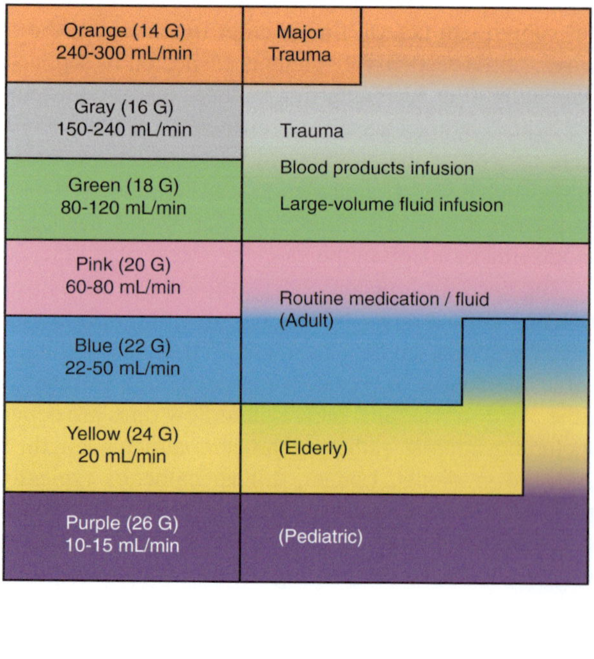

Fig. 11.1 Commonly used peripheral IV line gauges and their indications

placement at the antecubital fossa whenever possible. Intraosseous access should be considered when PIV access is unsuccessful or deemed to be infeasible [2]. However, the ACLS guidelines offer no specific guidance on how many PIV attempts should be made (or the duration of said attempts) prior to the decision to initiate IO access.

Most of the published literature on IO access for cardiac arrest highlights the use of proximal tibial IO placement, although this is a subdiaphragmatic location, and therefore appears to be suboptimal. Humeral or sternal IO catheters may be preferred, as these sites are associated with higher flow rates and are situated closer to the central circulation. Among neonates, umbilical venous cannulation is the preferred vascular access route in the delivery suite, although IO access may be attempted if the umbilical vein access is not available or the patient is being treated outside of the delivery room. Additional information about umbilical vein catheterization is provided in Chap. 8.

Patients with septic shock appear to enjoy improved mortality when receiving a central venous catheter (CVC) on the same day as admission, as compared to those who receive CVC placement later in their hospital course [3]. Of course, a diagnosis of septic shock requires that patients with sepsis fail to respond to an adequate (e.g., 30 mL/kg) resuscitative crystalloid fluid bolus and ultimately require vasopressors [4]. Many hypotensive patients presenting to the acute care provider are not yet differentiated, and some may respond to aggressive fluid resuscitation without the need for vasopressors. Thus, undifferentiated patients with hypotension, including those who are suspected of septic shock, should ideally receive adequate crystalloid fluid resuscitation through large-bore PIV cannulae before a central line is deemed to be required. Methods to assess the patient's intravascular volume status (e.g., collapsibility of the inferior vena cava on bedside ultrasound, response to leg lift, etc.) should be employed to gauge the patient's need for, and subsequent response to, fluid boluses. The management of hypotensive patients suspected of sepsis may therefore benefit from a staged response, including immediate placement of adequate large-bore peripheral vascular access, followed by central venous access as suggested by the patient's subsequent response to bolus fluid administration.

Indications for a central venous catheter are well-defined in the medical literature. In the emergent setting, the indications for CVC placement include inadequate peripheral venous access, need for continuous infusion of vasoactive medications, or need for hemodynamic monitoring. Of course, perceptions of the adequacy of peripheral access and need for hemodynamic monitoring are subject to provider interpretation.

Medication Characteristics

The need for intravenous medication infusion is another common indication for emergent vascular access. Although many medications can be administered safely via peripheral venous access, others may require central venous infusion. The *Infusion Nurses Society Standards of Practice* state that continuous infusions of medication with irritant or vesicant properties should be achieved with a CVC whenever possible [5]. For time-critical infusions of life-saving therapies, such as vasopressors, the infusion should be initiated with a PIV until a CVC can be safely inserted, preferably within 24–48 hours [5]. Hemodilution, the process by which potentially noxious medications are diluted in the bloodstream during infusion, is limited with infusion through peripheral veins. This can lead to injury to the vein or surrounding tissues when certain substances are infused through a peripheral vein, especially in the event of *infiltration* (i.e., infusate escaping from the vein/cannula into the surrounding tissue).

It is important to note the distinction between *venous irritants* and *vesicants* when assessing a patient's vascular access needs. Venous irritants cause pain or discomfort with infusion, while vesicants are agents capable of causing blistering, tissue sloughing, and soft tissue necrosis in the event of solute infiltration. Venous irritants may cause injury within the vessel lumen, including phlebitis and thrombophlebitis. *Extravasation* is the term generally used when describing infiltration of a vesicant solute, as opposed to less noxious (i.e., non-vesicant) solutes. Damage to the soft tissues due to vesicant extravasation can require aggressive management, including surgical debridement [5]. Common medications that qualify as venous vesicants are provided in Table 11.3.

Drugs that qualify as *venous irritants* can usually be safely administered via PIV with adequate monitoring, although central venous infusion is preferred when these medications are given as continuous infusions. Agents classified as venous irritants that should not generally be administered via PIV include potassium chloride ($\geq$20 mEq/100 mL), sodium chloride (23.4%), acyclovir >7 mg/mL, and long-term epoprostenol infusions. Of course, some venous irritant drugs are commonly given

Table 11.3 Common venous vesicants used in emergency care [5–7]

Drug	Recommended VAD
Adrenergic agents (e.g., dobutamine, dopamine, epinephrine, norepinephrine, vasopressin)	CVC
Aminophylline	CVC, monitor if PIV
Antiemetics (e.g., promethazine)	PIV (if proximal to wrist); may be given IM
Cardiovascular agents (e.g., amiodarone >2 mg/ml, digoxin, tromethamine)	CVC, monitor if PIV
Contrast (radiographic) agents	CVC, high-pressure injector midlines, monitor if PIV
Dantrolene	CVC, use PIV for emergencies
Diazepam	CVC, monitor if PIV
Electrolytes, high osmolarity (e.g., mannitol $\geq$5%, dextrose $\geq$10%, calcium chloride 10%, calcium gluconate 10%)	CVC, monitor if PIV
Methylene blue	CVC, monitor if PIV
Parenteral nutrition	CVC if contain >10% dextrose; use peripherally-compatible PN for PIV
Phenytoin	CVC, monitor if PIV

via PIV infusion under specific emergent circumstances such as dextrose (up to 50% solution, for severe hypoglycemia), calcium chloride 10% and amiodarone (in cardiac arrest), mannitol $\geq 5\%$ (for brain herniation), dantrolene (for malignant hyperthermia), and methylene blue (for methemoglobinemia or shock states) [5–7].

Vasopressors should generally be infused through a CVC, although these medications are occasionally provided through peripheral venous access. In one recent review, 85.3% of local tissue injury events were associated with vasopressor infusion through a PIV distal to the antecubital or popliteal fossae, and 96.8% occurred after 4 hours of infusion [7]. These results suggest that brief (<4 hours) vasopressor infusion may be considered through a proximal PIV (i.e., proximal or at the antecubital fossa) when the risk of delaying vasopressor initiation to obtain a CVC is high. It has been recommended that patients who require extended (duration >4 hr) vasopressor infusion should receive CVC placement to avoid such complications [5].

Providers may wish to administer *multiple medications through the same IV access*, utilizing secondary (piggyback) IV tubing. A typical IV tubing setup is illustrated in Fig. 11.2. The *primary set* is generally used for fluid infusion, although secondary lines of IV tubing can be linked into the primary tubing to facilitate simultaneous infusion of other fluids or medications through the same IV tubing system [8]. The *secondary set* used for piggybacking often features a shorter length of tubing than the primary set, typically without access ports or a backcheck valve. The bag attached to a secondary set is generally hung higher than the bag attached to the primary set, to increase the relative effect of gravity on infusion and overcome any flow obstruction imparted by the connection system. Piggyback bags are often smaller in volume than the primary bag, which can lead to reduced flow from the secondary set if both bags are held at the same height. Higher-volume bags will typically drain faster than lower-volume bags due to the effect of gravity on fluid flow, although different tubes from these infusion sets may have different inherent flow rates [9]. When needed, an extension hook may be used to drop the height of the primary set bag.

Extension adaptors are used to connect two or more tubing lines for piggybacking and other secondary line setup and may be found in a variety of shapes. The most commonly encountered forms are V-set, T-set, and Y-set connectors (Fig. 11.3). The Y-set and T-set connectors feature a "common space" where solutions from the two limbs can mingle before being drawn into the distal IV tubing, although V-sets lack this feature.

Certain medications may be incompatible with one another and should not be infused through the same VAD tubing at the same time. Incompatibilities are characterized by physical and/or chemical reactions that occur between two (or more) drugs when the solutions are combined in the same syringe, tubing, or bottle [10]. Such reactions can lead to reduced efficacy of the drugs, increase drug toxicity, or contribute to other adverse effects [10]. Many different incompatibilities exist, and the likelihood of these events should be assessed using a source such as Trissel's™ IV compatibility database [8]. However, some common examples of incompatible drug combinations are provided in Table 11.4.

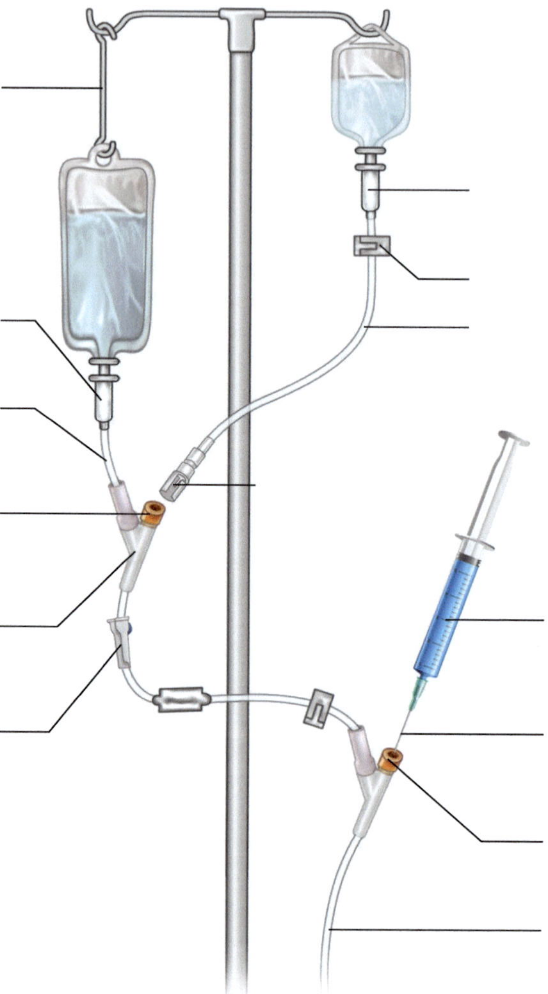

Fig. 11.2 Generic IV tubing setup, including Y-port

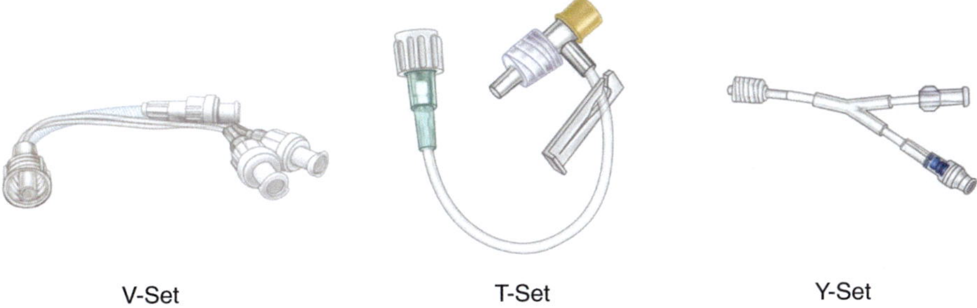

Fig. 11.3 V-set, T-set, and Y-set three-way connectors

Table 11.4 Common drug incompatibilities encountered in the care of critically ill patients [8, 10–11]

Drug + drug combinations	
Midazolam +	Cefepime
	Omeprazole
	Phenytoin
Hydrocortisone +	Midazolam
	Vancomycin
	Calcium chloride
	Vitamin B1
Vancomycin +	Cefepime
	Omeprazole
Phenytoin +	Ranitidine
	Noradrenaline
	Fentanyl
Sulfamethoxazole-trimethoprim +	Vancomycin
	Fentanyl
	Hydrocortisone
	Ranitidine
Lactated Ringer's +	Ciprofloxacin
	Cyclosporine
	Diazepam
	Ketamine
	Lorazepam
	Nitroglycerin
	Phenytoin
	Propofol

Provider-Specific Considerations

Providers should reflect on their own training and limitations prior to selecting a device or technique for use with an initial vascular access attempt. The provider's comfort and familiarity with placement techniques and devices are crucial to placement success. Thus, when establishing critical vascular access for an unstable patient, providers should generally refrain from selecting a new or unfamiliar technique. We suggest that providers learn new techniques when the "heat is off," so that they can refine their skills when the "heat is on." Provider-specific contributors to difficult vascular access are provided in Chap. 10, including distractibility, fatigue, stress, and lack of adequate experience. These factors will influence the provider's choice of vascular access device, and providers should be self-aware enough to recognize their own limitations and challenges that they bring to the vascular access effort.

Device Limitations

Traditionally, vascular access providers have been instructed to select the smallest-possible gauge required for the patient's care. Small-gauged devices take up less space in the vein, thus allowing increased blood flow around the device and theoretically reducing trauma to the vessel and surrounding tissues. This philosophy makes sense when considering stable patients with predefined indications for vascular access. However, such conservative strategies may be more challenging to employ in the earliest stages of patient resuscitation and stabilization, since the patient's future vascular access needs with subsequent care may not be apparent to the provider at the time of initial assessment. Providers must recognize this ambiguity in the emergent care of unstable patients and attempt to balance the need for selecting a minimally invasive device with the potential for inadequate access to meet the patient's needs.

A step-wise approach to vascular access device placement is therefore often indicated when managing undifferentiated patients with potential (or recognized) clinical instability. The concept of a "bridging device" is important here. In this context, *bridging devices* are vascular access devices that are understood *a priori* by the provider to be temporary vascular access points by which stabilizing interventions can be administered while planning or preparing for definitive vascular access device placement. A *definitive device* represents the ideal vascular access device needed (or anticipated) for optimal management of the patient's condition. If definitive device placement is the goal of the vascular access episode, bridging devices represent a means by which providers can achieve this goal for patients in whom definitive device placement is either impossible or unacceptably delayed. For example, IO or PIV catheter placement may be necessary to initiate bolus crystalloid fluid, blood product, or vasopressor infusion in an unstable (e.g., hypotensive) patient who cannot safely receive immediate and necessary CVC placement. The understood implication in placing a bridging device is that the initiation of intravenous infusion cannot be safely delayed while seeking definitive device placement. Although the circumstances surrounding the use of a bridging device may vary, they are often deployed when the provider has either failed definitive device placement or has determined that the time needed to achieve definitive access introduces greater risk than the decision to rely on suboptimal access to initiate therapy. *The perceived need for a bridging device results from a time-sensitive and subjective assessment by the vascular access provider.* In some cases, devices initially placed as a bridging device may ultimately serve as definitive access if the bridging device facilitates adequate clinical improvement so that the anticipated definitive access device is no longer required. For example, an undifferentiated hypotensive patient may be suspected of septic shock and receive PIV placement to initiate antibiotics and bolus fluid infusion while plans are made for CVC placement for continuous hemodynamic monitoring and vasopressor infusion. However, subsequent assessments may lead the provider to determine that the patient is merely dehydrated, which could obviate the need for CVC placement. As this example illustrates, decisions regarding specific vascular access needs for undifferentiated patients are dynamic and must be adjusted accordingly when the provider is faced with new clinical information.

Guidelines and Policies

Several published guidelines have been provided by proposed authorities on infusion therapy and acute care. Some of the more prominent guidelines are described below, including relevant guidance relating to emergent vascular access.

Michigan Appropriateness Guide for Intravenous Catheters (MAGIC) [12]

This reference focuses upon providing guidance on appropriate use of peripherally inserted central catheters (PICCs), including indications for insertion and duration of use. However, they have also opined on the use of other devices, especially as it relates to the duration of therapy and type of infusates to be administered. This multispecialty international panel concluded that *PICC lines are inappropriate for peripherally compatible solutions* when the proposed duration is ≤5 days. Patients requiring only peripherally compatible infusates for ≤5 days should ideally receive PIV placement in the dorsum of the hand (avoiding the forearm veins) if they are at risk for the need for dialysis (e.g., stage 3b chronic kidney disease or glomerular filtration rate <45 mL/min). This is intended to preserve veins for anticipated hemodialysis. The forearm insertion sites are preferred in patients with compatible infusions <5 days in non-renal patients, as placement in this area avoids joints and points of flexion.

Table 11.5 provides a summary of the MAGIC recommendations for peripherally compatible infusates, according to the duration of infusion.

For infusion of *non-peripherally compatible infusates*, central venous access is required. The MAGIC panel concluded that non-tunneled CVC is preferred in critically ill patient or if hemodynamic monitoring is needed for 6–14 days. Although PICC lines are considered appropriate for all proposed durations of therapy, tunneled catheters are equally appropriate for infusion durations of ≥15 days. Ports, tunneled catheter, and PICC lines are equally appropriate when the proposed duration of non-peripherally compatible infusion is ≥31 days. Ports should be considered as a first option unless there is a known complication with the device. However,

Table 11.5 MAGIC recommendations for peripherally compatible infusates, according to the duration of infusion [12]

Duration of infusion	Preferred device	Considerations
≤5 days	PIV or US-PIV	
6–14 days (non-critically ill)	US-PIV	US-PIV is preferred to PIV. Midline catheter is preferred to PICC
6–14 days (critically ill)	Non-tunneled CVC	If hemodynamic monitoring is needed for 6–14 days
15–30 days	PICC	PICC preferred to midline catheter, tunneled CVC, or port
≥30 days	Tunneled catheter or port	

the appropriateness of port use for emergent resuscitation is not addressed directly in these guidelines. It should be noted that tunneled catheters and ports are placed in the operating room or interventional radiology suite and are not options for emergent vascular access in the emergency department or other acute care environments. Placement of a PICC line, though recommended for various indications by the MAGIC guidelines, may also be impractical under emergent conditions. At many institutions, the placement of PICC lines is restricted to specific vascular access specialists, who may not be available when access is needed. Thus, guidance from the MAGIC guidelines and other resources should be balanced with the acute needs of the patient for immediate therapy.

Among patients with difficult vascular access (DVA), the MAGIC guidelines suggest that midline catheters and US-PIVs should be preferred to PICCs for duration of use between 6 and 14 days. However, in patients with stage 3b or greater chronic kidney disease (CKD), US-PIV is considered by the MAGIC panel to be inappropriate, due to the need to preserve forearm veins for future dialysis needs. They recommend placement of a small-bore tunneled central catheter instead for this population. External jugular (EJ) peripheral venous cannulation is appropriate for emergent situations when the duration of therapy is expected to be <96 hours. Placement of PIV lines in the lower extremities is considered inappropriate – except in rare emergency situations when other veins are unavailable. For the administration of IV contrast agents, panelists recommended the use of a proximal 16-, 18-, or 20-gauge PIV, rather than a PICC line.

Among critically ill patients, non-tunneled central venous catheters are preferred over PICC lines when the anticipated duration of use is ≤14 days. Among cancer patients who are likely to require irritant or vesicant infusion (e.g., chemotherapy), PICC lines were deemed appropriate, if the duration of therapy is ≤3 months.

Infusion Nurses Society (INS) Infusion Therapy Standards of Practice

This resource [5] offers comprehensive guidance to nurses and others who engage in vascular access placement and management and is updated every 5 years. The 8th edition (published in 2021) features 230 pages of material, including standards and practice recommendations with associated references. The scope of this resource is quite broad, although certain specific recommendations can be applied to the topic of emergent vascular access:

- *Short peripheral IV catheters.* In general, the INS standards recommend against "blind sticks," favoring vessels that can be directly visualized or palpated. The standards recommend that clinicians be allowed *"no more than two attempts"* to establish a PIV catheter, after which time the placement attempt should be escalated, "to a clinician with a higher skill level and/or consider alternative routes of medication administration." They also recommend that providers use the, *"smallest-gauge PIVC that will accommodate the prescribed therapy* and patient need," including a "20- to 24-gauge PIVC for most infusion therapies." Larger (>20-gauge) catheters are more likely to cause phlebitis but are recommended when rapid transfusion is required. Regarding continuous infusions of medications with irritant or vesicant properties, they suggest that "for time-critical infusions of lifesaving therapies, such as vasopressors, [providers may] *begin the infusion through a PIVC until a CVAD can be safely inserted.* Insert CVAD as soon as possible and within 24 to 48 hours." Avoid the cephalic vein whenever possible, to preserve future dialysis access.
- *Long peripheral IV catheters.* The INS standards recommend that long PIV catheters be used instead of short PIV when "all aspects of a short PIV are met, but the vessel is difficult to palpate or visualize with the naked eye; ultrasound guidance/near infrared technology is recommended. Evaluate depth of vessel when choosing a long PIVC to *ensure two-thirds of catheter lies within vein.*"
- *Midline catheters.* These devices are inserted into a peripheral vein of the upper arm (e.g., basilic, cephalic, brachial), with the terminal tip located at the level of the axilla. They differ from a central line in that the catheter *tip terminates in a proximal peripheral vein* rather than in a central vein. In neonates, these devices can be inserted into scalp veins or veins of the lower extremity as well. These should be used for infusates that are *peripherally compatible.* Further research is needed to establish the safety of using midline catheters for intermittent vesicant infusion. Avoid these devices in patients with history of thrombosis, hypercoagulability, decreased venous flow in the extremities, or end-stage renal disease requiring vein preservation. For PICC or midline catheters, ensure a catheter-to-vessel diameter ratio of <45%.
- *Intraosseous (IO) access.* The INS standards recommend that providers "anticipate use of the IO route in the event of adult or pediatric cardiac arrest if IV access is not available or cannot be obtained quickly" and "consider the IO route for emergent and non-emergent use in patients with *limited or no vascular access*; when the patient may be at risk of increased morbidity or mortality if access is not obtained, such as during shock, life-threatening or status epilepticus, extensive burns, major traumatic injuries, transfusion, or severe dehydration, and/or *when care is compromised without rapid vascular access.*"
- *Central venous catheters.* The INS standards recommend the use of ultrasound with CVC placement, "to increase success rates and decrease insertion-related

complications." They report that the IJ site is preferred for patients with *pre-existing respiratory compromise*, due to higher risk of pneumothorax with medial subclavian insertion. They further state that "if significant unilateral lung disease is present, ipsilateral insertion is recommended for IJ or SC cannulation to prevent further respiratory compromise with pneumothorax in lungs without injury or disease." Patients who have a *cardiovascular implantable electronic device* (e.g., pacemaker) should have either contralateral CVC placement or ipsilateral PICC line placement if central venous access is required. Patients who are actively anticoagulated should not receive SC line placement. Among patients who have *advanced kidney disease* and may ultimately require hemodialysis, it is recommended to avoid SC CVC or PICC lines due to increased risk of thrombosis and central vein stenosis; these patients should receive IJ, EJ, or femoral CVC placement instead of the SC site. Patients who present with an existing implanted port should have the port utilized as the "preferred IV route, in preference to insertion of an additional VAD."

Vessel Health and Preservation: The Right Approach for Vascular Access

This ebook [13] provides a practical approach to vessel health and preservation (VHP), including strategies for patient-specific vascular access assessment. The authors describe traditional vascular access methods as "reactive, painful, and ineffective, often resulting in the exhaustion of peripheral veins prior to consideration of other access options." The emphasis is on development of vascular access clinical pathways that can help to align VAD selection with the patient's medical condition, diagnosis, treatment plan, and vessel health. The "four quadrants of care" for the VHP model are (1) assessment/selection, (2) insertion, (3) management, and (4) evaluation.

Among the recommendations and observations provided in this resource are the following:

- Patients should be able to trust that "the VAD selected has the lowest risk for insertion location, device size not to exceed 33% of vein diameter, length, and number of lumen, and is the most appropriate to deliver the treatment." This 33% metric is intended to reduce the risk of venous thrombosis.
- Although placement of a PIV in the hand or antecubital fossa "is initially easier in most respects due to identification of veins visually and through palpation," these devices are also "uncomfortable for patients, and often fail in less than 72 hours" [14].
- "Optimal peripheral cannula site selection is one that allows ultrasound-guided needle access in a vein 2–4 mm in diameter or larger and 0.2–1.5 cm in depth" [15]. These measurements should be made in the veins' "native state," without a tourniquet.

Rapid Assessment of the Central Veins (RaCeVA) and Peripheral Veins (RaPeVA)

These resources from the Italian Group for Venous Access Devices (GAVeCeLT) are intended to help providers in evaluating the central (RaCeVA) and peripheral (RaPeVA) veins with ultrasound prior to attempting VAD insertion [16]. A thorough US assessment of the major veins prior to VAD insertion has been shown to reduce complications and improve placement success [17].

The *RaPeVA rapid peripheral vein assessment protocol* includes a systematic ultrasound evaluation of the peripheral veins, in the following sequence:

- Position 1 – *cephalic vein* at lateral cubital crease (antecubital fossa)
- Position 2 – *median cubital/basilic veins* at medial cubital crease
- Position 3 – *basilic vein* at bicipital humeral groove (upper arm)
- Position 4 – *brachial veins* (*venae comitantes*) at upper humerus
- Position 5 – *cephalic vein* at upper arm
- Position 6 – *cephalic vein* to intersection with *axillary vein*
- Position 7 – *subclavian/external jugular/internal jugular veins*

This assessment starts distally (at the antecubital fossa) and works proximally to the central veins. Vessels are evaluated for compressibility (lack of venous thromboses), size, and shape.

The *RaCeVA rapid central vein assessment protocol* includes a systematic ultrasound evaluation of the central veins, in the following sequence:

- Position 1 – *mid-neck* transverse US view of the *IJ vein* and carotid artery
- Position 2 – *low-neck* transverse US view of the *IJ vein* and carotid artery
- Position 3 – *sternal notch* transverse US view of *brachiocephalic vein*
- Position 4 – *supraclavicular* view of *subclavian/external jugular veins*
- Position 5 – *infraclavicular* view of *axillary/cephalic veins* in long axis
- Position 6 – *deltopectoral fossa* view of *axillary/cephalic veins* in long axis
- Position 7 – *second intercostal space* assessment of lung for pneumothorax

The purpose of this assessment is to systematically assess the peripheral and central veins for patency, suitability for cannulation, and presence of nearby anatomic structures (e.g., artery, nerve, lung) that should be considered in the cannulation attempt.

Guidelines for the Prevention of Intravascular Catheter-Related Infections

This reference [18] was published by the US Centers for Disease Control and Prevention (CDC) in 2011, with the targeted goal of reducing intravascular catheter-related infections through communication of best practices on catheter placement and management [18]. Select recommendations from this resource include the following:

- "Avoid using the femoral vein for central venous access in adult patients. Use a subclavian site, rather than a jugular or femoral site, in adult patients to minimize infection risk for nontunneled CVC placement. Avoid the subclavian site in hemodialysis patients and patients with advanced kidney disease, to avoid subclavian vein stenosis."
- "Use a sutureless securement device to reduce the risk of infection for intravascular catheters."
- "There is no need to replace peripheral catheter more frequently than every 72–96 hours to reduce risk of infection and phlebitis in adults. Replace peripheral catheters in children only when clinically indicated."
- "In adults, use of the radial, brachial, or dorsalis pedis [arterial cannulation] sites is preferred over the femoral or axillary sites of insertion to reduce the risk of infection. In children, the brachial site should not be used."

A Decision-Making Algorithm

Despite the abundance of guidance offered by reputable authorities on the topic, no adequate evidence-derived algorithm has yet been developed informing proper vascular access device selection for adult patients under emergent conditions. The lack of such a resource has traditionally impaired providers in seeking appropriate vascular access in the emergency department or similar pre-hospital or early in-hospital environment. Most existing algorithms relate to the placement of VADs in stable or ambulatory patients and include options such as PICC line placement, which is clearly not an option for critically unstable patients. Although VAD selection should be guided by the patient's specific clinical circumstances, and include consideration of national and international guidelines, algorithmic guidance on VAD selection may have value for specific medical and environmental conditions. Providers should determine whether their institution has an algorithm for VAD selection that encompasses emergent vascular access. If not, providers should consider creating such an algorithm, based upon existing evidence from the medical literature and incorporating their own institutional/professional policies and guidelines. Figure 11.4 shows an example of a VAD placement algorithm that might be considered for adult patients.

Conclusions

Decision-making is an underappreciated aspect of emergent vascular access, which deserves dedicated research and discussion in academic *fora*. Many factors must be considered in making decisions about the need for vascular access in critically ill and unstable patients. Device limitations and indications for use should be

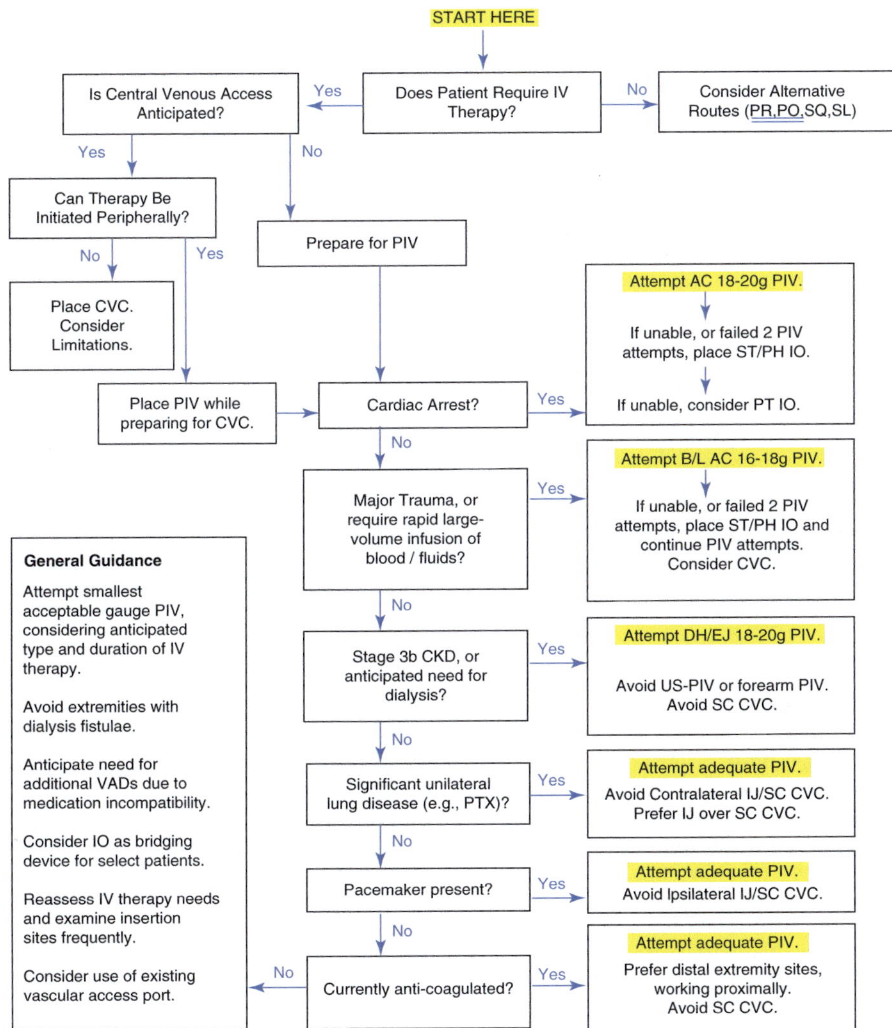

Fig. 11.4 Example of a VAD placement algorithm for adult patients. Notes: AC antecubital, CKD chronic kidney disease, CVC central venous catheter, DH dorsal hand, EJ external jugular, IJ internal jugular, IO intraosseous, PIV peripheral intravenous, PO per oral, PR per rectum, PTX pneumothorax, SC subclavian, SL sublingual, SQ subcutaneous, ST sternal, US-PIV ultrasound-guided peripheral intravenous

considered, as should potential immediate- and long-term complications from their use. Providers are inundated with myriad recommendations on how and why specific devices should be used, but much of this information relates to the management of stable, hospitalized patients and should be measured against the need for reliable and effective immediate vascular access in the setting of a medical emergency. Future research into the best practices for emergent vascular access device placement is needed.

Key Concepts
- Providers should establish a "game plan" for emergent vascular access prior to the acute episode of the access attempt, guided by their understanding of the patient's specific need for vascular access as well as the resources available to them with the attempt. This might include or be derived from an institutional algorithm guiding VAD selection.
- Best practices for emergent vascular access techniques should be determined, in part, by local institutional protocols, with consideration of evidence-based algorithms provided by reputable authorities.
- Decisions on optimal vascular access should be informed by familiarity with the recommendations endorsed by national and international guidelines on appropriate emergent vascular access.
- Current recommendations on the appropriateness of specific VADs for emergent patients should be viewed with an understanding of the applicability of these recommendations to the emergent patient. Recommendations pertaining to stable, hospitalized patients may not be universally applicable to patients requiring emergent vascular access.

References

1. American College of Surgeons. Committee on Trauma. Advanced trauma life support: student course manual. 10th ed. Chicago, IL: American College of Surgeons; 2018. p. 52.
2. Soar J, Maconochie I, Wyckoff MH, et al. 2019 international consensus on cardiopulmonary resuscitation and emergency cardiovascular care science with treatment recommendations: summary from the basic life support; advanced life support; pediatric life support; neonatal life support; education, implementation, and teams; and first aid task forces. Circulation. 2019;140:e826–80. https://doi.org/10.1161/CIR.0000000000000734.
3. Walkey AJ, Wiener RS, Lindenauer PK. Utilization patterns and outcomes associated with central venous catheter in septic shock: a population-based study. Crit Care Med. 2013;41(6):1450–7.
4. Singer M, Deutschman CS, Seymour CW, et al. The third international consensus definitions for sepsis and septic shock (sepsis-3). JAMA. 2016;315(8):801–10.
5. Gorski LA, Hadaway L, Hagle ME, et al. Infusion therapy standards of practice. J Infus Nurs. 2021;44(suppl 1):S1–S224.
6. Le A, Patel S. Extravasation of noncytotoxic drugs: a review of the literature. Ann Pharmacother. 2014;48(7):870–86.
7. Loubani OM, Green RS. A systematic review of extravasation and local tissue injury from administration of vasopressors through peripheral intravenous catheters and central venous catheters. J Crit Care. 2015;653:e9–e17.
8. Gorski LA, Phillips LD. Phillips's manual of I.V. Therapeutics. 7th ed. Philadelphia: FA Davis Company; 2018.
9. Lannoy D, Décaudin B, Dewulf S, et al. Infusion set characteristics such as antireflux valve and dead-space volume affect drug delivery: an experimental study designed to enhance infusion sets. Anesth Analg. 2010;111(6):1427–31.
10. Marsilio NR, da Silva D, Bueno D. Drug incompatibilities in the adult intensive care unit of a university hospital. Rev Bras Ter Intensiva. 2016;28(2):147–53.

11. Vallée M, Barthélémy I, Friciu M, et al. Compatibility of lactated Ringer's injection with 94 selected intravenous drugs during simulated Y-site administration. Hosp Pharm. 2019:1–7. https://doi.org/10.1177/0018578719888913.
12. Chopra V, Flanders SA, Saint S, et al. The Michigan appropriateness guide for intravenous catheters (MAGIC): results from a multispecialty panel using the RAND/UCLA appropriateness method. Ann Intern Med. 2015;163:S1–S39.
13. Moreau NL, editor. Vessel health and preservation: the right approach for vascular access. Cham: Springer; 2019. (eBook) Available at: https://doi.org/10.1007/978-3-030-03149-7. Accessed 15 March 2021
14. O'Grady NP, Alexander M, Burns LA, et al. Guidelines for the prevention of intravascular catheter-related infections. Am J Infect Control. 2011;39(4 Suppl):S1–S34.
15. Alexandrou E, Ray-Barruel G, Carr PJ, et al. Use of short peripheral intravenous catheters: characteristics, management, and outcomes worldwide. J Hosp Med. 2018;13. https://doi.org/10.12788/jhm.3039
16. Witting MD, Schenkel SM, Lawner BJ, Euerle BD. Effects of vein width and depth on ultrasound guided peripheral intravenous success rates. J Emerg Med. 2010;39:70–5.
17. Pittiruti M, Scoppettuolo G. GAVeCeLT manual of PICC and midline—indications, insertion, management. Edra S.P.A; 2017.
18. Pirotte T. Ultrasound-guided vascular access in adults and children: beyond the internal jugular vein puncture. Acta Anaesthesiol Belg. 2008;59:157–66.

The Future of Emergent Vascular Access

12

James H. Paxton, Nicholas J. Corsi,
and Bethanie Ann Szydlowski

Introduction

Establishing emergent vascular access will always challenge healthcare providers. Although tremendous effort and resources have already been deployed in the development of novel vascular access devices (VADs), humans are living longer than ever before with chronic diseases. It is only logical to assume that longer human life spans will mean more incidents of venous access over an average lifetime, leading to cumulative venous injury, ever-increasing the difficulty of subsequent vascular access attempts. In a recent prospective, observational study assessing stable patients (i.e., not acutely or critically-ill), one out of of every nine to ten adults in an urban ED met predefined criteria of "difficult vascular access," with significant associated comorbidities including intravenous drug abuse, diabetes mellitus, and sickle cell anemia [1]. Repetitive vascular trauma from a lifetime of intravenous cannulation leads to challenges for medical providers in accessing a scarred and stenotic vascular tree [1]. Within certain patient populations, vascular access is already very challenging. For example, end-stage renal disease patients may require a lifetime of vascular access procedures (e.g., catheters, fistulas, grafts, etc.) to receive uninterrupted life-sustaining hemodialysis. As a result, The Association of Vascular Access (AVA) released a position statement stressing the importance of

J. H. Paxton (✉)
Department of Emergency Medicine, Wayne State University School of Medicine,
Detroit, MI, USA
e-mail: james.paxton@wayne.edu

N. J. Corsi
Wayne State University School of Medicine, Detroit, MI, USA
e-mail: nicholas.corsi@med.wayne.edu

B. A. Szydlowski
Medline Industries, Inc., Mundelein, IL, USA
e-mail: BSzydlowski@medline.com

© Springer Nature Switzerland AG 2021
J. H. Paxton (ed.), *Emergent Vascular Access*,
https://doi.org/10.1007/978-3-030-77177-5_12

preservation of upper extremity peripheral veins to provide a vessel conduit for hemodialysis [2]. Recent epidemics of severe viral illnesses, including severe acute respiratory syndrome coronavirus 2 (SARS-CoV-2), have stressed the capacities of emergency departments and other care areas, further underscoring the need for rapid and effective vascular access techniques to treat critically ill patients.

Future advances in vascular access will likely be introduced in a variety of ways. Although there is certainly a role for new types of VADs in addressing society's increasingly complex vascular access needs, modifications and improvements to existing techniques and devices will also help to improve vascular access outcomes. Research into the best way to deploy existing devices, including focused efforts to improve first-attempt success rates, reduce complications from line placement and use (e.g., infection, extravasation, etc.), and "tailor" vascular access strategies to individual patients will likely guide the evolution of this field. Providers will also continue to explore under-utilized physiological techniques of leveraging the body's absorptive capacity for fluid and medication infusion through rectal, subdermal, intraosseous, sublingual, intranasal, and other routes.

This chapter aims to describe some of the recent advances in vascular access that will likely continue to influence the evolution of emergent vascular access techniques into the future.

The Future of Peripheral Intravenous Lines

Peripheral intravenous (PIV) infusion has been documented as far back as the 1600s and is considered today to be the gold standard method of infusing medications or fluids [3]. The first peripheral over-needle IV line, introduced by Zimmerman in 1945, was made of flexible polyvinyl chloride (PVC) [4]. Realizing that the firmness of PVC was suboptimal for intravascular applications, providers soon began utilizing polyurethane (PUR) catheters, which are firm enough to penetrate the vein but warm and soften at physiologic temperatures, reducing the risks of endothelial injury and extravasation [3]. Until recently, short (3–6 cm) PIV PUR catheters could not be left in place for more than 72–96 hours, to reduce risk of infection and phlebitis in adults [5]. However, the 2016 Infusion Nurses Society *Standards of Practice* no longer recommends maximum dwell times for short PIVs, stating instead that they should be discontinued "when clinically indicated, based on findings from site assessment and / or clinical signs and symptoms of systemic complications" [6]. Of course, this still effectively limits dwell time with conventional short PIV catheters to 1–7 days. Midlines (i.e., lines placed peripherally but terminating just distal to the axilla) can be safely left in place for several weeks due to their greater length and more proximal termination, but this extended dwell time comes at a cost. Midlines require ultrasound (US) imaging to place, and successful insertion is therefore user-dependent and subject to the availability of an US machine. The solution to this dilemma would appear to be creation of a longer polyurethane PIV that could be inserted like a traditional PIV. However, polyurethane may warm too quickly during the insertion attempt, making cannulation more difficult when the tip "crumples" before the line is even in place [7]. Polyurethane is also prone to stress fatigue with repeated bending, increasing the risk of catheter fracture with increased catheter length. Consequently, the need exists for longer PIV catheters that can be inserted quickly using external landmarks (rather than US imaging) possessing greater flexibility and crack resistance than polyurethane. Polyether-block-amide (PEBA) is a thermoplastic elastomer that may provide superior performance over PUR and is already being utilized with a new class of VAD – the "long peripheral catheter."

The *long peripheral catheter* (LPC) represents a hybridized form of vascular access that appears to incorporate the best attributes of midlines and short PIVs, offering extended dwell times (up to 4 weeks) and less risk of dislodgement than short PIVs, without the need for extensive soft tissue disruption/dilation or US guidance.

The "traditional" (direct) Seldinger technique, first described in 1953, involves cannulating the target vessel with a finder needle, then advancing a guidewire through the lumen of the needle, removing the needle, and then inserting the catheter over the guidewire before removing the guidewire [8]. Placement of LPCs is generally performed with an "accelerated" Seldinger (AS) technique, in which the guidewire is preloaded inside of the finder needle and catheter to facilitate rapid deployment. Commonly available LPC devices are compared in Table 12.1. The approach to LPC insertion is distinct from the "catheter over a needle" (CoN) technique traditionally used for short PIV insertion. Because LPCs insert superficially, they do not require tissue dilation. One recent trial compared the Powerwand® (Smiths Medical) LPC to a (so-called extended length) 4.78-cm long 20-gauge PIV for adult DVA patients in the ED with a target vein depth of 1.2–1.6 cm. This study found that the LPC was associated with a much longer median survival (4.6 vs. 1.3 days), longer time to insertion (8.66 vs. 5.37 min), and longer in-vein length (2.39 vs. 2.90-cm) [9]. Two examples of LPC catheters, the Endurance™ (Teleflex) catheter (Fig. 12.1) and the Powerwand® (Smiths Medical) catheter (Fig. 12.2), are shown.

Table 12.1 Comparison of selected long peripheral catheter (LPC) devices [10–13]

Device (manufacturer)	Features	Available lengths (cm)	Available gauges
Endurance™ catheter (Teleflex) [10]	Integrated extension line, max pressure 325 psi, max rate 8 mL/sec (using 11.8 cP viscosity), angled stabilization wings, nitinol guidewire	6, 8	18, 20, 22
AccuCath™ (Bard) [11]	Blood control valve, max pressure 325 psi, max rate 6 mL/sec, nitinol guidewire	3.2, 5.7	18, 20, 22
Leaderflex™ catheter (Vygon) [12]	Integrated extension tubing and wings, universal catheter for peripheral vein, central vein and arterial insertion	4, 6, 8, 20	22
Powerwand™ (Smiths Medical) [13]	Integrated extension line, max pressure 325 psi, max rate 8 mL/sec, ZERO EDGE™ transitions for atraumatic vessel entry	6	3-French (~20)

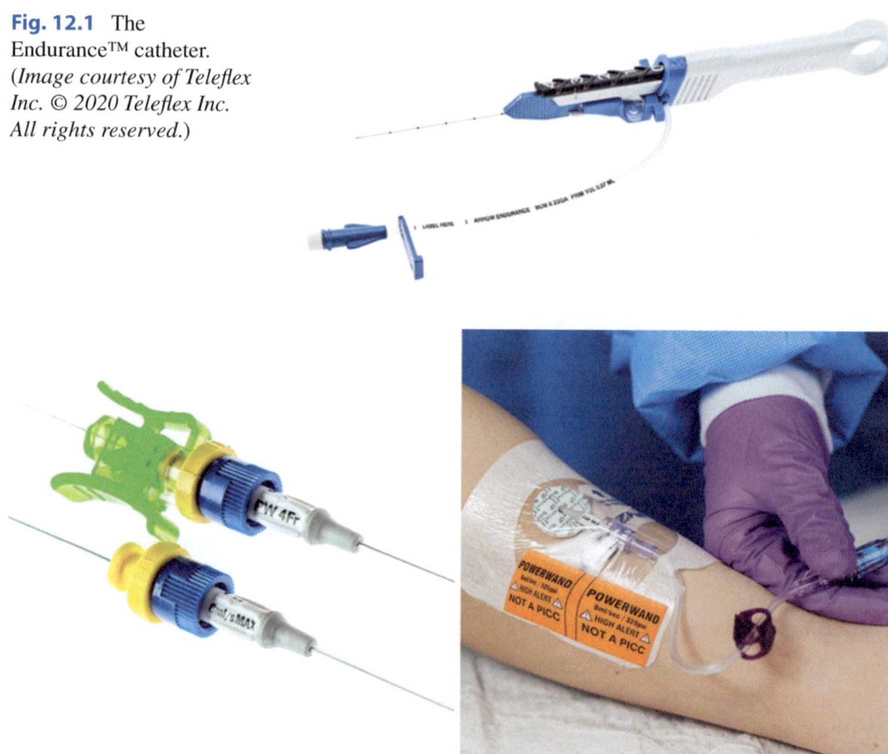

Fig. 12.1 The Endurance™ catheter. (*Image courtesy of Teleflex Inc. © 2020 Teleflex Inc. All rights reserved.*)

Fig. 12.2 The Powerwand® long peripheral catheter. (*Images courtesy of Smiths Medical. © 2020 Smiths Medical. All rights reserved.*)

Midline catheters, typically inserted into the basilic, cephalic, or median cubital veins, are usually between 15 and 25 cm long, with a high rate of first attempt placement for intravenous therapy of up to 6-week duration [14]. These catheters offer a comparable rate of device-related bloodstream infection to standard peripheral venous catheters, but a significantly decreased risk relative to PICC and CVC lines [15]. Midline catheters also carry a lower first failed attempt of insertion rate (3.2%) when compared to CVC lines (14%) [15]. Midlines are placed variably using the direct, accelerated, or "modified" Seldinger techniques. The modified technique often incorporates a peel-away tissue dilator, which dilates the soft tissue during the cannulation attempt but is removed after placement. A comparison of the LPC placement approach with other commonly-used venous access techniques is provided in Table 12.2.

Increased use of long peripheral and midline catheters may lead to improvement in the rates of complications seen with traditional PIVs. However, simply changing vascular access devices is unlikely to yield all the improvement that we are hoping for. Currently, PIV placement and use are associated with a wide range of complications, including thrombophlebitis, extravasation, hematoma formation, and pain [16]. A recent meta-analysis including 35 studies reported the incidence of phlebitis to be 30.7 per 100 catheters placed. The incidence of severe phlebitis was found to

Table 12.2 Features of various types of venous access devices

	Peripheral intravenous (PIV) catheter	Long peripheral catheter (LPC)	Midline catheter (MLC)	Peripherally inserted central catheter (PICC)	Central venous catheter (CVC)
Material	PTFE, PUR	PUR, PEBA	PUR, silicone	PUR, silicone	PUR, silicone
Length (cm)	3–6	6–15	15–25	20–60	15–60
Insertion technique	CoN	CoN, DS	DS, MS, AS	MS	DS, MS
Insertion site	At or distal to ACF	Forearm, ACF, UA	ACF, UA	UA, or mid-thigh	AX, IJ, FEM, SC
Catheter tip location	Distal circulation to axilla	Distal circulation to axilla	Axilla	SVC/IVC	SVC/IVC
Expected dwell time	<1 week	1–4 weeks	1–6 weeks	<1 year	Varies
Recommended osmolality (mOsm/kg H_2O) [6]	<900	<900	<900	n/a	n/a

Notes: *PTFE* polytetrafluoroethylene, *PUR* polyurethane, *PEBA* polyether-block-amide, *CoN* catheter-over-needle, *DS* direct Seldinger, *MS* modified Seldinger, *AS* accelerated Seldinger, *AX* axillary vein, *IJ* internal jugular vein, *FEM* femoral vein, *SC* subclavian vein, *SVC* superior vena cava, *IVC* inferior vena cava, *ACF* antecubital fossa, *UA* upper arm

be 3.6%. Lack of adequate standard aseptic precautions is believed to double the risk of thrombophlebitis [17], and the practice of multiple skin punctures with the same catheter is likely a major contributor [16]. Cultures of the intravascular portion of removed PIV catheters have found that 5–25% are colonized by skin flora at time of their removal [18]. Bacterial colonization of PIV catheters continues to represent a public health threat. Additionally, these concerns are compounded by the increased prevalence of antibiotic resistance [19]. Consequently, future research will need to focus on methods to reduce catheter contamination during placement and subsequent use. Given that PIVs placed by untrained personal have long been associated with higher risk of PIV infection [20], one approach to these problems is to develop an insertion bundle to identify appropriate site selection and appropriate device selection, which will ultimately increase the ease of catheter insertion and limit opportunities for user error, driving down infection risk.

Xact Medical's Fast Intelligent Needle Delivery (FIND™) is a new, non-FDA-approved, robotic ultrasound transducer that automates ultrasound-guided object placement in the body (Fig. 12.3). The robotic control has been created to simplify the task for the user by detecting a dynamic target zone, reducing human placement error. In simulated vessels, down to 5 mm in diameter, the device was assessed using a gel ultrasound phantom and demonstrated an accuracy of needle placement in up to >90% of attempts [21]. This type of automated line placement has the potential to not only improve accuracy of line placement, but to also reduce complications due to misplacement or repeated attempts at cannulation.

Four routes are generally recognized for contamination of venous catheters. The first (and most common for short-term catheters) is migration of skin organisms at

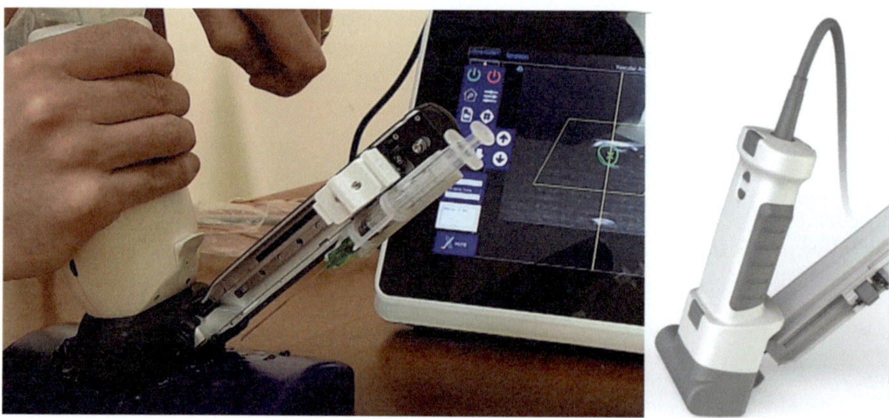

Fig. 12.3 Xact's Fast Intelligent Needle Delivery (FIND™) robot. (*Images courtesy of Xact Medical Inc. © 2020 Xact Medical Inc. All rights reserved.*)

the insertion site into the cutaneous catheter tract and along the surface of the catheter with colonization of the catheter tip. A second route is direct contamination of the catheter or catheter hub by contact with the provider's hands or contaminated fluids and/or devices. Less commonly, catheters may also become hematogenously seeded from another focus on infection. Rarely, insufflate contamination may lead to CRBSI [5]. Shortly after PIV insertion, a fibrin sheath begins to form around the catheter, which serves as a medium for bacterial growth and blocks circulating immune cells from eradicating the infection [22]. Catheter manufacturers have already begun to address these issues, and most of the central venous catheters being sold in the United States today have some antimicrobial and/or anti-thrombogenic features [23], including coating or extrusion with different active substances such as silver ions, antibiotics, and chlorhexidine. Providers appear to be moving away from silicone catheters due to reports that silicone instigates greater localized inflammation due to complement activation, and PVC and silicone both appear to be associated with increased risk of infection when compared to PUR or Teflon materials [24].

Utilizing an *in vitro* percutaneous catheter insertion model, ChronoFlex C® with BioGUARD™ (Access Scientific, LLC) has been shown to significantly inhibit bacterial attachment and biofilm formation when compared to standard polyurethane PIV catheter. This is attributed to the removal of surface additives from the material, thereby altering hydrophobicity to discourage microbe attachment [25]. AngioDynamics currently offers the BioFlo® midline catheter impregnated with Endexo® anti-thrombogenic additive, reducing thrombosis risk by resisting platelet aggregation. [26] The ARROWg+ard® Blue technology (Teleflex) coats the catheter's outer surface with chlorhexidine, while the ARROWg+ard® Blue PLUS technology coats both the outer and inner catheter surfaces [27].The Vantex® catheter (Medline Inc.) is extruded with Oligon (a silver, carbon and platinum polymer agent) to reduce risk of bacterial colonization.

Recent attention has also focused on adjunct medical devices that might reduce complications of PIV catheters. The Bard GuardIva® Antimicrobial Hemostatic IV dressing [28] combines chlorhexidine gluconate (CHG), which appears to have broad-spectrum antimicrobial and antifungal activity, with a hemostatic agent to prevent surface bleeding. In vivo animal studies show seven times less blood loss with the device [28]. Additionally, utilization of chlorhexidine-impregnated dressings over CVADs reduces infection risk when the extraluminal route is the primary source of infection. Other CHG dressings include Biopatch® (Johnson & Johnson) and Aegis ® (Medline), which is a hydrophilic foam disc impregnated with chlorhexidine gluconate (CHG) that reduces CLABSI, by inhibiting microorganisms on the dressings surface.

Disinfecting caps, which are placed over needleless connectors when not in use, may also help reduce infection risk. Researchers evaluated the 3M™ Curos™ disinfecting caps' ability to provide passive disinfection and a physical barrier to contamination for needless connectors. These caps utilize 70% isopropyl alcohol to reportedly disinfect in less than a minute, providing protection from infection for up to 7 days if left in place. One study found that using these caps as part of a PIV maintenance bundle reduced primary blood stream infections from 0.57 to 0.11 per 1000 patient days [29]. The use of passive disinfection caps containing disinfecting agents (e.g., isopropyl alcohol) has been shown to reduce intraluminal microbial contamination, decreasing rates of CLABSI. Additionally, use of disinfection caps on peripheral catheters has limited evidence but should be considered [6].

It is likely that future vascular access research will focus more upon patient-centered outcomes with PIV insertion and use. Cross-sectional studies across 25 different countries have shown that PIV access can be unduly stressful and anxiety-provoking in patients, especially in circumstances of IV failure and repeated attempts [30–32]. These complications are further exacerbated by the fact that 50% of first attempt insertions fail [33]. In the hospital setting, PIV access attempts are the leading cause of self-reported pain for children less than 5 years of age [34]. However, there are relatively few studies examining patient-centered outcomes for VAD placement in the context of emergencies. As we continue to improve upon existing techniques for PIV placement, it is likely that providers will ultimately recognize the need for improved understanding of patient perspectives and preferences regarding VAD placement.

The Future of Central Venous Catheters

More than five million central venous catheters (CVCs) are placed annually in the United States, with the global market for these devices growing at an annual rate of 4.88% and expected to reach $930 million by 2024 [35, 36]. However, 15% of all CVC placements are associated with some complication, such as device dysfunction, infection, and extravasation [37]. Health authorities and patients have become increasingly intolerant of these complications, and treatment of injuries attributable to these device complications (e.g., central line-associated bloodstream infections) are increasingly not being compensated by governmental payors. As a result, we will likely see continued improvements in the design of CVC lines, as well as how they are deployed.

Traditionally, chest radiographs have been the gold standard for confirmation of line placement and identification of pneumothorax with thoracic CVC (i.e., IJ or SC) line placement. However, this practice can delay emergent therapy and expose the patient to potentially unnecessary radiation and may delay identification of these complications if X-ray is not immediately available. Consequently, an increasing number of providers have begun exploring the use of ultrasound imaging to confirm vein entry, catheter tip placement, and the absence of pneumothorax. In one recent systematic review, the authors concluded that US had a pooled specificity and sensitivity of 98.9% and 68.2%, respectively, in detecting CVC malposition [38]. It seems likely that this low sensitivity of US may be increased with the development of improved techniques and greater experience with this technique. In addition, US offers the ability to detect complications *in real time* during the procedure and under sterile conditions, when providers may still have the chance to a remedy the problem. With the advent of portable US devices and electrocardiogram-synced line placement techniques, it seems likely that future providers will be able to prevent or correct complications of CVC placement while obviating the need for X-ray confirmation altogether.

Recognizing the superficial position and easy compressibility of the IJ vein, providers have also recently begun to explore the use of traditionally peripheral vascular access devices to cannulate this central vein [39]. Ultrasound-guided peripheral IV catheters require reduced access times when compared to traditional CVC or PICC lines, without any identified complications [40, 41]. However, to mitigate risk of spontaneous migration into the lumen, or complications such as a hematoma, the procedure must be performed by a well-trained vascular access specialist [41].

The central lines of the future will also likely integrate continuous monitoring capability, and precedents already exist. The Edwards Oximetry Central Venous Catheter® (Edwards Lifesciences) is the first central venous catheter to feature continuous central venous oxygen saturation (ScvO2) monitoring, which may allow for earlier identification of tissue malperfusion and hypoxia in the presence of normal vital signs [42]. Central venous oxygen saturation is already being used as a prognostic marker for patients with severe sepsis [43], acute heart failure [44], and acute hemorrhage [45]. Manufacturers are also investigating other "integrated sensors" which can be added to any catheter. Cikautxo Medical recently described efforts to develop an external flow-through "glucose sensor" that would be able to provide continuous monitoring of serum glucose levels when attached to an arterial, peripheral venous, or central venous line. This sensor acquires a fresh blood sample every 5–15 minutes before re-flushing the sample back into the patient [46]. Similar sensors could be used to monitor a wide variety of medical conditions.

Patients with thoracic central vein occlusions can provide a significant challenge to providers, often preventing CVC placement using traditional methods. The Surfacer® Inside-Out® Access Catheter System (Bluegrass Vascular) allows placement of a right internal jugular dialysis catheter from the "inside-out" (Fig. 12.4).

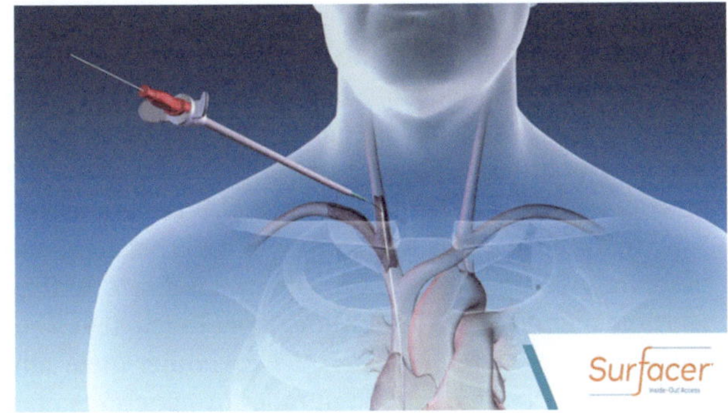

Fig. 12.4 The Surfacer® Inside-Out® Access Catheter System. (*Images courtesy of Bluegrass Vascular Inc. © 2020 Bluegrass Vascular Inc. All rights reserved.*)

Using this device, the provider cannulates the right femoral vein and advances the catheter over a guidewire through the inferior/superior vena cava and into the right internal jugular vein under fluoroscopy. The catheter then exits the internal jugular vein and through the skin. This retrograde approach to IJ central line insertion was developed to avoid left-sided central venous access for purposes of dialysis, since left-sided venous access is associated with lower blood flow rates, higher rates of venous stenosis, and increased vascular trauma than right-sided lines due to the tortuous route through the brachiocephalic vein [47, 48]. Although fluoroscopy is required with the current technique, this kind of retrograde central line insertion may show promise in the emergent placement of non-dialysis CVC lines, especially when femoral access may be available but suboptimal for patient care due to associated risks and complications of prolonged femoral catheter use [49, 50].

Ultrasound Guidance

First introduced in 1993, ultrasound guidance for central venous catheter placement has become increasingly popular, with reports of greater first-attempt success rates [51, 52]. However, there are also certain barriers to the use of ultrasound, including increased training requirements [53], difficulties obtaining ultrasound machines in a timely manner, increased time required to place the line, and difficulties in establishing ultrasound-guided line placement in agitated or uncooperative patients.

One prospective, randomized trial comparing real-time ultrasound-guided IJ cannulation versus external landmark method showed 100% US placement success rate, compared to 94.4% in the landmark group. Although the mean skin-to-vein access time was significantly lower in the landmark group (17.1 sec vs. 44 sec), the average number of attempts (1.1 SD 0.6 vs. 2.6 SD 2.9) trended toward higher values with the landmark-based approach [54]. Another prospective randomized trial found that two-dimensional ultrasound was significantly better than conventional guidance and reduced the number of failed internal jugular vein site cannulations from 35% to 0% [55]. Comparative studies show that real-time ultrasound guidance for CVC placement in "resource-poor" emergency department settings offers fewer complications and reduces the "flash time" (i.e., interval between skin puncture and the appearance of blood at the syringe hub) when compared to the traditional landmark-based technique [56].

Ultrasound guidance appears to offer a clear advantage over landmark methods regarding CVC line placement, although the benefits of US-guided PIV placement may be mixed. The use of bedside ultrasound techniques to place PIV lines presents additional obstacles, since the targets are generally deeper in the soft tissue than those veins targeted with external landmark methods. In one systematic review comparing the use of US guidance with conventional landmark PIV insertion techniques, the authors concluded that routine US guidance for PIV placement is *not recommended* [57]. Another meta-analysis found that ultrasound guidance has *no effect* on the number of punctures needed for successful cannulation or the time to successful cannulation [58].

However, as US devices and techniques continue to improve, it is likely that this technology will play an increasingly important role in PIV insertion for patients with difficult vascular access, especially those who can tolerate a delay in line placement. It is important to remember that US-guided VAD insertion is more than just US identification of the target vein. Ultrasound guidance should also be used to main continuous visualization of the catheter tip, including "walking" the tip into the vessel. Many organizations, including the Association for Vascular Access (AVA), Infusion Nurses Society (INS), and Society for Healthcare Epidemiology of America (SHEA) already recommend that US guidance should be used for patients with difficult vascular access (DVA). Providers should ensure that they are adequately proficient and competent with US insertion, not just US identification of the target vein for insertion. Many organizations support the "No Blind Stick" campaign, which suggests that providers should employ visualization of the target vein in all cases of venous cannulation, whether through direct visualization or US imaging.

Portable Ultrasound Devices

Portable ultrasound devices may offer a solution to some of the problems encountered with the US-guided approach [59]. These devices are gaining traction due to their ease of use for the operator, portability, and relatively low cost compared to standard US machines. One recent study compared the median time to achieve IJ venous puncture for emergency physicians in a simulated model comparing portable ultrasound device (PUD) to conventional ultrasound. They found no difference in the time to achieve venous access [60]. These PUDs can be broadly split into three categories: laptop (weighing 10–14 pounds), hand-carried (weighing 5–8 pounds), and handheld / hand-operated (weigh <1 pound) systems [61]. Some of the commercially available portable US systems are listed below in Table 12.3. Two examples of these devices, the Butterfly iQ® Portable Ultrasound System (Fig. 12.5) and the GE Vscan Extend R2 Portable Ultrasound System®(Fig. 12.6), are shown below.

Table 12.3 Commercially-available handheld portable ultrasound devices

Device	Weight	Functionality	Limitations	Cost	Manufacturer
Vscan Extend R2 with Dual Probe® [62]	0.85 lbs	First pocket-sized US with two transducers in single probe	–	$2995	GE Healthcare
Butterfly Basic® [63]	0.69 lbs	19 imaging presets. M-Mode, B-Mode, and Doppler. Compatible with iPhone 8 and tablet	5-hour recharge time for a full battery life of 2 continuous hours	$1999	Butterfly Network, Inc.
Sonoscanner U-Lite® (5th Generation) [64]	1.5 lbs	10 sec startup time, local archiving (store up to 1000 images), direct printing	–	$15,000	Sonoscanner
SonoQue® Linear Wireless Ultrasound Probe for iPhone and iPAD [65]	0.33 lbs	For emergency situations, clinics, and outdoors, waterproof, serves as Wi-Fi point	–	$1900	SonoQue

Note: Costs estimated from manufacturer websites [62–65]

Fig. 12.5 The Butterfly iQ® Portable Ultrasound System. (*Images courtesy of Butterfly Network Inc.* © *2020 Butterfly Network Inc. All rights reserved.*)

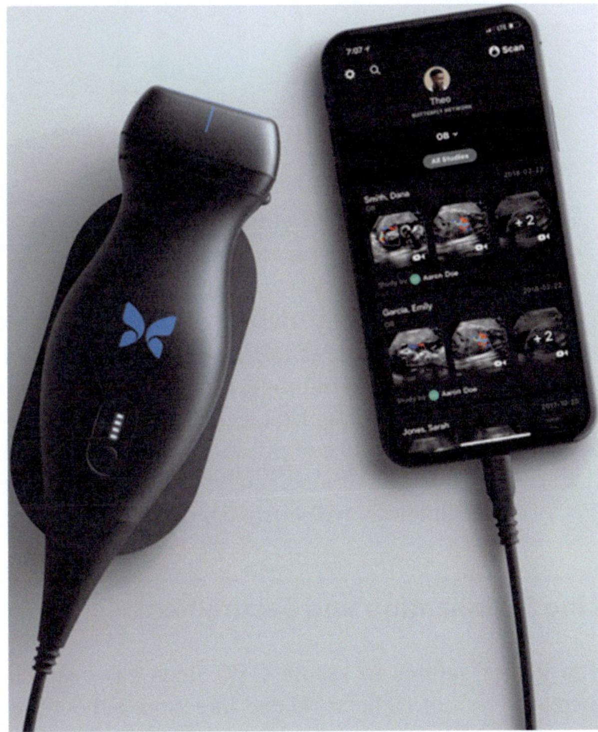

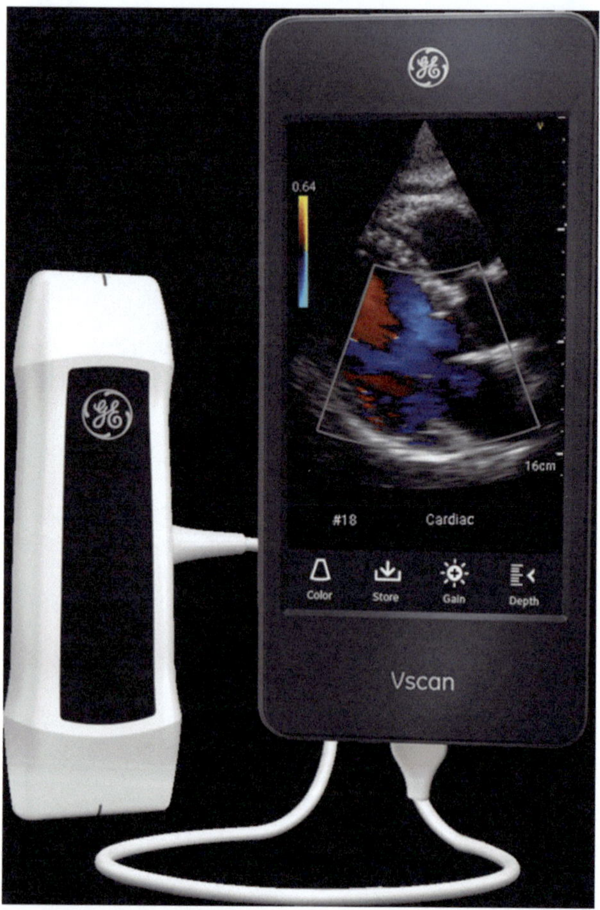

Fig. 12.6 The GE Vscan® Extend R2 Portable Ultrasound System. (*Images courtesy of GE Healthcare Inc. © 2020 GE Healthcare Inc. All rights reserved.*)

These PUDs offer many advantages to providers besides their portability, including the potential for more efficient image acquisition and data sharing. As software applications continue to improve, it is likely that providers may be able to generate three-dimensional imaging from handheld devices, or leverage machine intelligence to automatically identify complications or improper insertion techniques using real-time US monitoring. Although some of these devices are still rather expensive, the cost of this technology will likely continue to decline.

Line Stabilization and Securement

The use of sutures to secure CVC lines has been shown to be associated with increased risk of catheter-related infection, although evidence suggests that some providers still use sutures to guard against inadvertent line migration or dislodgement [66, 67]. This risk of dislodgement is very real, affecting an estimated 5–6%

of all lines placed [68]. Consequently, alternative methods are needed for the securement of short-term CVCs that will not increase the risk of catheter-associated infection. The FDA-approved SorbaView® SHIELD (Centurion Medical Products) is a one-step catheter securement system that combines enhanced dressing technology and improves vessel health and preservation [69]. The StatLock® stabilization device (Bard Medical) is an example of an adhesive-based device that can prevent dislodgement or migration without the need to penetrate the skin. Another novel approach is provided with SecurePortIV® (Adhezion Biomedical), a cyanoacrylate adhesive that is applied to the device and insertion site, is immediately water resistant, and can help to secure the catheter while sealing the insert site to prevent bacterial migration into the wound [20, 70]. Chlorhexidine-impregnated gel dressings have also been proposed, although early studies do not suggest any definite improvement in outcomes when compared to transparent polyurethane dressings [71].

The Future of Intraosseous Catheters

Intraosseous (IO) cannulation offers indirect access to the venous system, even under clinical conditions in which the venous system has collapsed due to hypovolemia or impaired cardiac function. Intraosseous infusion can be used for all age groups, can be established in less than 1 minute, and has more predictable absorption than the endotracheal route. Any drug that can be safely infused via PIV catheter can also be infused by the IO route. Although IO devices can be lifesaving for the right patient, many opportunities for improvement with their use exist, including limited dwell times, unpredictable pain control, and a limited understanding of how IO differs from IV infusion.

In 2010, the FDA approved the EZ-IO® (Teleflex, LLC) intraosseous infusion device for a dwell time of up to 24 hours. In 2011, the device received 72-hour dwell time in the European Union [72]. Because of these limited dwell times, it is currently recommended that IO catheters be removed as soon as alternate venous access has been achieved. Concerns about longer dwell times appear to revolve around the risk of infectious complications [73, 74]. However, studies have shown that osteomyelitis is extremely rare if the catheter is removed within 48 hours of insertion [75], and dwell times of up to 30 days have been tolerated without identified complications [76]. Considering this long track record of safety, it is likely that approved dwell times for IO catheters will continue to increase.

The pain experienced with IO insertion and infusion is modulated by the somatic pain receptors of the skin and bony periosteum, as well as visceral pain receptors within the intraosseous space. [77, 78]. Comparing the pain with IO insertion to that experienced during a PIV needlestick, providers do not generally anesthetize the patient's skin prior to IO insertion [79]. Once the catheter has been placed, slow (over 2 minutes) administration of 2% preservative-free and epinephrine-free lidocaine is given via syringe into the IO catheter as an intra-medullary anesthetic [80, 81]. This can be repeated as needed for pain, up to a maximum safe dose. The onset of anesthesia for lidocaine typically occurs within 2–5 minutes, although the duration of effect varies from 30 minutes to 2 hours for plain lidocaine [82, 83]. If the lidocaine is administered too rapidly, it will be taken up by the circulation and have little or no effect on local pain fibers. Pain scores have been found to be highest during the normal saline flush, and most volunteers (80%) require an additional dose of lidocaine to keep the pain level less than a 5 (1–10 scale) [84]. Prehospital surveys and UK military studies have found high levels of pain upon infusion even with high lidocaine dosing [85, 86]. Consequently, systemic pain medications or sedation may be required for those patients who do not experience adequate analgesia with lidocaine alone. Because of this unreliable analgesic response to IO lidocaine, new and different strategies must be sought to reduce the pain of IO insertion and infusion.

Alternative anesthetics may offer better pain control than lidocaine, but little research has been done on the subject. Bupivacaine, for example, causes a dose-dependent blockade of sodium channels and binds more strongly than lidocaine but is potentially cardiotoxic and can cause CNS effects in excess [87]. Differing doses of lidocaine may also offer some advantage, as IV lidocaine has already been shown to be effective in the treatment of acute hyperalgesia [88].

"Buffering" local anesthetics with sodium bicarbonate has been used in peripheral nerve blocks to decrease time to drug effect. This practice may also help to improve IO pain control. Some clinical trials have found a statistically significant improved time of anesthetic onset in an axillary block with the addition of sodium bicarbonate to mepivacaine [89], but others have found no statistical difference in time to motor blockade onset in brachial plexus anesthesia [90]. It has been speculated that "buffering" the IO lidocaine bolus with 8.4% sodium bicarbonate (1 mEq/mL) prior to IO infusion may offer similar benefits, but only anecdotal reports have surfaced on the subject.

Regional nerve blocks could also theoretically be utilized to prevent and reduce the pain of IO insertion and infusion. Through an ultrasound-guided technique, a transducer can help identify and anesthetize spinal nerve roots C5 through C7, as well as the superficial cervical plexus. An interscalene nerve block serves as a powerful analgesic agent for any form of invasive procedure on the distal clavicle and shoulder. It should also sufficiently anesthetize the proximal humerus, which is a frequently accessed site for IO infusion. However, this block is contraindicated in patients with compromised respiratory function due to a high likelihood of ipsilateral phrenic nerve block and diaphragm hemiparesis [91]. Additionally, interscalene nerve blocks may not be practical under emergent conditions, as the time from the start of administration of the anesthetic until initiation of procedure has been shown to average 28 minutes [92].

Pain with IO infusion appears to be related to increased pressure within the medullary space during pressurized infusion [93, 94]. Consequently, it may be possible that spaces with larger medullary cavities, or with higher rates of outflow from the medullary space, may be associated with lower pain scores. Certain studies have assessed pain levels in relation to the anatomical site of infusion. The greatest reported pain was associated with the left tibia (7.9 ± 2.8), whereas the least reported pain was the humerus (4.6 ± 2.9) [84]. Using IO flow rate as a surrogate for increased medullary space, we can speculate that pain may vary inversely with flow rate between IO insertion sites at a constant infusion pressure. In other words, pain may be greatest when outflow is the most limited, leading to higher intramedullary pressures and greater stretch on the pain fibers. Flow rates with bolus infusion appear to be greatest at the sternum, approximately 1.6 times greater than the proximal humerus, and 3.1 times greater than the proximal tibia in a human cadaveric model [95]. Future studies will likely further illuminate this relationship between anatomic insertion site, infusion rate, infusion pressure, and pain perception.

Another difficulty that providers may face in assessing the risk-benefit ratio for IO infusion is the lack of contemporary data, regarding both patient-specific complications and equivalency with IV medication/fluid infusion. Case reports have reported instances of acute tibial osteomyelitis caused by an intraosseous access 3 months after initial resuscitation [96]. Other instances of adverse events in the adult population include vasopressor extravasation and threatened limb perfusion [97]. Although several reviews and meta-analyses of IO complications have been performed previously, most include historical data (from as far back as the 1940s), combine data from a range of different devices, and group adult and pediatric subjects together. Considering the great advances that have occurred regarding infection prevention, device manufacturing, and the use of disposable (versus reusable) trocars, it is likely that these historical data do not reflect the actual risks associated with IO use in the modern era. Furthermore, it also seems likely that the risks of IO use in a pediatric subject are not the same as those in an adult subject. Adults have larger bones, potentially different comorbidities, and very likely different intraosseous anatomy and physiology. It is therefore difficult, if not impossible, to understand what the risks of IO use will be for a specific patient (whether adult or pediatric). Further study will be needed in these areas, to help providers understand the "actual" risks of IO use, considering modern devices and techniques.

Additional research is also needed to confirm the bioavailability and efficacy of medications that are currently considered safe and effective for IO infusion. Teleflex reports that over 105 different infusates have been delivered via the IO route and referenced in clinical literature (e.g., atropine, phenytoin, vecuronium) [80]. Clinical and preclinical studies demonstrate that most drugs and fluids via IO reach central circulation with similar concentrations [80]. For instance, results of prospective, randomized studies show no significant differences in the pharmacokinetic profiles between intraosseous and intravenous administration of morphine sulfate [98]. Additionally, a large randomized, placebo-controlled clinical trial compared the differences in survival to hospital to hospital discharge in patients that were randomized by emergency medical services (EMS) to an antiarrhythmic drug, Amiodarone, versus placebo, when stratified by intravenous vs. intraosseous route. There was no significant effect modification by drug administration route for amiodarone or lidocaine compared to placebo during out-of-hospital cardiac arrest [99].

Subcutaneous Injection

Needless hypodermic injection ("hypospray") technology has been in use since the 1950s but remains largely under-utilized in the care of human patient [100–102]. One recent study of a needle-free, jet injection device demonstrated effective sub-dermal medication delivery in under a millisecond. Researchers could deliver greater than 90% of a 100-microliter volume to a site 3 mm deep with a highly controllable handheld device in a rabbit model [103]. Other biomedical researchers have created micro-jet devices that can penetrate the human epidermis and assess quantitative delivery of insulin in vitro [104]. These devices eliminate the hazard of needles and decrease needlestick injury for healthcare providers. The Tropis Needle-Free Injector® (PharmaJet) is a spring-powered device that has been shown to deliver an inactivated poliovirus vaccine in one-tenth of a second [105, 106]. This FDA-cleared technology can be used for injectable fluids up to 0.5 mL in volume. Consequently, such devices are not able to infuse large volumes of fluid but may be effective for use in quickly administering highly potent drugs.

Hypodermoclysis (or "dermoclysis") is the injection of fluids or medications into the subcutaneous space. Subcutaneous infusion by hypodermoclysis was first introduced in the 1940s but has subsequently been used for the administration of a variety of drugs and fluids [107, 108]. Unfortunately, the flow rate with this technique is also quite slow, with recommended subcutaneous fluid infusion rates of no more than 1 mL/min at each site [109]. Although multiple infusion sites can be used simultaneously, the total amount of fluid administered should be limited to 3000 mL over a single 24-hour period [110]. The simplicity of hypodermoclysis (as compared to vascular access device placement) allows this technique to be administered by non-medical personnel, and it has been studied in the home hospice setting due to its cost-effectiveness and relative safety [111].

Proctoclysis

While oral hydration is often contraindicated due to concerns for aspiration in critically ill patients, providers have begun to remember that the colon is able to absorb a great deal of water. Proctoclysis (rectal infusion) is already being explored for patients who are unable to receive oral fluid and have difficulties receiving peripheral intravenous infusion. The rectum is an underutilized administration point [112]. In patients with hypovolemic shock, rectal fluid resuscitation was studied during the Korean War and WWI for mass casualty situations, even in animal models [113]. The Macy Catheter® (Hospi Corporation) for rectal infusion has been approved by the FDA since 2014 and may be the leading device for rectal infusion of fluids or medications on the market today (Fig. 12.7).

The catheter is inserted past the anal sphincter, and fluids or medication are administered via slow infusion with gravity tube feeding bag, at infusion rates of 250–400 mL/hour [114, 115]. Future studies are needed to determine if faster rates of infusion may be safely tolerated. The Macy Catheter® allows for repeat drug

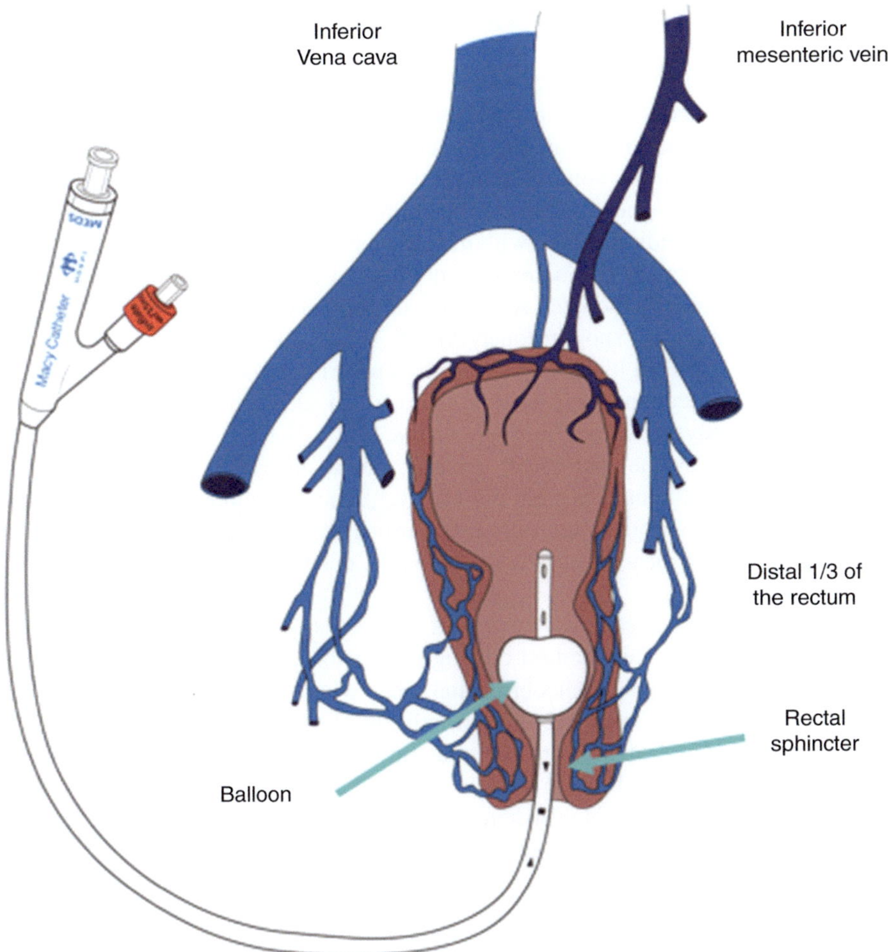

Fig. 12.7 The Macy Catheter® for rectal infusion. (*Images courtesy of Hospi Corporation. © 2020 Hospi Corporation. All rights reserved.*)

administration without re-penetration of the rectal vault. In the setting of hospice or palliative care, rectal catheters can be used up to 28 days with adequate early absorption [116]. Certain drugs absorption profiles have been shown to surpass the oral absorption levels, suggesting that certain drugs partially avoid first-pass metabolism by the liver [117]. Proctoclysis has shown to be very useful in nursing home settings and in emergency pre-hospital care [118]. Case reports have highlighted the effectiveness of proctoclysis in the absence of intravenous access in rural and remote settings, such as a patient in a trekking expedition with lifesaving fluid resuscitation [119]. Studies have utilized tap water for rectal hydration due to its low cost and ready availability [114], although normal saline or lactated Ringer's solution may also be administered via this route [120].

Other Anatomic Sites for Venous Access

Trauma researchers have investigated the penis as an alternative route for emergent venous access in males as well as animal models [121]. In acute settings, the penis venous drainage system has unique advantages, as the vein is always available regardless of the patient's volume status and has high capacity of drainage in short time [122]. There is no need for emergent venous cut-down. The corpora cavernosa injection has been studied in men with massive burns, sclerotic veins from repeated injections, and extensive limb trauma for blood transfusion or fluid hydration. Reported complications included subcutaneous penile hematoma (2 patients, out of the 15) which resolved spontaneously [123]. While this technique may deserve future attention, it is not likely to gain much popularity in the acute care world.

Intracardiac injections have been studied as an alternative route of vascular access. Commonly performed throughout the 1960s, the use of cardiac injection fell out of favor by the mid-1970s as safer and easier routes of administration emerged [124]. Challenges present with this approach, including the risk of lacerating the heart or coronary arteries. Intracardiac injection should be considered only when no other forms of access are available, due to the risk of serious complications [125].

Another anatomic site for venous access is the use of endotracheal medication in cardiac emergencies. This method of drug absorption and drug delivery occurs at the distally level of the tracheobronchial tree, where most efficient absorption occurs at the alveolar level [126]. Currently, the endotracheal administration of drugs is only recommended for the administration of naloxone, atropine, vasopressin, lidocaine, and epinephrine in the setting of pediatric advanced life support when peripheral vascular access is insufficient [127]. The recommended dose is 2.0–2.5 times the IV dose, although little evidence support this practice. Drugs administered via endotracheal tube should be diluted in water or 0.9% normal saline solution.

The nasal mucosa is utilized by the Mad-100® (Teleflex, LLC), a nasal drug delivery device. This device produces a fine mist-like spray that targets mucosal regions even out in austere conditions in first responders in the field, appropriate for advanced life support [128]. While the nasal route is not appropriate for large-volume infusions, it is likely that intranasal formulations of new and familiar drugs will likely to be explored into the future, considering the rapid uptake of medications using this route and the ease of infusion.

Other potentially useful anatomic sites for drug administration are through the sublingual or buccal route. Sublingual drug absorption appears to be faster than buccal delivery due to the thinner epithelial layer in this space, and this route avoids first-pass metabolism by the liver. Nanoparticulate systems have already been shown to increase uptake, accumulation, and absorption of drugs via the GI tract, and these nanoparticulates are currently being explored for the sublingual route. Nanoparticulates increase permeability of drug across the epithelial membrane [129] and ultimately lead to a higher bioavailability for systemic absorption [130]. This pharmacological development has a potential to help achieve therapeutic treatment quicker for acutely ill patients.

Guidelines

The Infusion Nurses Society (INS) released its first evidence-based practice standards, the "Infusion Nursing Standards of Practice," in 1980. The sixth revision of these practice standards, renamed the "Infusion Therapy Standards of Practice," was released in 2016 [6]. Over the last 40 years, much has changed in the world of vascular access and infusion, including the introduction of new materials, devices, approaches, and guidelines for the placement and maintenance of VADs. Some of the recent trends endorsed by the INS are the creation of designated infusion teams to place and manage VADs, the use of vessel visualization devices (e.g., US, near-infrared light devices, and visible light (trans-illumination) devices), and so-called VAD planning, in which the "appropriate VAD is selected to accommodate the patient's vascular access needs based on the prescribed therapy or treatment regimen; anticipated duration of therapy; vascular characteristics; and patient's age, comorbidities, history of infusion therapy, preference for VAD location, and ability and resources available to care for the device" [6]. In general, the "Standards" endorse use of the least-invasive VAD with the fewest number of lumens and the smallest outer diameter that will suffice for the patient's specific needs [6]. As the leading authority in VAD management, the INS has guided the evolution of vascular access with a goal of improving VAD placement success and reducing the risk of complications from to their use. It is likely that the guidelines produced by organizations like the INS will continue to shape the future of vascular access for years to come.

In addition to the INS "Standards," many other organizations have introduced guidance for vascular access providers. The American College of Emergency Physicians (ACEP) [131], Emergency Nurses Association (ENA) [132], and the Association For Vascular Access (AVA) [133] have issued policies on the management of difficult vascular access, suggesting that the use of US-guided and intraosseous techniques should be considered when other forms of peripheral venous access are not available. However, determinations on when to initiate these alternate techniques are largely left to the provider. The INS "Standards" do offer some guidance on the permitted number of PIV attempts, suggesting that only two attempts should be made by the same provider, with no more than four total attempts on the patient before considering alternative methods for venous access [6].

As peripherally inserted central catheter (PICC) lines have gained popularity over the past several years, there has been a growing need to define the indications for insertion, maintenance, and care of these lines. The Michigan Appropriateness Guide for Intravenous Catheters (MAGIC) endorsed by the ImprovePICC group (www.improvepicc.com) provides guidance for PICC usage through a multispecialty panel, with the goal of increasing patient safety and reducing adverse outcomes. This panel is multidisciplinary and representative, including specialists from vascular access nursing, internal medicine, nephrology, and surgery. The panel utilizes a RAND Corporation/University Appropriateness Method to create criteria for appropriate use of PICCs and VADs. After reviewing relevant guidelines such as the INS Standards for Practice and the Centers for Disease Control and Prevention/

Healthcare Infection Control Practices Advisory committee, the study extensively reviewed 665 scenarios. They concluded that 288 (43%) cases were considered to include inappropriate PICC utilization for 5 or fewer days. Interestingly, panel members suggested that the decision to place a PICC is frequently seen as dichotomous, without adequate consideration of other devices [134]. This finding suggests that additional options for vascular access are needed. This study also illustrates the changing field of thought surrounding the utilization of ultrasound for difficult peripheral access. In the absence of other indications of venous access for general medical or critically-ill patients, panelists rated US-guided peripheral intravenous catheters as more appropriate than use of a PICC.

Intraosseous (IO) access continues to be recognized as a critical tool in the emergency medical provider's toolkit in providing care in advanced life support. In the 2015 American Heart Association (AHA) Guidelines Update for Cardiopulmonary Resuscitation and Emergency Cardiovascular Care position on Pediatric Advanced Life Support (PALS) [135], the authors reported that IO provides a safe, effective, and acceptable route for access in children, referencing a Class I recommendation level. Furthermore, in 2016, the AHA Guidelines for Cardiopulmonary Resuscitation and Emergency Cardiovascular Care stated IO cannulation is appropriate for providing access to the non-collapsible venous plexus found in the bone marrow space, thus enabling drug delivery like that achieved by direct peripheral venous access. The PALS cardiac arrest algorithm now also supports IO vascular access as the initial vascular access in cases of cardiac arrest [4, 10]. Beyond its utility in the resuscitative setting, initiation of IO vascular access is considered appropriate even in non-emergent situations when IV access cannot be obtained, and the patient would be compromised without the medications or solutions prescribed [1, 11–14]. The 2018 AHA PALS update included intraosseous access in the pediatric cardiac arrest algorithm, in the workflow for asystole/pulseless electrical activity [136].

Conclusions

As new vascular access devices emerge on the market, there should be shared responsibility between first responders, emergency medicine providers, and device manufacturers in evaluating their safety and efficacy. Future research should strive for consistency and standardization of device utilization in vascular access practice, considering the most up-to-date, evidence-based practices. This will require increased collaboration between researchers and the disparate organizations that generate the clinical guidelines and performance metrics that are used to evaluate vascular access providers, with a focus upon improving patient outcomes and disseminating best practices. Recognizing that vascular access is a crucial step in providing safe and effective care for critically ill patients, the medical community must decide to allocate adequate effort, funding, and other needed resources to advance vascular access research in a systematic, evidence-driven manner, rather than relying upon device manufacturers and other private-sector interests to advance the field.

Individual providers must continue to reflect upon their selection of device for each unique patient scenario in obtaining peripheral or central vascular access, and good decisions in this regard can be facilitated through education. Simulation training, for example, may help health professionals to identify early complications of VAD placement and improve outcomes for patients [137, 138]. Input from all members of the vascular access care team, including prehospital providers, nurses, technicians, and physicians, should be utilized in the development of research protocols and the translation of study results to clinical practice. After all, nurses and technicians are most often responsible for the insertion, use, and care of VADs [139]. It has been suggested that in order to move the needle forward in collaborative care, there must be a strong intersection between research evidence and clinical practice [139]. This will require a multidisciplinary collaboration between vascular access nurses and physician-scientists, united with a focus on patient care. It has been shown that dedicated vascular access teams reduce infections in intensive care units [140]. However, similar studies have not yet been adequately performed in other clinical care environments. It is likely that intraosseous access will play an increasingly large role in the resuscitation of critically ill patients in the future. Greater attention should be paid to how intraosseous as well as peripheral venous access is achieved in the prehospital and emergency department environments, especially for time-critical conditions such as cardiac arrest [141, 142].

Given the challenges that emergency care providers face daily in obtaining rapid venous access, there is an imminent need for innovation and creativity in developing novel ways to achieve and optimize vascular access. Future technological advances will likely focus on the exploration of new devices, new techniques for line placement, and new (or previously underutilized) physiologic routes for medication and fluid infusion. Although direct intravenous infusion will likely always be the preferred route for administration of therapeutic substances, vast potential exists for new and innovative means of introducing life-saving interventions for critically ill patients. While the future of emergent vascular access remains unknown, we believe that the approaches described in this chapter represent at least a portion of the leading technologies that will likely define the vascular access techniques of the future.

Key Concepts

1. New and innovative methods are needed to improve vascular access efficiency and outcomes for patients.
2. Although polyurethane and silicone materials are still widely utilized, the use of novel synthetic materials for catheter construction, including materials impregnated with antibiotic and anti-thrombotic substances, may help to reduce the risks of infection, phlebitis, thrombosis, and catheter fracture.
3. The long peripheral catheter represents a promising, hybridized form of venous access leveraging the strengths of both midline and short PIV catheters. These devices may allow for extended dwell times and reduced risk of complications.

4. In the future, providers and device developers will continue to leverage the body's untapped absorptive capacity through a multitude of underutilized routes, including, but not limited to, subdermal, rectal, intraosseous, and intranasal infusion.

5. Assistive technologies, such as handheld portable ultrasound devices (PUDs), will continue to grow in popularity and accessibility, providing opportunities for more rapid data acquisition and complication management.

6. High-quality evidence evaluating the efficacy of new vascular access devices and techniques is lacking. Future research in these areas, especially incorporating patient-centered outcomes, is critically important to the future of this field.

Bibliography

1. Fields JM, Piela NE, Au AK, Ku BS. Risk factors associated with difficult venous access in adult ED patients. Am J Emerg Med. 2014;32(10):1179–82.
2. AVA Board of Directors. Association for Vascular Access: Position Statement on Preservation of Peripheral Veins in Patients with Chronic Kidney Disease [Internet]. www.avainfo.org. 2011 [cited 16 March 2020]. Available from: https://cdn.ymaws.com/www.avainfo.org/resource/resmgr/Files/Position_Statements/Preservation_of_Peripheral_V.pdf.
3. Rivera AM, Strauss KW, van Zundert A, Mortier E. The history of peripheral intravenous catheters: how little plastic tubes revolutionized medicine. Acta Anaesthesiol Belg. 2005;56(3):271–82.
4. Dudrick SJ. History of vascular access. J Parenter Enter Nutr. 2006;30(1 Suppl):S47–56.
5. O'Grady NP, Alexander M, Burns LA, Dellinger EP, Garland J, Heard SO, et al. Guidelines for the prevention of intravascular catheter-related infections. Clin Infect Dis. 2011;52(9):e162–93.
6. Gorski LA. Infusion nursing standards of practice. J Infus Nurs. 2007;30(3):151–2.
7. Bierman S. A New Tool for the Vascular Access Toolbox | Infection Control Today [Internet]. 2017 [cited 2020 Feb 3]. Available from: https://www.infectioncontroltoday.com/infusion-vascular-access/new-tool-vascular-access-toolbox.
8. Seldinger SI. Catheter replacement of the needle in percutaneous arteriography: a new technique. Acta Radiol. 1953;39(5):368–76.
9. Bahl A, Hang B, Brackney A, Joseph S, Karabon P, Mohammad A, et al. Standard long IV catheters versus extended dwell catheters: a randomized comparison of ultrasound-guided catheter survival. Am J Emerg Med. 2019;37(4):715–21.
10. Arrow® Endurance™ Extended Dwell Peripheral Catheter System | US | Teleflex [Internet]. [cited 2020 Jun 18]. Available from: https://www.teleflex.com/usa/en/product-areas/vascular-access/peripheral-access/arrow-endurance-extended-dwell-peripheral-catheter-system/index.html.
11. AccuCath® Ace Intravascular Catheter System | Peripheral IV Catheters | BD [Internet]. [cited 2020 Jun 18]. Available from: https://www.bardaccess.com/products/peripheral/accucath-ace.
12. http://www.vygon.com. [Internet]. [cited 2020 Jun 18]. Available from: http://www.vygon.com.
13. EDC - Access Scientific [Internet]. [cited 2020 Jun 18]. Available from: https://accessscientific.com/edc/.
14. Ludeman K. Choosing the right vascular access device. Nursing (Lond). 2007;37(9):38–41.

15. Adams DZ, Little A, Vinsant C, Khandelwal S. The midline catheter: a clinical review. J Emerg Med. 2016;51(3):252–8.
16. Johann DA, Danski MTR, Vayego SA, Barbosa DA, Lind J. Risk factors for complications in peripheral intravenous catheters in adults: secondary analysis of a randomized controlled trial. Rev Lat Am Enfermagem. 2016;24:e2833.
17. Lv L, Zhang J. The incidence and risk of infusion phlebitis with peripheral intravenous catheters: a meta-analysis. J Vasc Access. 2020;21(3):342–9.
18. Tagalakis V, Kahn SR, Libman M, Blostein M. The epidemiology of peripheral vein infusion thrombophlebitis: a critical review. Am J Med. 2002;113(2):146–51.
19. Lewis R. The rise of antibiotic-resistant infections. FDA Consum. 1995;29(1)
20. Zhang L, Cao S, Marsh N, Ray-Barruel G, Flynn J, Larsen E, et al. Infection risks associated with peripheral vascular catheters. J Infect Prev. 2016;17(5):207–13.
21. Doellman D, Mecoli M, von Allmen D. Leading the Way: The Use of Robotics for Ultrasond Guided Vascular Access in Pediatric Patients [Internet]. [cited 2020 Mar 15]. Available from: https://ava2019-ava.ipostersessions.com/default. aspx?s=50-14-E5-FD-0E-5B-E3-AD-3E-D7-5A-30-BA-71-19-B5.
22. Tobin CR. The Teflon intravenous catheter: incidence of phlebitis and duration of catheter life in the neonatal patient. J Obstet Gynecol Neonatal Nurs. 1988;17(1):35–42.
23. On point: Trends and developments in vascular access devices and antimicrobials [Internet]. Medical Plastics News. 2016 [cited 2020 Mar 16]. Available from: https:// www.medicalplasticsnews.com/news/medical-devices/on-point-trends-and-developments-in-vascular-access-devices–/.
24. O'Grady MD N. Guidelines for the Prevention of Intravascular Catheter-Related Infections, 2011 [Internet]. [cited 2020 Jun 16]. Available from: https://www.cdc.gov/hai/pdfs/bsi-guidelines-2011.pdf.
25. Pathak R, Bierman SF, d'Arnaud P. Inhibition of bacterial attachment and biofilm formation by a novel intravenous catheter material using an in vitro percutaneous catheter insertion model. Med Devices (Auckl). 2018;11:427–32.
26. AngioDynamics. BioFlo Midline Catheter with Endexo Technology [Internet]. [cited 2020 Mar 15]. Available from: https://www.angiodynamics.com/img/resources/BioFlo_Midline_ Brochure-386139.pdf.
27. Central Venous Catheters | LA | Teleflex [Internet]. [cited 2020 Jun 18]. Available from: https://www.teleflex.com/la/en/product-areas/vascular-access/central-venous-catheters/.
28. GuardIVa® Antimicrobial Hemostatic IV Dressing | Procedural Accessories | BD [Internet]. [cited 2020 Mar 15]. Available from: https://www.bardaccess.com/products/procedural/ guardiva.
29. Duncan M, Warden P, Bernatchez SF, Morse D. A bundled approach to decrease the rate of primary bloodstream infections related to peripheral intravenous catheters. JAVA. 2018;23(1):15–22.
30. Cooke M, Ullman AJ, Ray-Barruel G, Wallis M, Corley A, Rickard CM. Not "just" an intravenous line: Consumer perspectives on peripheral intravenous cannulation (PIVC). An international cross-sectional survey of 25 countries. PLoS One. 2018;13(2):e0193436.
31. Robinson-Reilly M, Paliadelis P, Cruickshank M. Venous access: the patient experience. Support Care Cancer. 2016;24(3):1181–7.
32. Song C, Oh H. Burn patients' experience of peripherally inserted central catheter insertion: analysis of focus group interviews from a South Korean burn center. Burns. 2016;42(7):1439–44.
33. Schults J, Rickard C, Kleidon T, Paterson R, Macfarlane F, Ullman A. Difficult peripheral venous access in children: an international survey and critical appraisal of assessment tools and escalation pathways. J Nurs Scholarsh. 2019;51(5):537–46.
34. Cummings EA, Reid GJ, Finley GA, McGrath PJ, Ritchie JA. Prevalence and source of pain in pediatric inpatients. Pain. 1996;68(1):25–31.
35. American News Hours. Central Venous Catheter Market 2019 Key Players Analysis, Business Growth, Development Status, Sales Revenue Forecast to 2024 – MarketWatch [Internet]. 2019 [cited 2020 Mar 14]. Available from: https://www.marketwatch.com/press-release/

central-venous-catheter-market-2019-key-players-analysis-business-growth-development-status-sales-revenue-forecast-to-2024-2019-08-26.

36. PR Newswire. Central Venous Catheters Market to Reach USD 2,234.1 Million by 2026 | Reports And Data [Internet]. [cited 2020 Mar 14]. Available from: https://www.prnewswire.com/news-releases/central-venous-catheters-market-to-reach-usd-2-234-1-million-by-2026%2D%2Dreports-and-data-300940550.html.

37. McGee DC, Gould MK. Preventing complications of central venous catheterization. N Engl J Med. 2003;348(12):1123–33.

38. Smit JM, Raadsen R, Blans MJ, Petjak M, Van de Ven PM, Tuinman PR. Bedside ultrasound to detect central venous catheter misplacement and associated iatrogenic complications: a systematic review and meta-analysis. Crit Care. 2018;22(1):65.

39. Butterfield M, Abdelghani R, Mohamad M, Limsuwat C, Kheir F. Using ultrasound-guided peripheral catheterization of the internal jugular vein in patients with difficult peripheral access. Am J Ther. 2017;24(6):e667–9.

40. Polderman KH, Girbes ARJ. Central venous catheter use. Part 2: infectious complications. Intensive Care Med. 2002;28(1):18–28.

41. Teismann NA, Knight RS, Rehrer M, Shah S, Nagdev A, Stone M. The ultrasound-guided "peripheral IJ": internal jugular vein catheterization using a standard intravenous catheter. J Emerg Med. 2013;44(1):150–4.

42. Reinhart K, Kuhn H-J, Hartog C, Bredle DL. Continuous central venous and pulmonary artery oxygen saturation monitoring in the critically ill. Intensive Care Med. 2004;30(8):1572–8.

43. Rady MY, Rivers EP, Martin GB, Smithline H, Appelton T, Nowak RM. Continuous central venous oximetry and shock index in the emergency department: use in the evaluation of clinical shock. Am J Emerg Med. 1992;10(6):538–41.

44. Ander DS, Jaggi M, Rivers E, Rady MY, Levine TB, Levine AB, et al. Undetected cardiogenic shock in patients with congestive heart failure presenting to the emergency department. Am J Cardiol. 1998;82(7):888–91.

45. Nebout S, Pirracchio R. Should we monitor ScVO(2) in critically ill patients? Cardiol Res Pract. 2012;2012:370697.

46. Inside information: The benefits of integrated sensors in catheters - Medical Plastics News [Internet]. 2018 [cited 2020 Mar 15]. Available from: https://www.medicalplasticsnews.com/news/opinion/inside-information/.

47. Salik E, Daftary A, Tal MG. Three-dimensional anatomy of the left central veins: implications for dialysis catheter placement. J Vasc Interv Radiol. 2007;18(3):361–4.

48. Kundu S. Central venous obstruction management. Semin Intervent Radiol. 2009;26(2):115–21.

49. Ebner A, Gallo S, Cetaro C, Gurley J, Minarsch L. Inside-Out Upper Body Venous Access [Internet]. Endovascular Today. 2013 [cited 2020 Mar 16]. Available from: https://evtoday.com/articles/2013-june/inside-out-upper-body-venous-access.

50. Reindl-Schwaighofer R, Matoussevitch V, Winnicki W, Kalmykov E, Gilbert J, Matzek W, et al. A novel inside-out access approach for hemodialysis catheter placement in patients with thoracic central venous occlusion. Am J Kidney Dis. 2020;75(4):480–7.

51. Lau CSM, Chamberlain RS. Ultrasound-guided central venous catheter placement increases success rates in pediatric patients: a meta-analysis. Pediatr Res. 2016;80(2):178–84.

52. Bowdle A. Vascular complications of central venous catheter placement: evidence-based methods for prevention and treatment. J Cardiothorac Vasc Anesth. 2014;28(2):358–68.

53. Portable Ultrasound Devices in the Pre-Hospital Setting: A Review of Clinical and Cost-Effectiveness and Guidelines. Ottawa (ON): Canadian Agency for Drugs and Technologies in Health; 2015.

54. Karakitsos D, Labropoulos N, De Groot E, Patrianakos AP, Kouraklis G, Poularas J, et al. Real-time ultrasound-guided catheterisation of the internal jugular vein: a prospective comparison with the landmark technique in critical care patients. Crit Care. 2006;10(6):R162.

55. Mallory DL, McGee WT, Shawker TH, Brenner M, Bailey KR, Evans RG, et al. Ultrasound guidance improves the success rate of internal jugular vein cannulation. Chest. 1990;98(1):157–60.

56. Kunhahamed MO, Abraham SV, Palatty BU, Krishnan SV, Rajeev PC, Gopinathan V. A comparison of internal jugular vein cannulation by ultrasound-guided and anatomical landmark technique in resource-limited emergency department setting. J Med Ultrasound. 2019;27(4):187–91.

57. Liu YT, Alsaawi A, Bjornsson HM. Ultrasound-guided peripheral venous access: a systematic review of randomized-controlled trials. Eur J Emerg Med. 2014;21(1):18–23.

58. Stolz LA, Stolz U, Howe C, Farrell IJ, Adhikari S. Ultrasound-guided peripheral venous access: a meta-analysis and systematic review. J Vasc Access. 2015;16(4):321–6.

59. Savino K, Ambrosio G. Handheld ultrasound and focused cardiovascular echography: use and information. Medicina (Kaunas). 2019;55(8)

60. Chetioui A, Masia T, Claret P-G, Markarian T, Muller L, Lefrant JY, et al. Pocket-sized ultrasound device for internal jugular puncture: a randomized study of performance on a simulation model. J Vasc Access. 2019;20(4):404–8.

61. Hope B. What's next for portable ultrasound machines. Imag Technol News. 2012;3

62. General Electric Company Healthcare. Buy Vscan Extend R2 w/ Sector Probe | GE Healthcare US Store [Internet]. [cited 2020 Jun 4]. Available from: https://store.gehealthcare.com/en-us/products/point-of-care/vscan-extend-r2-sector-probe.

63. Butterfly Network, Inc. Butterfly iQ - Butterfly Store [Internet]. [cited 2020 Jun 4]. Available from: https://store.butterflynetwork.com/us/en/iq/configure/.

64. Sonoscanner. Pocket handheld ultrasound scanner | Sonoscanner [Internet]. [cited 2020 Jun 4]. Available from: https://www.sonoscanner.com/en/products/u-lite/.

65. SonoQue. L3 Portable Linear Transducer Wireless Ultrasound Probe Machine [Internet]. [cited 2020 Jun 4]. Available from: https://www.sonoque.com/s/l3-wireless-ultrasound-probe/.

66. Marschall J, Mermel LA, Fakih M, Hadaway L, Kallen A, O'Grady NP, et al. Strategies to prevent central line-associated bloodstream infections in acute care hospitals: 2014 update. Infect Control Hosp Epidemiol. 2014;35(7):753–71.

67. Karpanen TJ, Casey AL, Whitehouse T, Timsit J-F, Mimoz O, Palomar M, et al. A clinical evaluation of two central venous catheter stabilization systems. Ann Intensive Care. 2019;9(1):49.

68. Ullman A, Marsh N, Rickard C. Securement for vascular access devices: looking to the future. Br J Nurs. 2017;26(8):S24–6.

69. SorbaView SHIELD – CATHETER SECUREMENT SOLUTION [Internet]. [cited 2020 Jun 17]. Available from: http://www.sorbaviewshield.com/.

70. Simonova G, Rickard CM, Dunster KR, Smyth DJ, McMillan D, Fraser JF. Cyanoacrylate tissue adhesives – effective securement technique for intravascular catheters: in vitro testing of safety and feasibility. Anaesth Intensive Care. 2012;40(3):460–6.

71. Margatho AS, Ciol MA, Hoffman JM, Dos Reis PED, Furuya RK, Lima DAFS, et al. Chlorhexidine-impregnated gel dressing compared with transparent polyurethane dressing in the prevention of catheter-related infections in critically ill adult patients: a pilot randomised controlled trial. Aust Crit Care. 2019;32(6):471–8.

72. Medgadget Editors. Vidacare EZ-IO Intraosseous Injection System Gets Expanded CE Mark Approval | Medgadget [Internet]. Medgadget. 2011 [cited 2020 Mar 15]. Available from: https://www.medgadget.com/2011/05/vidacare-ez-io-intraosseous-injection-system-gets-expanded-ce-mark-approval.html.

73. Fiser DH. Intraosseous infusion. N Engl J Med. 1990;322(22):1579–81.

74. Rosetti VA, Thompson BM, Miller J, Mateer JR, Aprahamian C. Intraosseous infusion: an alternative route of pediatric intravascular access. Ann Emerg Med. 1985;14(9):885–8.

75. Rosovsky M, FitzPatrick M, Goldfarb CR, Finestone H. Bilateral osteomyelitis due to intraosseous infusion: case report and review of the English-language literature. Pediatr Radiol. 1994;24(1):72–3.

76. Valdes MM. Intraosseous fluid administration in emergencies. Lancet. 1977;1(8024):1235–6.

77. Miller L, Kramer GC, Bolleter S. Rescue access made easy. JEMS. 2005;30(10):suppl 8–18; quiz suppl 19.

78. Ross MH, Romrell LJ, Kaye GI. Histology: a text and atlas. Baltimore; 1995. p318. 18.

79. Nutbeam T, Daniels R. ABC of practical procedures. 1st ed. John & Sons, Incorporated: Wiley; 2009.

80. Teleflex. 2017 The Science and Fundamentals of Intraosseous Vascular Access [Internet]. www.teleflex.com. [cited 2020 Mar 16]. Available from: https://www.teleflex.com/usa/en/clinical-resources/ez-io/documents/EZ-IO_Science_Fundamentals_MC-003266-Rev1-1.pdf.

81. Vizcarra C, Clum S. Intraosseous route as alternative access for infusion therapy. J Infus Nurs. 2010;33(3):162–74.

82. Stantonhicks M. Local anesthesics – pharmacology and clinical applications. Hospital Formulary. 1987;22(2)

83. Kennedy RM, Luhmann JD. The "ouchless emergency department". Getting closer: advances in decreasing distress during painful procedures in the emergency department. Pediatr Clin N Am. 1999;46(6):1215–47, vii.

84. Philbeck TE, Miller LJ, Montez D, Puga T. Hurts so good. Easing IO pain and pressure. JEMS. 2010;35(9):58–62. 65

85. Schalk R, Schweigkofler U, Lotz G, Zacharowski K, Latasch L, Byhahn C. Efficacy of the EZ-IO needle driver for out-of-hospital intraosseous access–a preliminary, observational, multicenter study. Scand J Trauma Resusc Emerg Med. 2011;19:65.

86. Davidoff J, Fowler R, Gordon D, Klein G, Kovar J, Lozano M, et al. Clinical evaluation of a novel intraosseous device for adults: prospective, 250-patient, multi-center trial. JEMS. 2005;30(10):suppl 20–3.

87. OpenAnesthesia. Bupivacaine toxicity Rx [Internet]. [cited 2019 Dec 12]. Available from: https://www.openanesthesia.org/bupivacaine_toxicity_rx/.

88. Eipe N, Gupta S, Penning J. Intravenous lidocaine for acute pain: an evidence-based clinical update. BJA Educ. 2016;16(9):292–8.

89. Quinlan JJ, Oleksey K, Murphy FL. Alkalinization of mepivacaine for axillary block. Anesth Analg. 1992;74(3):371–4.

90. Bedder MD, Kozody R, Craig DB. Comparison of bupivacaine and alkalinized bupivacaine in brachial plexus anesthesia. Anesth Analg. 1988;67(1):48–52.

91. Zisquit J, Nedeff N. Interscalene block. StatPearls. Treasure Island, FL: StatPearls Publishing; 2020.

92. Brown AR, Weiss R, Greenberg C, Flatow EL, Bigliani LU. Interscalene block for shoulder arthroscopy: comparison with general anesthesia. Arthroscopy. 1993;9(3):295–300.

93. Niv D, Gofeld M, Devor M. Causes of pain in degenerative bone and joint disease: a lesson from vertebroplasty. Pain. 2003;105(3):387–92.

94. Lemperg RK, Arnoldi CC. The significance of intraosseous pressure in normal and diseased states with special reference to the intraosseous engorgement-pain syndrome. Clin Orthop Relat Res. 1978;136:143–56.

95. Pasley J, Miller CHT, DuBose JJ, Shackelford SA, Fang R, Boswell K, et al. Intraosseous infusion rates under high pressure: a cadaveric comparison of anatomic sites. J Trauma Acute Care Surg. 2015;78(2):295–9.

96. Chalopin T, Lemaignen A, Guillon A, Geffray A, Derot G, Bahuaud O, et al. Acute Tibial osteomyelitis caused by intraosseous access during initial resuscitation: a case report and literature review. BMC Infect Dis. 2018;18(1):665.

97. Greenstein YY, Koenig SJ, Mayo PH, Narasimhan M. A serious adult intraosseous catheter complication and review of the literature. Crit Care Med. 2016;44(9):e904–9.

98. Von Hoff DD, Kuhn JG, Burris HA, Miller LJ. Does intraosseous equal intravenous? A pharmacokinetic study. Am J Emerg Med. 2008;26(1):31–8.

99. Daya MR, Leroux BG, Dorian P, Rea TD, Newgard CD, Morrison LJ, et al. Survival after intravenous versus intraosseous amiodarone, lidocaine, or placebo in out-of-hospital shock-refractory cardiac arrest. Circulation. 2020;141(3):188–98.

100. Mogey GA. Centenary of hypodermic injection. Br Med J. 1953;2(4847):1180–5.

101. Contreras V, Schmid FR, Ziff M. Use of the hypospray jet injector for the intra-articular and local administration of hydrocortisone acetate. Ann Rheum Dis. 1956;15(3):227–32.

102. Hughes GR. The use of the hypospray in the treatment of minor orthopaedic conditions. Proc R Soc Med. 1969;62(6):577.
103. Taberner A, Hogan NC, Hunter IW. Needle-free jet injection using real-time controlled linear Lorentz-force actuators. Med Eng Phys. 2012;34(9):1228–35.
104. Arora A, Hakim I, Baxter J, Rathnasingham R, Srinivasan R, Fletcher DA, et al. Needle-free delivery of macromolecules across the skin by nanoliter-volume pulsed microjets. Proc Natl Acad Sci U S A. 2007;104(11):4255–60.
105. Resik S, Tejeda A, Mach O, Fonseca M, Diaz M, Alemany N, et al. Immune responses after fractional doses of inactivated poliovirus vaccine using newly developed intradermal jet injectors: a randomized controlled trial in Cuba. Vaccine. 2015;33(2):307–13.
106. Daly C, Molodecky NA, Sreevatsava M, Belayneh AD, Chandio SA, Partridge J, et al. Needle-free injectors for mass administration of fractional dose inactivated poliovirus vaccine in Karachi, Pakistan: a survey of caregiver and vaccinator acceptability. Vaccine. 2020;38(8):1893–8.
107. Champoux N, Du Souich P, Ravaoarinoro M, Phaneuf D, Latour J, Cusson JR. Single-dose pharmacokinetics of ampicillin and tobramycin administered by hypodermoclysis in young and older healthy volunteers. Br J Clin Pharmacol. 1996;42(3):325–31.
108. Mace SE, Harb G, Friend K, Turpin R, Armstrong EP, Lebel F. Cost-effectiveness of recombinant human hyaluronidase-facilitated subcutaneous versus intravenous rehydration in children with mild to moderate dehydration. Am J Emerg Med. 2013;31(6):928–34.
109. Saganski GF, de Souza Freire MH. Safety and effectiveness of hypodermoclysis compared to intravenous fluid infusion for rehydrating children with mild to moderate dehydration: a systematic review protocol. JBI Database System Rev Implement Rep. 2019;17(7):1270–6.
110. Sasson M, Shvartzman P. Hypodermoclysis: an alternative infusion technique. Am Fam Physician. 2001;64(9):1575–8.
111. Vidal M, Hui D, Williams J, Bruera E. A prospective study of hypodermoclysis performed by caregivers in the home setting. J Pain Symptom Manage. 2016;52(4):570–574.e9.
112. Macygin KMC, Kulstad E, Mokszycki RK, Goldsmith M. Evaluation of the Macy Catheter®: a rectal catheter for rapid medication and fluid administration. Expert Rev Med Devices. 2018;15(6):407–14.
113. Foëx BA, Dark P, Rees DR. Fluid replacement via the rectum for treatment of hypovolaemic shock in an animal model. Emerg Med J. 2007;24(1):3–4.
114. Bruera E, Pruvost M, Schoeller T, Montejo G, Watanabe S. Proctoclysis for hydration of terminally ill cancer patients. J Pain Symptom Manag. 1998;15(4):216–9.
115. Honasoge A, Lyons N, Hesse K, Parker B, Mokszycki R, Wesselhoff K, et al. A novel approach for the administration of medications and fluids in emergency scenarios and settings. J Vis Exp. 2016;117
116. Lam YWF, Lam A, Macy B. Pharmacokinetics of phenobarbital in microenema via macy catheter versus suppository. J Pain Symptom Manag. 2016;51(6):994–1001.
117. van Hoogdalem E, de Boer AG, Breimer DD. Pharmacokinetics of rectal drug administration, Part I. General considerations and clinical applications of centrally acting drugs. Clin Pharmacokinet. 1991;21(1):11–26.
118. Tremayne V. Proctoclysis: emergency rectal fluid infusion. Nurs Stand. 2009;24(3):46–8.
119. Grocott MPW, McCorkell S, Cox ML. Resuscitation from hemorrhagic shock using rectally administered fluids in a wilderness environment. Wilderness Environ Med. 2005;16(4):209–11.
120. Wolf CJ. Book review. Clinical physiology of acid-base and electrolyte disorders. N Engl J Med. 1990;322(15):1092.
121. Abolyosr A, Sayed MA, Elanany F, Smeika MA, Shaker SE. Blood transfusion and resuscitation using penile corpora: an experimental study. Urology. 2005;66(4):888–91.
122. Godec CJ, Cass AS. The penis-a possible alternative emergency venous access for males? Ann Emerg Med. 1982;11(5):266–8.
123. Shafik A, El Sibai O, Shafik IA, Shafik AA. Corpora cavernosa as an alternative route for transfusion. Front Biosci. 2006;11:2535–7.

124. Reichman EF. Emergency medicine procedures. 2nd ed. New York, Mcgraw-Hill Education/Medical; 2013.

125. Beavers CJ, Pandya KA. Pharmacotherapy considerations for the management of advanced cardiac life support. Nurs Clin North Am. 2016;51(1):69–82.

126. Greenberg MI. The use of endotracheal medication in cardiac emergencies. Resuscitation. 1984;12(3):155–65.

127. Committee on Drugs. Drugs for pediatric emergencies. Pediatrics. 1998;101(1):e13.

128. Corrigan M, Wilson SS, Hampton J. Safety and efficacy of intranasally administered medications in the emergency department and prehospital settings. Am J Health Syst Pharm. 2015;72(18):1544–54.

129. Morales JO, Brayden DJ. Buccal delivery of small molecules and biologics: of mucoadhesive polymers, films, and nanoparticles. Curr Opin Pharmacol. 2017;36:22–8.

130. Hua S. Advances in nanoparticulate drug delivery approaches for sublingual and buccal administration. Front Pharmacol. 2019;10:1328.

131. https://www.acep.org/globalassets/new-pdfs/policy-statements/alternative-methods-to-vascular-access-in-the-emergency-department.pdf. [Internet]. [cited 2020 Jun 18]. Available from: https://www.acep.org/globalassets/new-pdfs/policy-statements/alternative-methods-to-vascular-access-in-the-emergency-department.pdf.

132. 2011 ENA Emergency Nursing Resources Development Committee, Crowley M, Brim C, Proehl J, Barnason S, Leviner S, et al. Emergency Nursing resource: difficult intravenous access. J Emerg Nurs. 2012;38(4):335–43.

133. 2020 Resource Guide for Vascular Access - Association for Vascular Access [Internet]. [cited 2020 Jun 18]. Available from: https://www.avainfo.org/page/resourceguide.

134. Chopra V, Flanders SA, Saint S, Woller SC, O'Grady NP, Safdar N, et al. The Michigan Appropriateness Guide for Intravenous Catheters (MAGIC): results from a multispecialty panel using the RAND/UCLA appropriateness method. Ann Intern Med. 2015;163(6 Suppl):S1–S40.

135. de Caen AR, Berg MD, Chameides L, Gooden CK, Hickey RW, Scott HF, et al. Part 12: pediatric advanced life support: 2015 American Heart Association guidelines update for cardiopulmonary resuscitation and emergency cardiovascular care. Circulation. 2015;132(18 Suppl 2):S526–42.

136. Duff JP, Topjian A, Berg MD, Chan M, Haskell SE, Joyner BL, et al. 2018 American Heart Association focused update on pediatric advanced life support: an update to the american heart association guidelines for cardiopulmonary resuscitation and emergency cardiovascular care. Circulation. 2018;138(23):e731–9.

137. Davidson IJA, Lok C, Dolmatch B, Gallieni M, Nolen B, Pittiruti M, et al. Virtual reality: emerging role of simulation training in vascular access. Semin Nephrol. 2012;32(6):572–81.

138. Davis L, Owens AK, Thompson J. Defining the specialty of vascular access through consensus: shaping the future of vascular access. JAVA. 2016;21(3):125–30.

139. Meyer BM, Chopra V. Moving the needle forward: the imperative for collaboration in vascular access. J Infus Nurs. 2015;38(2):100–2.

140. Legemaat MM, Jongerden IP, van Rens RMFPT, Zielman M, van den Hoogen A. Effect of a vascular access team on central line-associated bloodstream infections in infants admitted to a neonatal intensive care unit: a systematic review. Int J Nurs Stud. 2015;52(5):1003–10.

141. Gonvers E, Spichiger T, Albrecht E, Dami F. Use of peripheral vascular access in the prehospital setting: is there room for improvement? BMC Emerg Med. 2020;20(1):46.

142. Reades R, Studnek JR, Vandeventer S, Garrett J. Intraosseous versus intravenous vascular access during out-of-hospital cardiac arrest: a randomized controlled trial. Ann Emerg Med. 2011;58(6):509–16.

Arterial Catheters

13

Brendan F. Mullan and James H. Paxton

Introduction

The ability to obtain rapid access to the arterial blood supply is an essential skill for providers who manage critically ill patients presenting to the emergency department, intensive care unit, and other in-hospital settings. Although medications are not generally infused into the arterial system (outside of the interventional administration of thrombolytic agents), the effects of medical interventions are frequently assessed with the analysis of arterial blood gases or other serum laboratory studies derived from arterial blood. Arterial catheter placement can facilitate continuous monitoring of blood pressure and cardiac output, as well as the collection of serial arterial blood specimens without requiring repeated arterial puncture. This allows providers to accurately monitor hemodynamic changes in response to treatment with vasoactive drugs and to monitor the condition of critically ill patients deemed to be at high risk for clinical deterioration. The purpose of this chapter is to introduce the reader to the indications for arterial access, key anatomic considerations, and commonly utilized techniques for catheter placement. The underlying principles of emergent arterial access described in this chapter will be of value to most clinicians who routinely access the arterial system of their patients for therapeutic or diagnostic purposes.

B. F. Mullan
Wayne State University School of Medicine, Detroit, MI, USA
e-mail: brendanfmullan@wayne.edu

J. H. Paxton (✉)
Department of Emergency Medicine, Wayne State University School of Medicine, Detroit, MI, USA
e-mail: james.paxton@wayne.edu

© Springer Nature Switzerland AG 2021
J. H. Paxton (ed.), *Emergent Vascular Access*,
https://doi.org/10.1007/978-3-030-77177-5_13

Arterial Anatomy

The arterial blood supply is generally outlined in Chap. 2, including the major anatomical structures relevant for a discussion of the arterial system. These structures are provided here again in Fig. 13.1. Historically, a wide variety of anatomic sites have been utilized to gain arterial vascular access, including the brachial, ulnar, radial, axillary, femoral, dorsalis pedis, posterior tibial, and temporal arteries. However, the two most commonly utilized anatomic sites for arterial vascular access are the *radial artery* and the *femoral artery*. These two arteries are most commonly accessed by emergency care providers because of their relatively high safety profile, convenient anatomic landmarks, ease of cannulation, and familiarity to those who care for critically ill patients. As this chapter is meant to serve as an introduction to

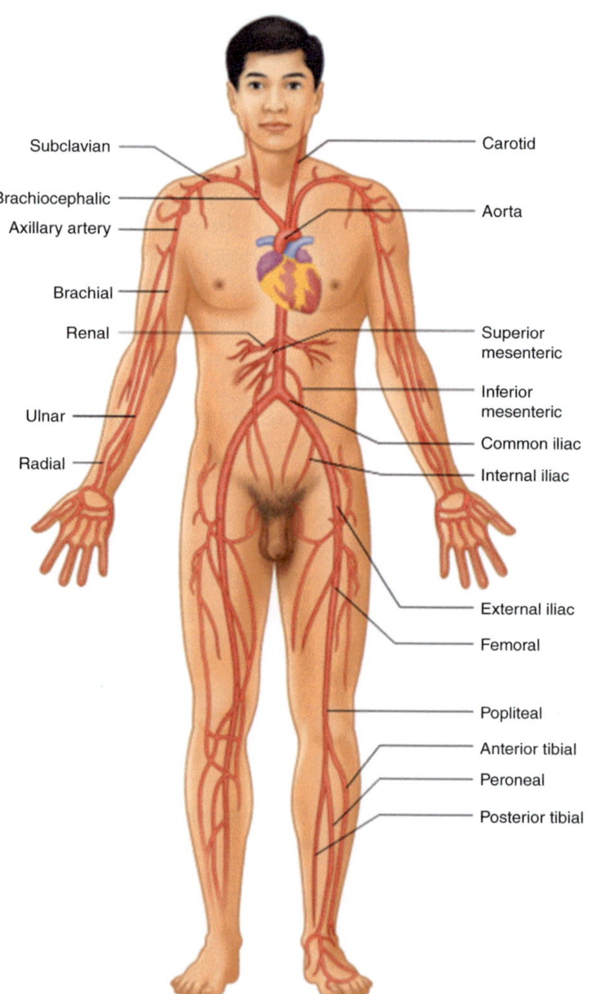

Fig. 13.1 The human arterial system

the principles of emergent arterial access, we have limited the discussion to the major arteries of the wrist (i.e., radial and ulnar arteries) and the femoral artery, which we feel are adequate to illustrate the major learning points. While this chapter does not specifically address potential cannulation of other major arteries (e.g., brachial artery), the underlying principles of arterial access described herein will provide the reader with a basic understanding of the primary considerations for puncture and cannulation of the arterial blood supply.

Arteries of the Wrist

The *radial artery* is the largest artery supplying the distal forearm and hand. It originates as a branch of the brachial artery at the level of the cubital fossa, just medial to the biceps tendon. The artery then travels distally along the lateral forearm toward the styloid process of the radius to perfuse the hand through a network of arches anastomosing with the ulnar artery. Anatomical variation in the radial artery exists in up to 30% of patients [1]. However, the radial artery insertion site is typically found just medial and proximal to the radial styloid process and lateral to the *flexor carpi radialis* tendon, 1–2 cm proximal to the wrist crease. The cannulation site should be at least 1 cm proximal to the styloid process of the radius to avoid puncture of the superficial branch of the radial artery and the flexor retinaculum. This site also minimizes kinking of the catheter following insertion with patient wrist flexion. Care should be taken to avoid damage to the superficial branch of the *radial nerve*, which runs lateral and deep to the radial artery at this site. The relevant anatomy for the radial artery insertion site is illustrated in Fig. 13.2. The anatomic relationship between the radial styloid process and the proper insertion site is shown in Fig. 13.3.

The *ulnar artery* is the "other" main artery of the distal forearm and hand and has been utilized for arterial puncture and cannulation with great success. However, it is seldom used in the emergent setting due to concerns about its deeper location within the forearm and risk of iatrogenic injury to the *ulnar nerve*. This increased risk of nerve injury may be attributed to the fact that the ulnar nerve and ulnar artery are often *found at the same depth*, unlike the radial nerve (which is usually found deep to its corresponding artery). However, recent reports have suggested that the ulnar artery may be a suitable first cannulation site for those patients with a strong ulnar pulse [2], although it is not recommended when the ulnar pulse is weak. Among patients with a strong ulnar pulse, complication rates with proper insertion technique appear to be similar to those for the radial artery insertion site [2].

When considering radial or ulnar artery puncture and cannulation, the clinician is expected to first assess for collateral circulation between the radial and ulnar arteries, though the methodology and the necessity of this assessment remain controversial. Generally, this is done using the *modified Allen test* (Fig. 13.4). The modified Allen test differs from the traditional Allen test in that the traditional test evaluates both radial arteries at the same time, followed by assessment of both ulnar arteries at the same time. The modified Allen test (which has almost universally replaced the traditional Allen test in clinical practice) evaluates the radial and ulnar

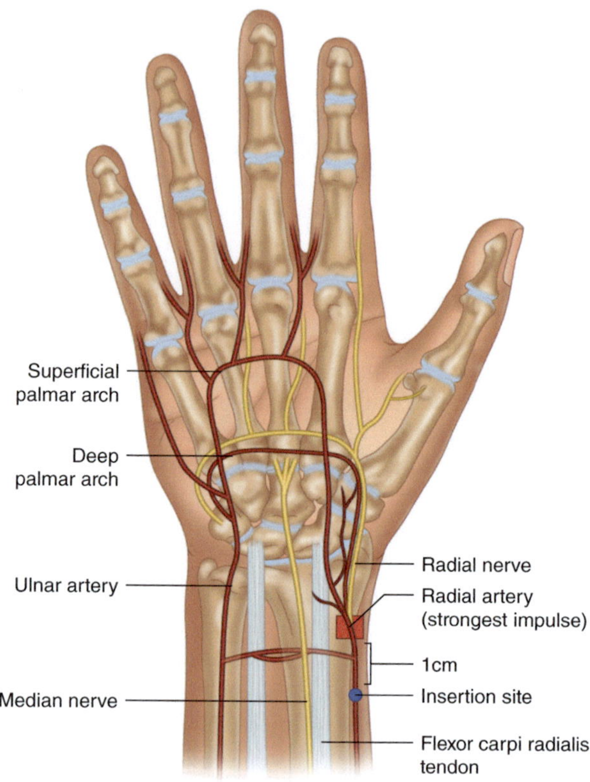

Fig. 13.2 Relevant anatomy of the radial artery insertion site

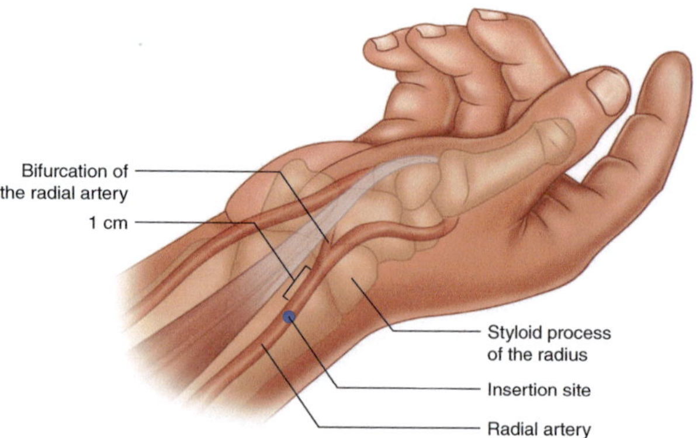

Fig. 13.3 Relationship between the radial insertion site and the styloid process

arteries on one hand followed by assessment of the radial and ulnar arteries on the other hand. The modified Allen test assesses the relative contributions of the radial and ulnar arteries to the anastomotic network of arteries (including the superficial and deep palmar arches) that supply blood flow to the hand. The modified Allen test is performed by first having the patient flex their arm at the elbow and "make a fist."

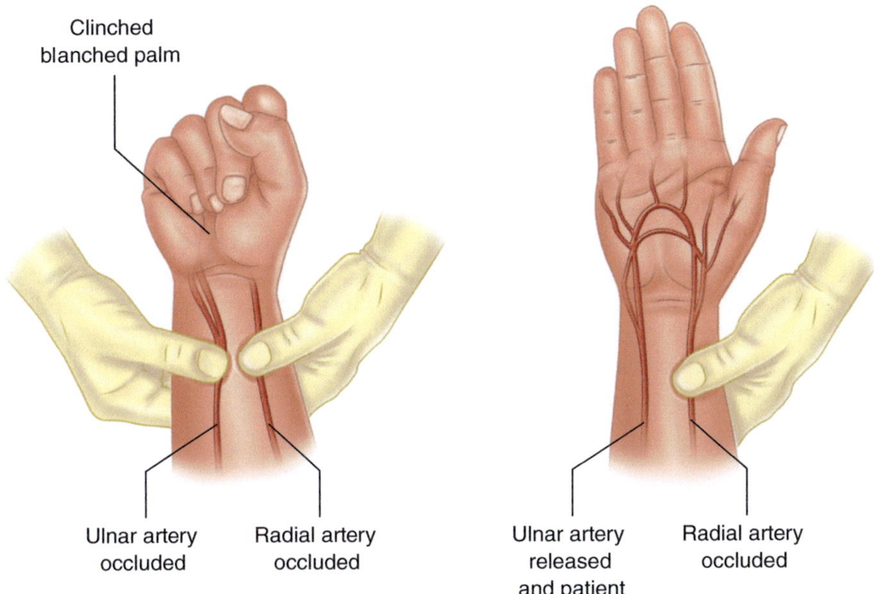

Fig. 13.4 Allen's test for collateral circulation of the hand

At the level of the wrist, and proximal to the expected cannulation site, the examiner then *simultaneously occludes both the radial and ulnar arteries* with direct pressure. The patient is then asked to "relax the fist," after which time the hand should appear pale due to reduced perfusion while both arteries are occluded. Next, the examiner will *release pressure only on the ulnar artery* (while still compressing the radial artery) to assess the return of blood flow to the entire hand through the ulnar artery. If capillary perfusion does not return to normal within 10 seconds, the examiner should suspect compromised flow of blood through the ulnar artery and its associated vascular beds. *Compromised ulnar arterial flow suggests that the radial artery is required to maintain adequate perfusion of the hand due to an incomplete palmar arch network.* In this setting, radial artery cannulation is not recommended, since it could lead to ischemia of the hand if the radial artery is occluded, thrombosed, or transected during the cannulation attempt. Multiple studies have shown that a physiologically incomplete superficial palmar arch is present in 10–12% of patients [3–5].

In those cases when the ulnar artery is selected for insertion, the procedure is modified and reversed to feature continued compression of the ulnar artery with release of the radial artery. Although the modified Allen's test is widely recommended to assess "collateral circulation" of the hand, it has been shown to be of poor diagnostic accuracy and does not objectively predict the risk of ischemic complications from radial or ulnar artery cannulation attempts [6]. Other techniques can be incorporated in conjunction with the Allen's test to add objectivity to the interpretation of collateral circulation including pulse oximetry, plethysmography, and Doppler ultrasound [7].

Since the radial artery is often the dominant artery of the hand, a patient's radial pulse is usually stronger than the ulnar pulse in the same arm [2]. Success rates for arterial cannulation at these sites may be best predicted by the strength of the pulse appreciated by the clinical provider [2]. Thus, preference for selection of either the radial or ulnar artery as the first attempted site should be determined by the strength of the appreciated pulse rather than a priori concerns about nerve injury. Although failed radial artery cannulation has traditionally been considered a contraindication for ulnar artery attempts on the same extremity, this is not an absolute contraindication. One large retrospective review failed to show any serious complications from ipsilateral ulnar artery cannulation after failed radial artery cannulation when appropriate assessment has been performed [8–10].

Femoral Artery

The *femoral artery* (at the recommended insertion site, more properly termed the *common femoral artery* (CFA)) is the largest artery commonly cannulated in clinical practice and may therefore be the easiest to access for patients experiencing hypotension or shock. In fact, the CFA is the largest artery in the lower extremity, originating from the *external iliac artery* and entering the thigh within the *femoral sheath* deep to the *inguinal ligament*, midway between the *anterior superior iliac spine* (ASIS) and the *pubic symphysis*. The external iliac artery changes its name to the CFA after it passes posterior to the inguinal ligament, and the CFA should ideally be cannulated approximately 3 cm (two finger widths) distal to the ligament. Cannulation attempts superior to this site are associated with increased risk of retroperitoneal hemorrhage, while more distal cannulation is associated with increased risk of pseudoaneurysm, arteriovenous fistula (AVF), hematoma, and limb ischemia.

Within the femoral sheath, the femoral artery lies lateral to the *femoral vein* and medial to the *femoral nerve*. The femoral artery travels inferiorly down the thigh for 4–5 cm before bifurcating into the *superficial femoral artery* (SFA) and *deep femoral artery* (DFA), although there have been some documented cases of this division occurring as close as 2.5 cm distal to the inguinal ligament.

The insertion site for the femoral artery is located within the so-called femoral triangle, which is defined by its three borders: the *inguinal ligament*, the *sartorius muscle*, and the *adductor longus muscle*. The femoral triangle also contains the *femoral nerve*, *femoral vein*, and lymphatic vessels. The relative position of these structures (from most lateral to medial) is predicted by the acronym: *NAVEL* (*nerve, artery, vein, empty space, lymphatics*). Thus, if one of these structures is identified, the provider can predict the likely location of the other structures using this mnemonic. Keep in mind that these structures are mirrored on the contralateral side. In other words, the femoral artery is generally lateral to the femoral vein at the level of the inguinal ligament, regardless of which body side is examined. The relevant anatomy at the femoral artery insertion site is illustrated in (Fig. 13.5).

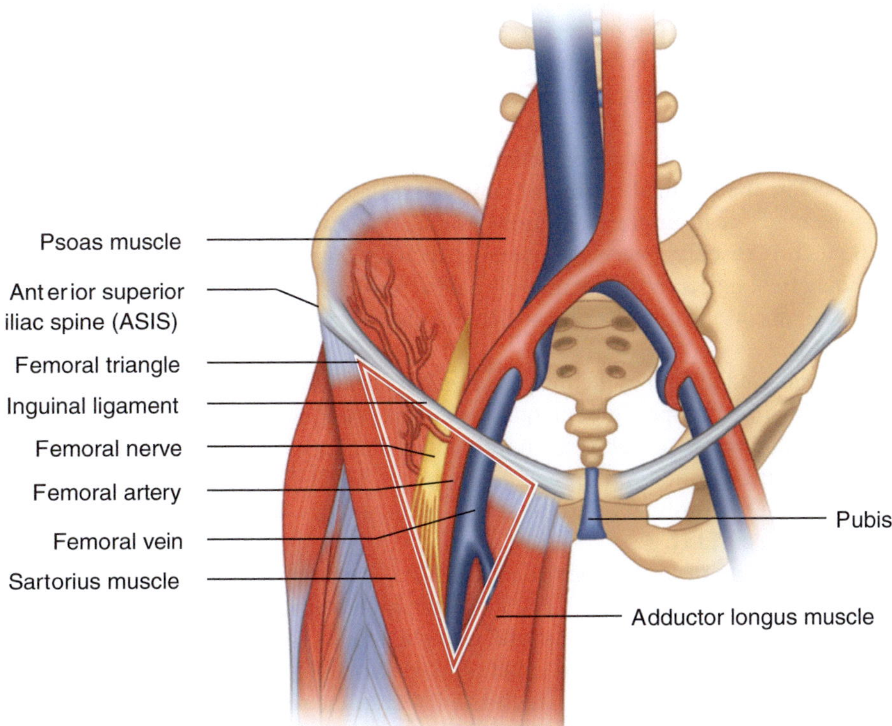

Fig. 13.5 Relevant anatomy of the femoral artery insertion site

One recent study found that, on average, the femoral artery lies 17.1 mm (SD 6.4) below the skin surface at the insertion site, which is more superficial than the femoral vein (22.0 mm, SD 6.7) at this level [11]. In the same study, the femoral artery and vein were approximately 2.6 mm (SD 2.0) apart [11]. The mean diameter of the femoral artery in adults appears to be between 8 and 9 mm, only slightly smaller than the femoral vein (about 9.5 mm) [11]. It should be noted that the femoral artery's depth below the skin is highly dependent upon the patient's body mass index (BMI) and adipose distribution pattern, while the artery's diameter appears to be correlated with patient height [11]. The strength of femoral pulse felt by the clinician is a product of multiple factors, including BMI, the patient's systolic blood pressure, previous surgery, arteriosclerosis and other comorbidities, and distance from the inguinal ligament [11].

As the femoral artery travels more distally from the inguinal ligament within the femoral triangle, it becomes more superficial and smaller in diameter, although the changes are only a few millimeters in scale and almost imperceptible [12]. While the femoral vessels only overlap (i.e., artery immediately superficial to the vein) partially in about 30% of patients at the level of the inguinal ligament, the femoral artery will ultimately completely overlap the femoral vein as it travels distal to the inguinal ligament, with nearly 100% of patients having some degree of overlap (and 50% with complete overlap) at 4 cm distal to the inguinal ligament. Thus, as one travels distally from the ligament, the likelihood of the femoral vein lying underneath the femoral artery is greatly increased [12]. By contrast, the femoral vein rarely overlaps the femoral artery [12]. These facts underscore the importance of selecting the proper site of insertion for femoral artery cannulation, as the traditionally defined "safe" distance for femoral artery cannulation (i.e., in a range from 2 to 4 cm below the inguinal ligament) may still realize a high likelihood of iatrogenic venous injury with imprecise arterial cannulation attempts. Many older textbooks still cite this vascular overlap to occur up to 10 cm from the inguinal ligament, and this historical inaccuracy may provide a false sense of security to the clinician when selecting an insertion site near or distal to the 4-cm mark from the inguinal ligament [13].

The precise location of the inguinal ligament can be difficult to identify on external landmarking, especially in obese patients. Among the commonly available external landmarks palpable to the clinician, the *femoral head* may be the best marker for the location of the inguinal ligament, as the bifurcation of the CFA into the SFA and the profunda femoris artery (PFA) occurs below the femoral head in 77% of subjects [14].

The ideal site of CFA puncture is therefore near to the midpoint of the femoral head [14]. Cannulation of the CFA above the inguinal ligament, or too far distal to this site, is associated with significant complications [14]. Caudal artery punctures below the bifurcation occur outside the structural stability of the femoral sheath and lack underlying bony support, which can increase the risk of bleeding, hematoma, and pseudoaneurysm formation [15, 16]. Moreover, smaller arterial diameter below the bifurcation increases the risk of cannulation-related injury [16], including AVF formation as branches of the femoral vein can cross over the SFA. Cannulation *above* the inguinal ligament introduces the risk of retroperitoneal hemorrhage, due to the inability to provide effective direct compression of the insertion site [17]. Similarly, accessing the femoral artery just below the inguinal ligament could be problematic as the taught nature of the inguinal ligament can prevent effective compression of the artery. Thus, *the optimal location for CFA cannulation is 2–3 cm distal to the inguinal ligament*, where the artery can be easily palpated and compressed as needed [14].

"Rupp's rule" defines the ideal site for CFA cannulation to be 1 cm lateral to the most medial aspect of the femoral head, midway between its superior and inferior borders [18]. Providers may have difficulty identifying the femoral head, as it is a deep bony structure. However, the midpoint of the femoral head and other relevant anatomic landmarks can be roughly estimated by external palpation. Firm pressure on the anterior aspect of the pelvis laterally will identify the ASIS, while pressure on the lateral aspect of the hip will identify the *greater tubercle* of the femur. The most superior aspect of the *greater tubercle of the femur* likely corresponds to the midpoint of the femoral head, as illustrated in Fig. 13.6.

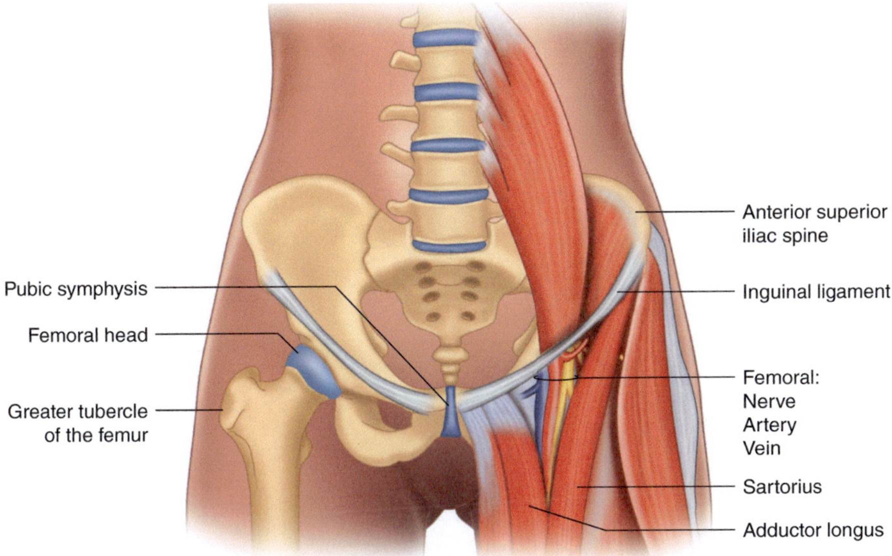

Fig. 13.6 Anatomic location of the femoral head

Another commonly used method of identifying the proper location for femoral artery/vein cannulation is the so-called V Technique, which utilizes the clinician's hand to predict the location of the femoral vessels. With this method, the clinician places their contralateral hand on the patient (e.g., provider's left hand on the right side of the patient), with the clinician's index finger on the ASIS and the clinician's thumb on the *pubic symphysis*. The femoral vein (and artery) should be located at the apex of the "V" formed by the first web space of the provider's hand, as illustrated in Fig. 13.7.

Although the "V Technique" may not always predict the precise location of the femoral vessels, it can be used to estimate the general location of the femoral artery prior to cannulation under emergent conditions characterized by hypotension, when a pulse may not be felt.

When considering CFA cannulation, a comprehensive history should be acquired focusing upon the presence of conditions that may complicate femoral artery access, including peripheral vascular disease, diminished femoral pulse, history of iliofemoral bypass graft, prior femoral arterial access with closure devise, complications from prior femoral arterial cannulation, active groin infection, prior groin surgery, known aneurysms of the iliofemoral or aortoiliac system, the inability to lie flat for prolonged periods of time, or morbid obesity [14]. While these conditions are not absolute contraindications to femoral artery cannulation, their presence should suggest consideration of the radial or other peripheral arteries for cannulation rather than the femoral artery.

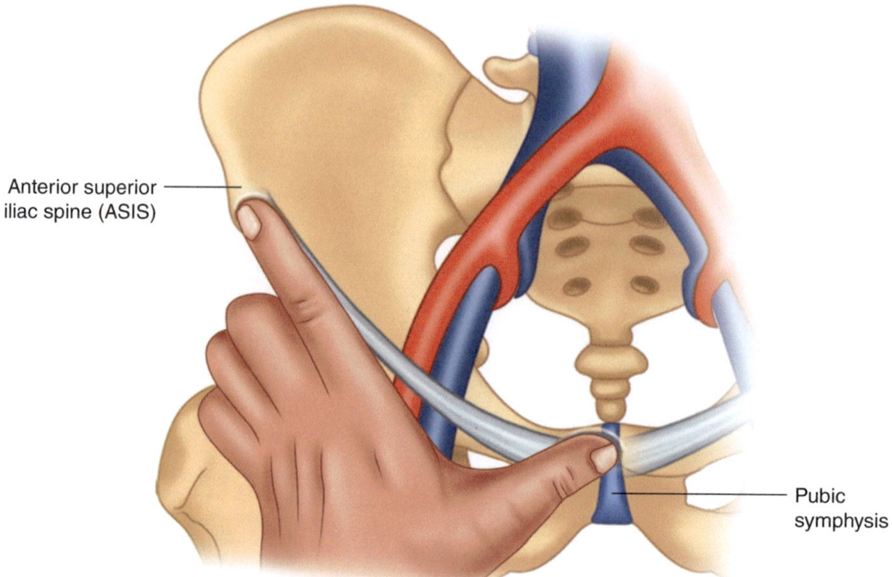

Fig. 13.7 The "V Technique" for identification of the femoral vessels, utilizing the provider's hand to estimate the location of the femoral vessels

Insertion Site Selection

As mentioned above, the most common sites utilized for arterial puncture or cannulation are the *radial artery* and the *common femoral artery*. As discussed above, the *ulnar artery* may also be a good choice, especially if the patient has a stronger pulse at the ulnar artery than at the radial artery. The carotid artery is not recommended for arterial cannulation due to perceived increased risk of embolic or thrombotic complications affecting cerebral blood flow. Other options for arterial cannulation include the subclavian artery, the brachial (antecubital) and axillary arteries of the upper extremity, and the posterior tibial and dorsalis pedis arteries of the foot.

While providers may be tempted to cannulate deep arteries utilizing ultrasound techniques, it is generally recommended that *superficial arteries* be sought first as they may be at less risk of complications, including iatrogenic injury to adjacent structures (e.g., nerves, veins), line kinking, catheter dislodgement, or procedural failure. However, the selection of an appropriate site for arterial puncture and cannulation should be informed and guided by a host of factors, including anatomical considerations, feasibility, and clinician experience.

The radial artery is the most commonly selected site for arterial puncture or cannulation, due to the associated low rate of serious complications and ease of placement [19]. It is a superficial artery and is easily palpable and identifiable in non-hypotensive patients [20]. However, providers must remember that peripheral (e.g., radial, ulnar; posterior tibial; etc.) arterial pressure monitoring *may not provide an accurate estimate of corresponding central arterial pressures* [19]. This appears to be especially true for patients receiving high doses of inotropic or vasopressor support [21–23]. When properly placed, femoral artery catheters offer the additional advantages of decreased line placement failure and increased catheter longevity, as compared to radial arterial lines [24, 25]. It has been suggested that up to one line failure could be prevented for every four times that a femoral line is selected over a radial cannulation [25].

Given the available evidence, we suggest that the *radial artery* be selected for first attempt in patients with normal or elevated blood pressure who are unlikely to become hypotensive or require vasopressor support. This might include patients with respiratory failure but otherwise stable vital signs who require arterial line placement primarily for frequent arterial blood sampling.

However, patients who have been resuscitated from cardiac arrest (and are therefore susceptible to hypotension, subsequent cardiac arrest, and additional ACLS intervention), or who are anticipated to require aggressive correction of hypotension (e.g., sepsis, cardiogenic shock; etc.) including vasopressors or inotropes, may achieve more accurate blood pressure monitoring with a *femoral arterial line*. While each patient's unique presentation (and available anatomy) should always dictate appropriate site selection, it is important to consider the patient's future hospital course and anticipate the patient's needs later in the hospitalization when selecting the proper arterial catheter insertion site.

Along with selection of a site for the initial insertion attempt, the provider should also develop a "game plan" for subsequent arterial line insertion sites if their initial attempt fails. Knowing what to do if one's initial attempts fail *before* starting the initial attempt will streamline the process of ultimately obtaining arterial access. This anticipation of future needs will allow assistants or colleagues to gather the necessary supplies (e.g., catheter kits, ultrasound machine, sterile supplies, etc.) for another attempt in the same area, or to even begin prepping a new site while the failed attempt is being managed (e.g., pressure held to attempt site; etc).

Some patients may require interventional endovascular procedures for treatment of neurological or cardiac conditions, and the femoral or radial arteries may both be used as access points for such procedures. When feasible, providers should become familiar with the preferred access sites for interventionalists at their institution for such procedures. Since arterial lines are generally placed in the emergency department or an inpatient setting, it may be possible to solicit from the interventionalists at the provider's institution whether they typically have a preference to preserve either the left or right side artery for use with interventional procedures. Interventionalist preferences for the femoral or radial artery may also exist. If such a preference exists, it may be preferable to use the contralateral arteries for puncture and cannulation of an arterial catheter. This will allow uninterrupted arterial monitoring in the event that the patient is found to require an endovascular procedure.

Indications for Arterial Cannulation

In general, arterial line placement has value for patients who require *continuous blood pressure monitoring* (e.g., hypotension or hypertension requiring aggressive titration of vasoactive medications) or who require *repeated, frequent arterial blood sampling* due to respiratory failure with ongoing concerns about arterial blood oxygenation. However, the ultimate decision to place an arterial line is complex and depends upon a variety of factors, including (perhaps most importantly) the predicted course of the patient in the hours and days that follow the immediate need for arterial cannulation. Ideally, arterial catheters should only be placed when strictly needed for blood pressure or arterial blood sampling. Conditions that may benefit from arterial line placement include (but are not limited to) hypertensive emergency, stroke, shock, shock requiring the titration of vasoactive medications, and patients undergoing complex surgical procedures [26]. Arterial catheterization can be especially beneficial in cases where careful blood pressure monitoring is essential but sphygmomanometric (e.g., blood pressure cuff) monitoring is expected to be inaccurate, such as critically ill patients who are morbidly obese, thin, or extremely burned [27, 28].

Contraindications

Arterial vascular access is generally considered a safe procedure. However, relative contraindications should be considered when assessing potential anatomic insertion sites. First and foremost, arterial catheterization is not recommended if there is an absent pulse at the proposed cannulation site (suggesting limb ischemia) or if the patient has *thromboangiitis obliterans* (Buerger disease), Raynaud syndrome, or other evidence of inadequate circulation or insufficient collateral perfusion of the targeted extremity [28]. Other site-specific contraindications include adjacent infection (e.g., abscess, cellulitis), burns overlying the proposed cannulation site, evidence of previous surgery in the area (suggesting scar formation and/or distorted anatomy), or the presence of synthetic arterial or vascular grafts. When feasible, arterial cannulation should be performed at the site with the strongest palpable pulse and avoided at sites with a relatively weaker pulse. The presence of a weaker pulse at a single extremity suggests that arterial flow may be compromised or that the artery is situated deeper at this site than on the contralateral side. Special care should also be taken with patients receiving anticoagulation or thrombolytic therapy or who present with coagulopathy. These patients will be at higher risk of hemorrhage and hematoma with unsuccessful attempts and may benefit from ultrasound-guided line placement, when possible.

Table 13.1 Incidence rates of complications related to radial and femoral artery cannulation [24, 33–42]

Site	Radial	Femoral
Complication	Incidence range (%)	Incidence range (%)
Permanent ischemic damage	0–2 [33, 34]	0–0.31 [35, 36]
Local site infection	0–4.8 [37, 38]	0–1.8 [35, 39]
Compartment syndrome	Rare	Rare
Nerve injury	Rare	Not documented
Sepsis	0–1.5 [24, 38]	0–1.8 [24, 35]
Bleeding from insertion site	0.51–0.56 [24, 39]	0–3.5 [24, 39]
Transient occlusion of vessel	1.5–35 [24, 40]	0–4.7 [24, 41]
Hematoma	3.8–31 [33, 41]	3.1–11.8 [41, 42]

Complications

The risks of serious delayed complications from indwelling arterial catheters increases with increasing duration of the catheter, though these risks are rare when catheters are removed within 12 hours [29]. Serious complications, though uncommon, include permanent ischemic damage to the distal extremity, local site infection, compartment syndrome, nerve injury, and sepsis [19, 30, 31]. These complications are relatively rare when proper aseptic technique is practiced during the procedure. More commonly, minor immediate complications include pain, bleeding from the insertion site, transient occlusion of the vessel, and hematoma [19, 32]. Proper training, preparation, and awareness of these common complications can mitigate and correct the problem before they cause serious injury. The rates of previously reported complications associated with radial and femoral arterial line placement are provided in Table 13.1.

Procedural Approaches

The technique should be decided prior to starting the procedure. The technique will depend on the kit provided as some kits have guidewires separate from needle and catheter, while other kits feature a single apparatus incorporating the guidewire, needle, and catheter. In this section, we describe three frequently used techniques for obtaining radial or femoral artery vascular access: the *Seldinger technique* (i.e., catheter-over-wire), *modified Seldinger technique*, and *catheter-over-needle technique*.

The Seldinger (i.e., catheter-over-wire) and modified Seldinger techniques both involve the use of a needle to gain initial entry into the artery, a guidewire that is inserted through the needle into the artery, and a catheter which is introduced over the wire into the artery [43]. These techniques are generally preferred for deeper arteries (i.e., femoral artery) but can be used for superficial arteries (i.e., radial artery). It should be noted that these techniques are discouraged for radial artery cannulation in neonatal and infant patients as their small arteries make proper guidewire insertion difficult.

The catheter-over-needle technique is recommended for superficial arteries, including the radial artery. This technique may be most familiar to providers, as it is similar to peripheral intravenous catheter placement. With this method, an introducer needle with an integrated catheter is introduced into the lumen of the artery, the catheter is advanced over the needle, and the needle is removed. If cannulation using the catheter-over-needle technique is ineffective, the procedure may be salvaged with the use of a guidewire [44].

General Procedural Preparation

Although each of these three techniques entails specific differences, the process of preparing for arterial line placement is generally the same for all insertions. The steps involved in a generic arterial line placement include:

1. Provider preparation
2. Selection of insertion site
3. Insertion site positioning
4. Sterilization of insertion site
5. Local anesthetic infiltration
6. Arterial puncture with needle
7. Catheter insertion and dressing
8. Catheter securement and tubing attachment

1. *Provider Preparation*

Informed consent should be obtained from the patient, including a thorough discussion of the risks (e.g., complications) and benefits (e.g., indications) of the procedure. Written consent from the patient or their legally authorized representative should be documented when possible, although emergent implied consent may be required if informed consent cannot be obtained. A proper "time-out" should be held prior to starting the procedure, to confirm the site and laterality of the procedure. This will also allow members of the care team an opportunity to voice any concerns about the site selected for arterial cannulation.

Once consent has been obtained and documented, the provider should gather all equipment needed to complete the procedure, ensure that an ultrasound machine is available (when appropriate), and make preparations for an arterial pressure transducer line setup (including all necessary tubing and priming of the system). If nursing staff are preparing the arterial line setup, they will need time to prepare it. Providers should wash their hands, don the appropriate personal protective equipment (e.g., sterile gown, cap, mask, sterile gloves), and enlist any additional assistants needed to complete the procedure. It is always advisable to have a non-sterile assistant at the bedside throughout the procedure, to avoid interruptions in the procedure when additional supplies, equipment, or help from ancillary staff are needed.

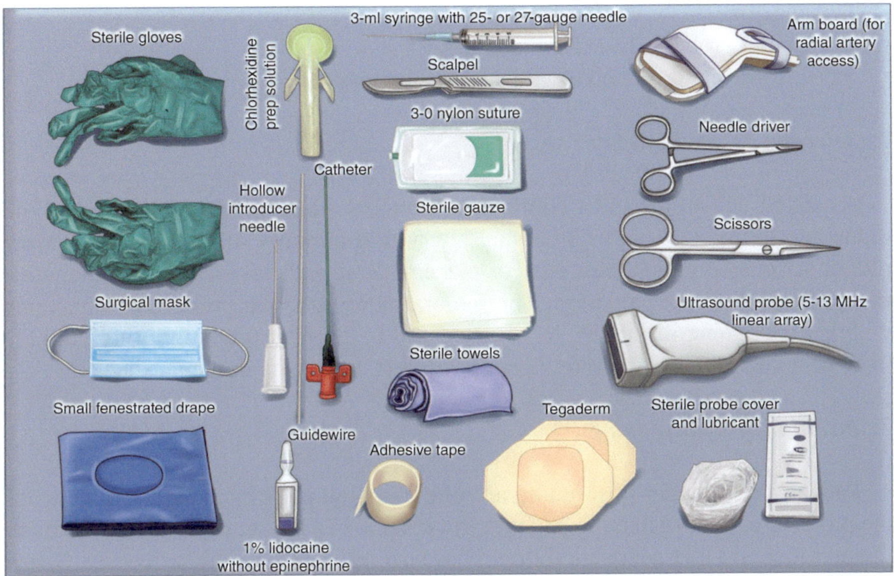

Fig. 13.8 Supplies required for arterial catheterization. (The image above is a placeholder)

The supplies needed to insert an arterial catheter are illustrated in Fig. 13.8 and include:

- Sterile gloves and fenestrated drapes
- Skin preparation solution (e.g., povidone-iodine or chlorhexidine)
- 18-, 20-, or 22-gauge introducer needle
- Arterial catheter of appropriate gauge and length
- Guidewire (if using Seldinger or modified Seldinger techniques)
- 5-ml vial of 1% lidocaine without epinephrine
- 3-ml syringe with 25- or 27-gauge needle for subcutaneous administration of lidocaine
- #11 scalpel blade
- 3–0 or 4–0 nylon or other nonabsorbable suture
- Needle driver
- Sterile gauze (2 × 2 and 4 × 4 inches)
- Sterile towels
- Adhesive tape
- Tegaderm® or other sterile dressing
- Biopatch® protective disc
- Three-way stopcock
- Sterile 10-mL saline syringes
- Pressure transducer kit with all IV lines, transducer cables, and monitor setup
- Pressure tubing
- Size-appropriate arm board (if accessing radial artery)

- T-connector
- Ultrasound probe 5–13 MHz linear array
- Sterile ultrasound probe kit with sterile lubrication

2. *Selection of Insertion Site*

As stated above, the most common anatomical sites for arterial access are the radial and femoral arteries. The radial artery is commonly selected due to its low rate of serious complications, ease of placement, superficial location, and identifiability through direct palpation. The femoral artery may be preferred for patients with hemodynamic instability or when central blood pressure monitoring is likely to be of higher clinical value (e.g., cardiac arrest, sepsis, cardiogenic shock).

3. *Insertion Site Positioning*

Patient and provider positioning are of paramount importance to the success of the procedure. Ensure that the patient's stretcher is at a height that is comfortable to the provider and that adequate lighting has been provided for the procedure. When

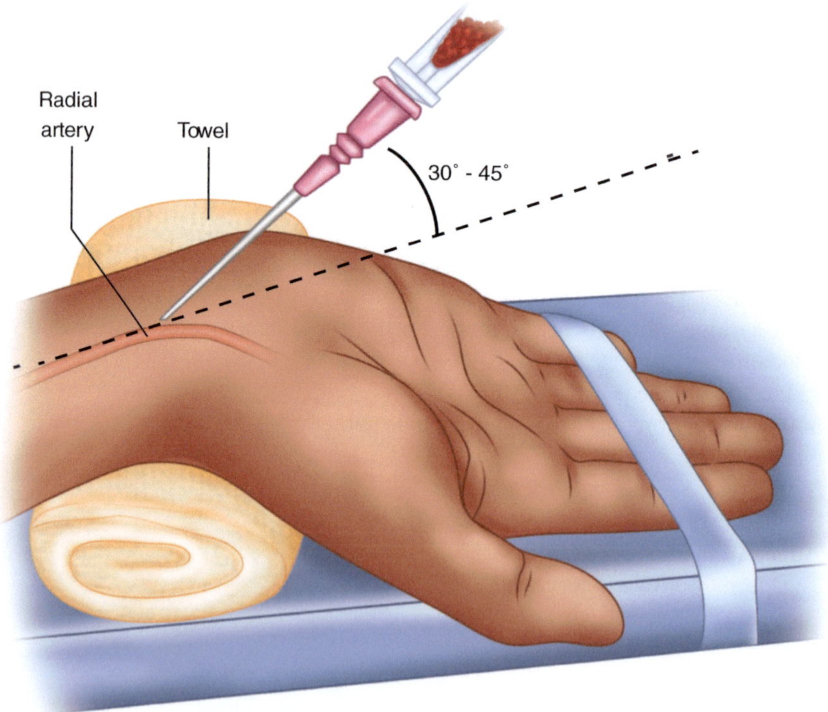

Fig. 13.9 Wrist position and angle of needle insertion with radial artery cannulation

placing a radial catheter, it is important to abduct the arm away from the patient and secure the arm to prevent inadvertent movement during the procedure. To maximize exposure during a radial artery attempt, place the patient's body and nondominant hand both in a supine position and extend the wrist 45° from neutral position, supported by a rolled sterile towel roll placed under the wrist, as depicted in Figure 13.9 [45]. It may be necessary to secure the patient's arm and hand with tape to an arm board and/or Mayo stand to minimize movement of the wrist during the procedure. Arm boards may be kept in place after placement has been completed for select (e.g., pediatric, noncompliant) patients who are prone to excessive wrist flexion, which can cause kinkage and occlusion of the catheter after placement. Locate the optimal arterial insertion site through direct palpation of the arterial pulse or through ultrasound guidance prior to preparing the sterile field, as the sterile field should be centered on the insertion site.

For femoral artery cannulation, the patient should also be in a supine position with the ipsilateral hip externally rotated. The femoral artery should be identified through direct palpation or ultrasound guidance before establishing a sterile field, and the insertion site should be disinfected and draped as described above for the radial artery.

The provider should be positioned on the same side of the stretcher as the targeted artery, to avoid strain associated with reaching over the patient to access the insertion site. When ultrasound is used, the ultrasound machine should be positioned on the contralateral side of the patient, so that the target vessel and the monitor are within the same direct line of sight from the provider. Be sure to adjust ambient lighting and place your Mayo stand with needed supplies close to the work space to avoid excessive stretching or reaching for items during the procedure. The provider should plan to use their dominant hand to insert the catheter, so adjustments may need to be made to this arrangement to facilitate provider comfort during the procedure. In general, the key here is to maximize the ergonomic arrangement of needed devices and supplies to avoid excessive interruption or awkward straining by the provider during line placement.

4. *Sterilization of Insertion Site*

Once the insertion site has been selected and the limb positioned, a sterile field must be created for the procedure. The sterile field should be centered on the targeted insertion site, but the fenestration in the sterile drape should also frame an area larger than the initially targeted insertion site, to allow for more proximal puncture if the initial puncture attempt is not successful. The provider should cleanse the skin thoroughly with chlorhexidine gluconate or povidone-iodine solution and frame the area of insertion with sterile drapes. Proper sterile technique should be used to reduce the risk of line-associated bloodstream infections [19]. It is advisable to thoroughly clean the target area prior to skin sterilization, to remove any visible soiling or debris. Once the area has been cleaned and sterilized, great care should be taken to avoid re-contaminating the area by touching or through contact with non-sterile items. When an ultrasound probe is to be used, the provider must include the entire probe and connecting transducer lead/cable that may come into contact with the sterile field in a sterile cover. Anything that touches the sterile field (i.e., insertion site and drape) should be sterile.

5. *Local Anesthetic Infiltration*

To alleviate the pain associated with arterial line placement, providers should infiltrate 1–2 ml of 1% lidocaine in the skin directly overlying the insertion site to create a small (5-mm) wheal. It is important that the wheal not be too large, as it may distort the relevant anatomy and reduce the strength of the pulse that is appreciated. Gentle rubbing of the wheal prior to skin puncture may help mitigate this effect.

6. *Arterial Puncture with Needle*

Arterial walls contain a layer of vascular smooth muscle that contracts with injury. The resultant vasospasm following arterial injury may cause vasoconstriction and reduce the cross-sectional diameter of the target vessel. This reduces the strength of the pulse at that site and makes subsequent cannulation attempts increasingly difficult. Thus, the *first attempt at arterial puncture and cannulation is a provider's best shot* at achieving procedural success, and this effect is especially injurious when attempting cannulation of the radial artery, which may already be a very small cross-sectional target. The tailor's adage of "measure three times, cut once" is relevant here. If the first attempt is not successful, the provider should reassess the pulse. If the strength of the pulse has not diminished, and no hematoma or other complication is noted, additional attempts may be warranted at the same site. However, if vasospasm is suspected at the initial targeted site, the provider should assess adjacent *more proximal portions* of the same artery to determine if cannulation may be feasible and safe. Portions of the artery that are distal to the site of vasospasm are likely to have a similarly reduced pulse, making cannulation more difficult.

When inserting the needle, providers should confirm that the bevel (angled tip of the needle) is facing "up" (i.e., toward the ceiling) to avoid the needle tip obstructing the guidewire or catheter in subsequent steps. The direction of needle insertion should be along the predicted path of the artery's course within the extremity. The goal is to position the orifice of the needle tip precisely at the middle of the arterial lumen, pointing directly down the center of the lumen. Once the provider has received a "flash" of arterial blood indicating arterial entry, it may be necessary to slightly reposition the angle of the needle to achieve maximal blood flow through the needle. When using a traditional puncture needle, maximal blood flow is suggested when arterial blood "spurts" out of the needle hub with each heartbeat. The stronger the "spurt," the better the position. Visualizing dark blood dribbling out of the hub suggests venous entry, as venous blood pressures are much lower than arterial blood pressures and venous blood is darker than arterial blood due to deoxygenation. However, bright red blood dribbling (and not spurting) out of the hub suggests that the provider has accessed the artery but the needle tip is not currently in the center of the lumen or the bevel is not properly positioned in the upward direction.

Gently rotating the needle to a bevel up position or advancing/withdrawing the needle tip by 1–2 mm may result in a better position of the needle tip, which should improve the strength of the pulsatile blood stream. It is important to avoid large (>1–2 mm) movements of the needle tip once the artery has been accessed. Making such micro-movements requires a steady hand and a great deal of practice to perfect. If the provider is using a newer arterial access device with an "all-in-one" integral wire guide, the strength of the pulse blood stream may not be evident.

Introducer needles are usually 18-, 20-, or 22-gauge in diameter and typically come packaged with a compatible guidewire of a slightly smaller diameter than the introducer needle. However, providers should test to ensure that the guidewire glides freely inside the hollow introducer needle before attempting arterial puncture, especially when combining components from different kits.

Guidewires used for arterial access are usually constructed of stainless steel (possibly with a nitinol core) and come in a variety of lengths. The length of guidewire required will depend upon the depth of the target vessel and the length of the catheter to be used. In all cases, the guidewire must be longer than the catheter and should be inserted at least as far as the catheter is to be inserted. Guidewires have a flexible tip on one end, which is intended to prevent inadvertent penetration of the opposing artery wall, creation of a false passage in the soft tissues surrounding the vessel, or advancement of the wire into a side branch of the artery. This flexible tip may be "J"-shaped (Fig. 13.10) or straight but should be distinguished from the stiff end of the guidewire. It is not recommended to advance the stiff end of the guidewire first into the introducer needle, as this increases the risk of complications and does not improve success rates. Inability to advance the guidewire

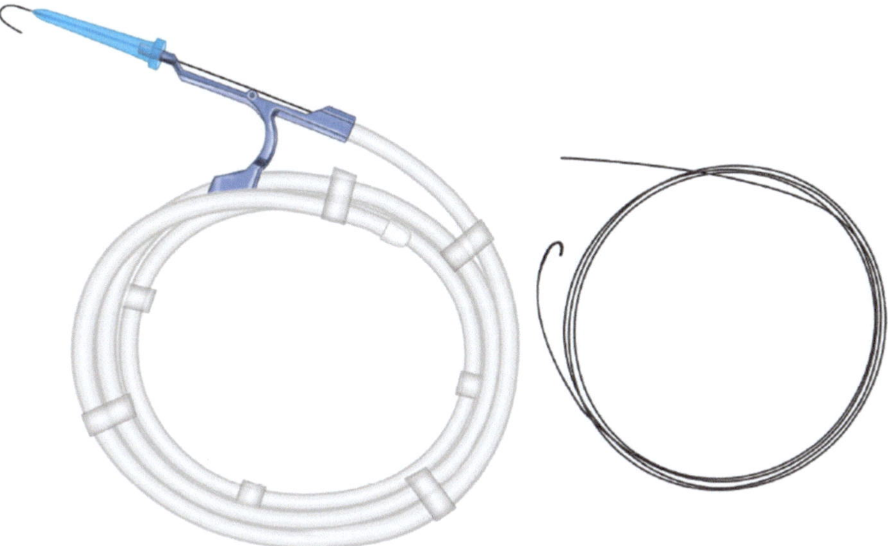

Fig. 13.10 Traditional flexible "J" tip guidewire, with and without casing

through the introducer into the artery suggests malposition of the needle tip, and this problem is only exacerbated by use of the wrong end of the guidewire. In rare cases, the guidewire tip (regardless of which type of flexible tip is used) may become impaled on the needle tip, or the stiff portion of the wire may become kinked inside of the vessel; both of these complications can prevent the guidewire from being withdrawn from the needle after deployment. In these cases, the provider should remove the introducer needle-guidewire complex en masse to avoid shearing the guidewire tip or causing additional injury to the artery during the attempt to remove the guidewire.

Arterial catheters range in diameter from 18 to 24 gauge, although the diameter and length of catheter required will vary depending upon the age and weight of the patient, as well as the targeted arterial insertion site. Radial catheters range from 2.5 cm to 5 cm in length, while femoral catheters are usually much longer. In adults, the radial artery catheter is usually 20 gauge and 4.5–5 cm in length, while femoral catheters are typically 18 gauge and 12–20 cm long.

The process of inserting an introducer needle begins with palpation of the target artery with the second and third fingers of the nondominant hand just proximal to the desired skin puncture site. Then, with the bevel facing upward, the provider uses the dominant hand to grasp the needle barrel and advances the needle tip through the skin at a 30–45° angle (relative to the plane of the skin surface) toward the pulsation felt under the fingertips of the nondominant hand (Fig. 13.9). As stated before, the needle shaft should be angled in the anticipated direction of the artery's path.

Once the introducer needle has penetrated the vessel wall and been confirmed to be in good position within the artery, next steps will depend upon which technique

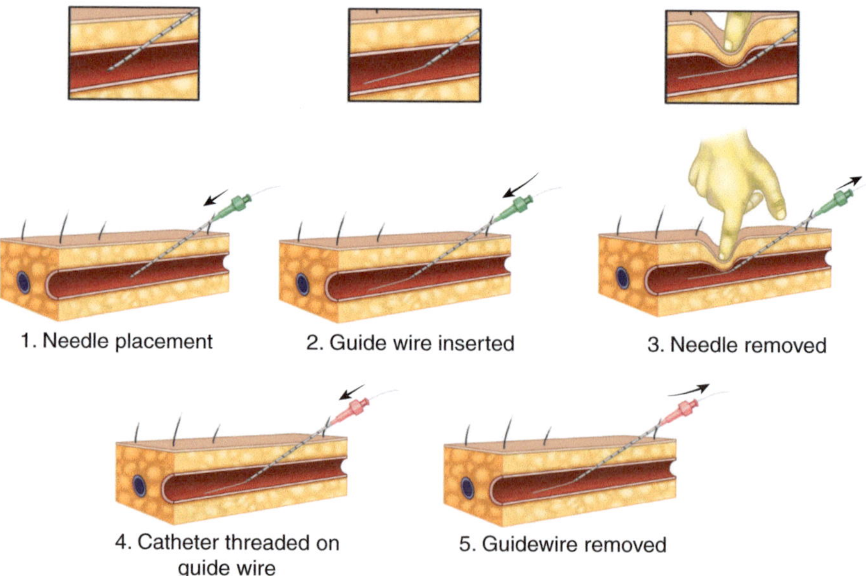

Fig. 13.11 Seldinger (catheter-over-wire) technique

for catheter insertion has been selected: the Seldinger technique, modified Seldinger technique, or catheter-over-needle technique.

Seldinger Technique

Using this technique, the introducer needle is placed (Fig. 13.11, Step 1), and a separate guidewire of appropriate length is then advanced through the lumen of the introducer needle and into the vessel (Step 2). If the guidewire encounters resistance, the provider may exert minimal pressure to advance the guidewire past this resistance but should not force the guidewire excessively. After the guidewire has been advanced easily into the lumen of the artery, the needle is removed (Step 3), leaving the guidewire in the vessel. Finally, the catheter is advanced over the guidewire until it is hubbed (Step 4), and the guidewire is then removed (Step 5). At this point, the provider should see arterial blood flowing from the catheter. If no blood is flowing from the catheter, the catheter tip may not be in the arterial lumen, and the catheter may be retracted slightly to see if this improves blood flow. If not, the catheter should be removed, pressure held to the arterial puncture site to control hematoma formation, and a new arterial puncture attempt made.

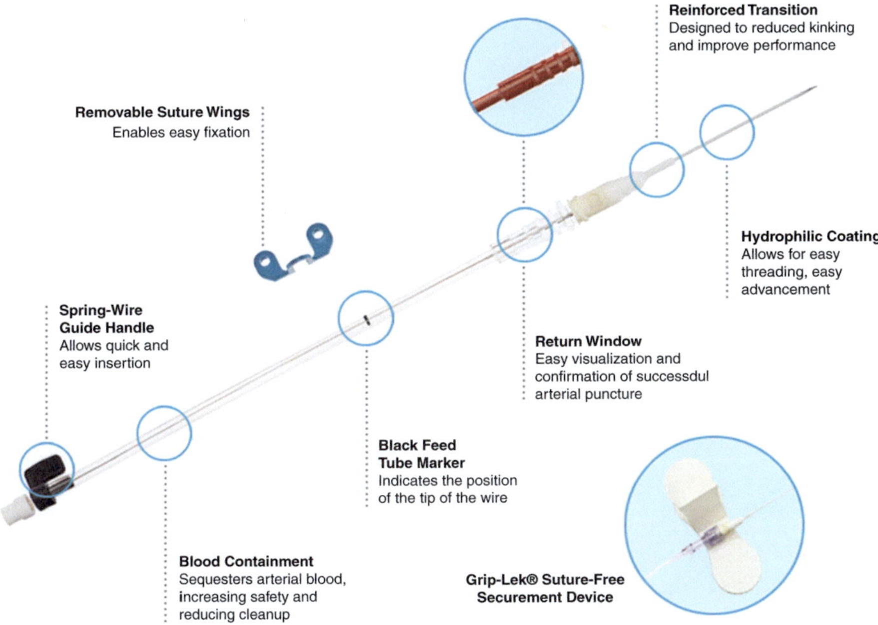

Fig. 13.12 The Arrow® Integrated Arterial Catheter system (*Image courtesy of Teleflex Inc. © 2020 Teleflex Inc. All rights reserved.*)

Modified Seldinger Technique

This technique is similar to the traditional Seldinger technique, with the *caveat* that all of the cannulation components (i.e., introducer needle, guidewire, and catheter) are fitted together as a single integrated unit [46]. One example of a device used with the modified Seldinger technique is the Arrow® Integrated Arterial Catheter (Fig. 13.12).

Catheter-Over-Needle Technique

The catheter-over-needle technique may be more technically simple than the Seldinger or modified Seldinger techniques and is especially useful for the cannulation of superficial arteries (e.g., radial artery). This technique utilizes an apparatus consisting of a hollow introducer needle situated inside of an integrated catheter (Fig. 13.13). As this technique is not dependent on a guidewire, it may be preferred for patients with exceedingly small arteries, including neonates and infants. As with the other techniques, the needle is inserted through the skin and advanced toward the artery at a 30–45° angle with the bevel facing upward (Fig. 13.9, Step 1). Arterial access is identified once a strong pulsatile blood flow is noted through the catheter hub. At this point, the needle-catheter device complex is lowered to an angle of 10–20° (relative to the skin surface), and the

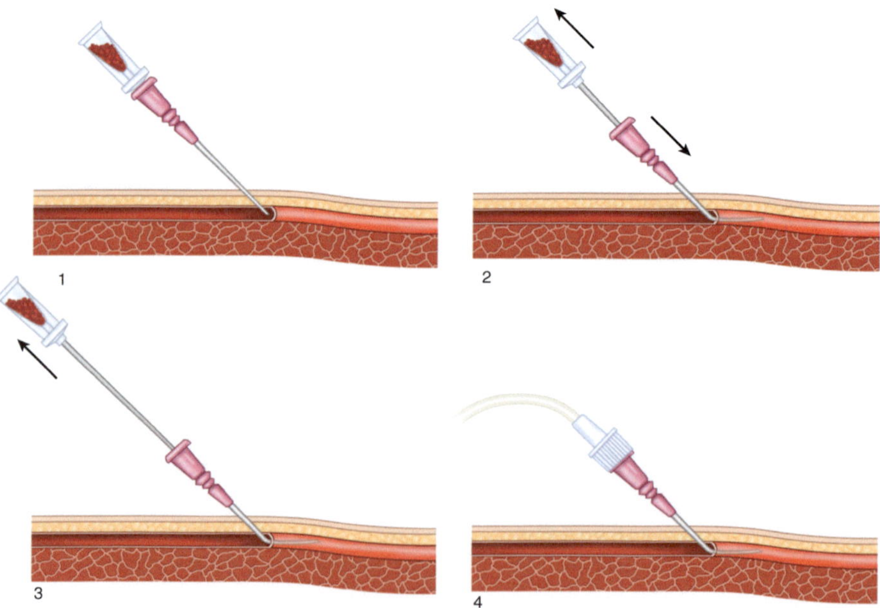

Fig. 13.13 Catheter-over-needle technique

complex is advanced 1–2 mm further (Step 2). This ensures that the catheter tip has fully entered the arterial lumen. The catheter can then be fully advanced into the vessel until the hub of the catheter is contacting the skin (Step 3). If at any time resistance is felt while advancing the catheter, the needle can be shifted slightly and additional attempts made to advance the catheter once appropriate blood flow resumes. Providers should never retract the catheter back onto the needle once it has been advanced, as this can shear the tip of the catheter leading to embolization into the artery or loss of the catheter tip within the subcutaneous tissues. Once the catheter is able to be advanced fully, the needle is removed, the catheter is secured, and any needed transducer tubing is attached to the catheter hub (Step 4).

7. *Catheter Insertion and Dressing*

The most challenging part of arterial line placement is often appropriate placement of the guidewire. After this stage, catheter insertion should progress uneventfully, although care must be taken to prevent avoidable complications. When utilizing the Seldinger technique, it is important to maintain the sterility of the guidewire, avoiding contact between the guidewire and other objects in the environment that may not be sterile. Especially with the femoral approach, it is also important to keep a significant portion of the guidewire outside of the patient and to maintain control of this external portion, to avoid the rare complication of a "lost" guidewire inside of the patient. This complication appears to be a greater risk with venous cannulation but is not impossible with arterial cannulation if an inappropriately short guidewire is used or if the guidewire is advanced excessively into the patient. In general, the guidewire should be advanced into the patient approximately the same distance as the length of the catheter to be inserted. The guidewire should be firmly held between two fingers of the nondominant hand while loading the catheter on the guidewire to prevent inadvertent advancement of the wire while advancing the catheter into the patient. The ability to advance the guidewire should (hopefully) serve as a surrogate indicator of the ability to advance the catheter, and inability to advance the guidewire into the patient to an adequate depth suggests that the catheter may not be able to be advanced either. Given the flexibility and smaller diameter of a guidewire, as compared to that of the arterial catheter, it is better to identify obstructions preventing proper placement at the guidewire stage (thus enabling selection of a new site, as needed) than to identify obstructions after the catheter has already been inserted and the arteriotomy has been dilated with the catheter.

After stabilization of the guidewire with the nondominant hand and removal of the introducer needle, the dominant hand is used to thread the arterial catheter onto the guidewire. The catheter is then advanced into the artery until it is "hubbed" (i.e., catheter hub touches skin), as in Fig. 13.13. If there is difficulty with catheter advancement, a rotating motion can be incorporated as the catheter is pushed over the guidewire into the artery. Once the catheter is sufficiently inside the artery, the provider should remove the guidewire and apply pressure to the artery proximal to the site of catheter insertion, to aid in temporarily occluding blood flow from the catheter until the tubing can be attached to the hub of the catheter (Fig. 13.11). Pulsatile blood flow out of the hub of the catheter prior to pressure being applied suggests proper catheter positioning within the artery.

After the catheter has been fully inserted, the provider must connect it to the pressure transducer tubing. This step can be challenging, since many tubing products are not sterile and risk contamination of the sterile field. At this point, it is helpful to have an assistant who is able to handle the non-sterile tubing without contaminating the sterile field. If no assistant is available, it is recommended for the provider to change sterile gloves before recontacting the insertion site to place the sterile dressings. Especially with radial line insertion, it is easy to lose control of the catheter when connecting the transducer tubing, which could lead to catheter dislodgement. For this reason, many providers will connect a sterile 10-mL syringe (usually included in the kit) to the Luer-lock end of the arterial catheter immediately after placement, which will prevent continued bleeding from the catheter while the catheter is being secured. This will also allow to facilitate blood sampling from the line. Once the catheter is sutured or otherwise anchored at the insertion site, the syringe is removed and the transducer tubing is connected.

Many methods exist for securing the arterial catheter after placement, including the use of sutures, adhesive stickers, clamps, adherent dressings, and tape. Most arterial catheters include an integrated *suture wing*, which is meant to facilitate anchoring of the catheter close to the insertion site (Fig. 13.14). Although 3–0 or 4–0 nylon sutures have classically been used to anchor the suture wings to the patient's skin, less-invasive stickers and adhesive dressings are also available. As with venous catheters, chlorhexidine gluconate (CHG)-impregnated sponges, such as the Biopatch® protective disc, may help to reduce the risk of local soft tissue or bloodstream infection for up to a week after placement.

Dressing of the insertion site should also include a sterile transparent dressing (e.g., Tegaderm®), which should be *centered on the puncture site* to maximize its

Fig. 13.14 Standard femoral arterial catheter with integrated suture wing

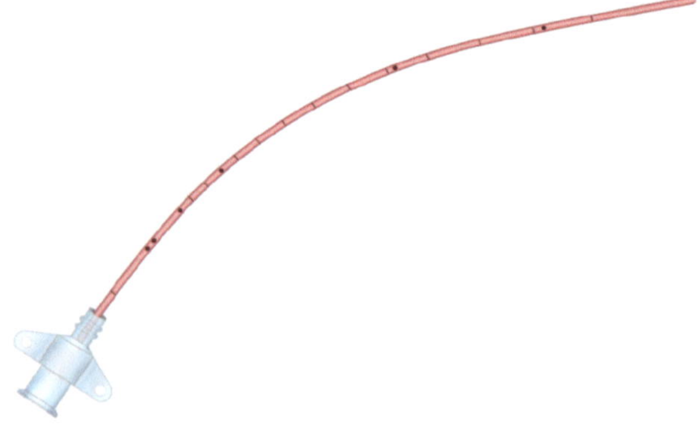

effectiveness at preventing site contamination. Prior to placing a transparent dressing, the skin to be covered should be thoroughly (and sterilely) dried and cleansed of any blood that may have oozed from the puncture site, as blood or other fluids may serve as a nidus for bacterial growth. Thorough removal of residual ultrasound gel from the site will also improve adherence of the dressing to the skin surface.

8. *Catheter Securement and Tubing Attachment*

Once the catheter has been sutured in place or otherwise anchored at the insertion site, and the insertion site has been sterilely dressed, additional securement of the catheter and tubing is recommended to avoid inadvertent migration or dislodgement of the catheter. Many methods for tubing securement exist, and no clear evidence exists to suggest advantages with any specific method. Whichever method is suggested, it is essential that the provider secure the tubing before leaving the bedside. In this chapter, we will suggest one method that appears to perform adequately, but the provider should feel free to modify this technique as needed.

Once the three-way stopcock and transducer tubing have been attached and the insertion site is covered with sterile dressings, the provider's attention should then be turned to securement of the transducer tubing to the patient's extremity. At the radial site, the tubing can be looped around the thumb (coming from the palmar

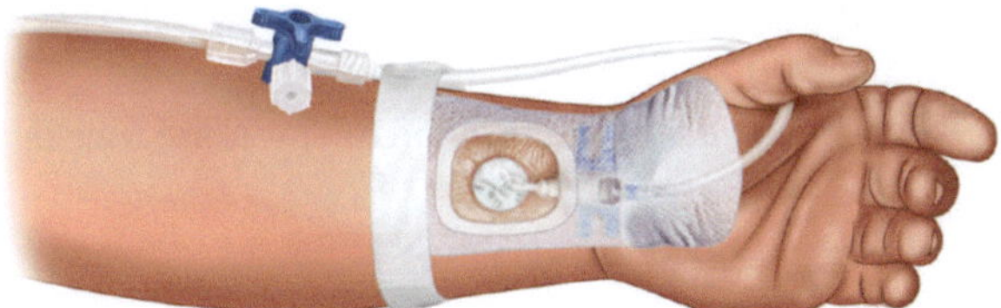

Fig. 13.15 Technique for securement of transducer tubing following radial arterial line placement

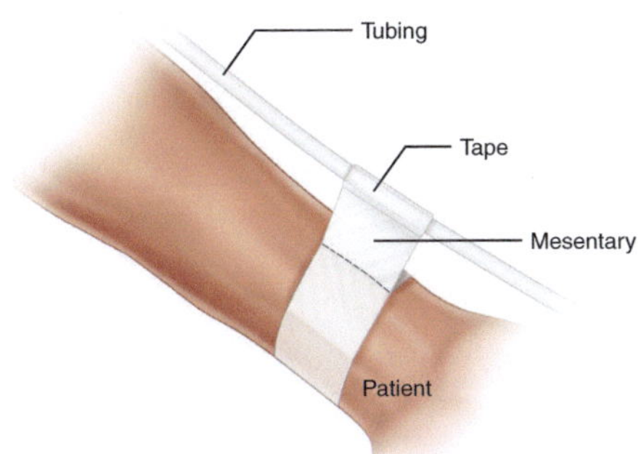

Fig. 13.16 Creation of a "mesentery" tape attaching transducer tubing to the extremity

side) and secured to the radial side of the wrist and forearm. Care should be taken to make this loop loose enough to avoid excessive tension on the tubing with thumb or wrist movement. A gentle curve is recommended, to avoid creating kinks in the tubing. The tubing can be secured to the patient with surgical silk tape (e.g., 3M Durapore™) and/or additional Tegaderm® dressings. One technique for radial artery cather securement is illustrated in Fig. 13.5, which includes securement of the transducer tubing around the patient thumb and radial side of the forearm.

When securing tubing to the patient, it is important to avoid circumferential taping (i.e., looping the tape completely around the circumference of the extremity) to reduce the risk of limb ischemia. This is especially important with radial lines or when the patient has significant extremity edema. The creation of a tape "mesentery" (Fig. 13.16) further down the extremity (away from the insertion site) may also be advantageous, allowing for some freedom in tubing movement while still anchoring the tubing effectively to the extremity.

Pressure Transducer Setup

A pressure transducer system is used to continuously monitor the patient's blood pressure through the arterial catheter. The pressure transducer kit includes non-compressible tubing, a three-way stopcock used for zeroing, and transducer cable that attaches to the monitor [47]. Additional supplies that are needed include an IV pole and transducer mount, 500 ml of normal 0.9% saline, a pressurized infusion cuff, and cardiac monitor with associated cables.

Steps involved with setting up the pressure transducer system include:

Fig. 13.17 Blood pressure transducer system

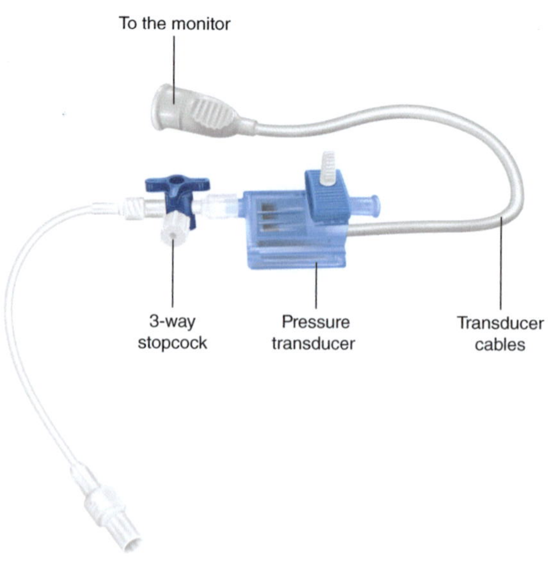

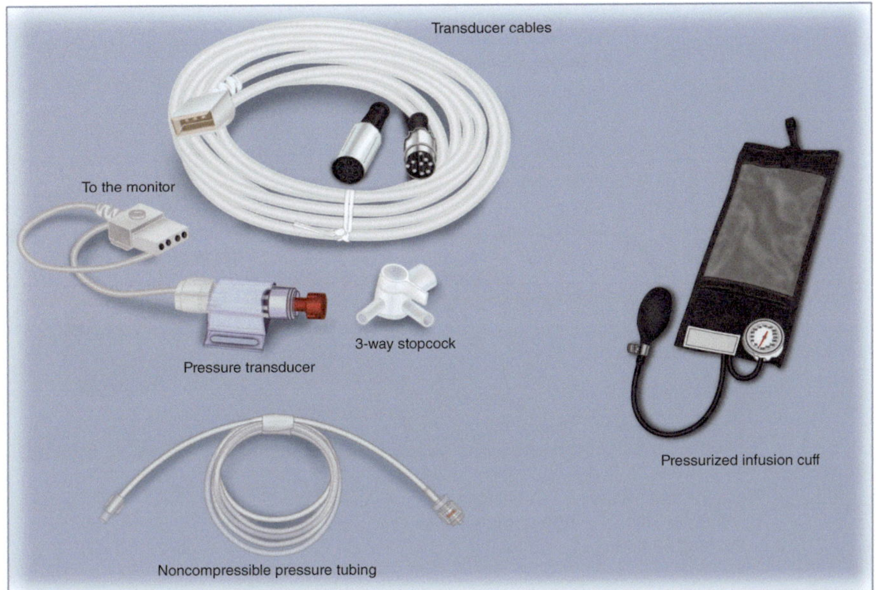

Fig. 13.18 Transducer cable, pressure transducer system, pressure tubing, and infusion cuff required for arterial pressure monitoring

- Turn on the cardiac monitor, and attach the reusable cabling.
- Remove the transducer system from its packaging, and ensure that all connections are adequately tightened. A standard blood pressure transducer with three-way stopcock and cabling is shown in Fig. 13.17.

- Connect the transducer cable to the monitor cable, making sure that the connection is secure.
- Attach the saline line with drip chamber to the saline bag, place the saline bag into the pressure infusion cuff, hang it onto the IV pole, and squeeze the drip chamber, filling to approximately half full. The cabling, pressurized tubing, and pressurized infusion cuff are depicted in Fig. 13.18.

- Prime the line by flushing saline through all of the tubing, ensuring that there is no air trapped inside the tubing. Air trapped within the tubing risks creating an air embolus within the patient's vasculature. The liquid (saline) medium also allows for proper propagation of the fluid pressure wave, which is dampened by retained air within the system. To prime the line, open the roller clamp near the drip chamber and activate the flush device near the transducer. The type of flush device will depend on the specific transducer kit provided at your institution. There are two common flush devices: (1) squeeze flush devices, in which the

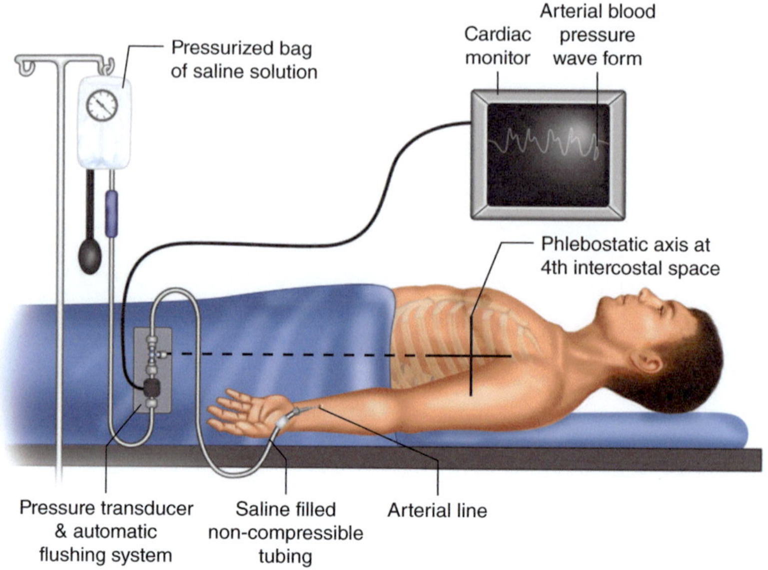

Fig. 13.19 Pressure transducer system setup

provider squeezes a compression tab to allow fluid flow, and (2) pull-tab flush devices, in which the provider pulls the pigtail to allow fluid flow. Flush the system until fluid flows through the open port on the zeroing stopcock, then turn the zeroing stopcock off to the zeroing port, and cover with non-vented cap. Use the flush device to flush the remaining line through to connector which will soon attach to the patients catheter and then close the connector with a non-vented cap.

- Pressurize the saline bag to 300 mmHg and close the pressure cuff clamp. Make sure the drip chamber does not fill completely during pressurization. Pressurizing the systems ensures there is no back flow of blood into the pressure transducer.
- Calibrate ("zero") the system at the level of the patient's phlebostatic axis located at patient's fourth intercostal space, mid-axillary line as illustrated in Figure 13.19 [48]. This is achieved by bringing the transducer to the same horizontal level of this point on the patient and turning the handle of the zeroing stopcock off toward the patient's end of the tubing and removing the non-vented cap from the zeroing port. This will open the transducer to atmospheric pressure.
- Calibrate the cardiac monitor according to monitor manufacturer's instructions.
- Close the zeroing stopcock and tighten the non-vented cap on the zeroing port.

At this point, the patient's catheter tubing is ready to be connected to the pressure monitoring system. To ensure that there are is no air trapped at the end of the tubing, the provider should activate the flush device and watch saline flow and drop out of the tubing while it is being attached. Once all of the tubing is attached, the patient is ready for hemodynamic monitoring of arterial pressures.

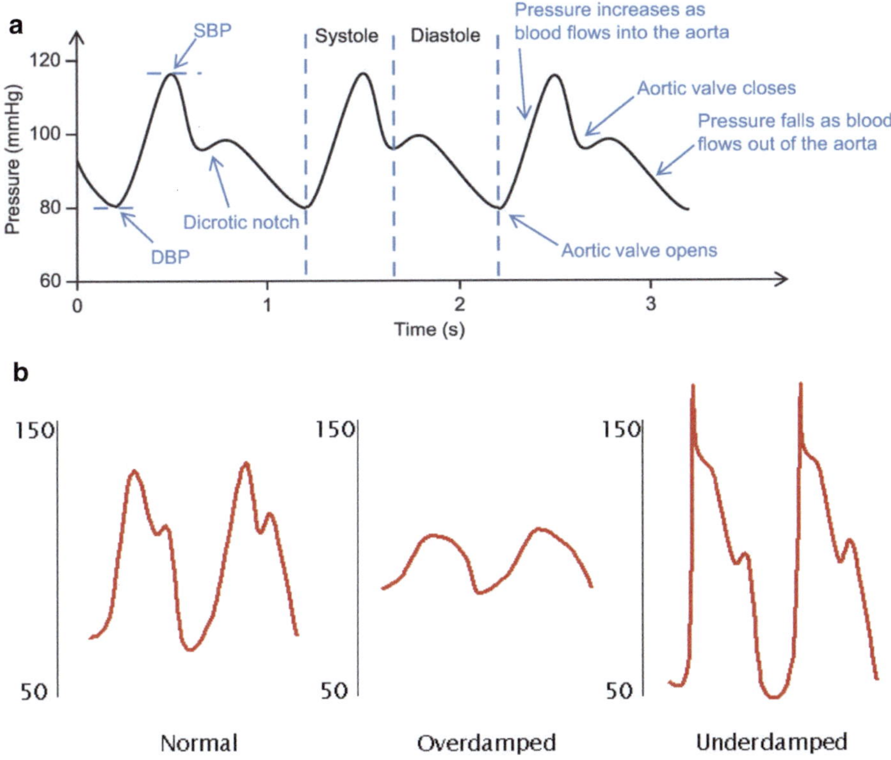

Fig. 13.20 Arterial pressure waveform including key features (**a**); and illustrations of waveform damping (**b**)

Interpreting Arterial Pressure Waveforms

The arterial pressure waveform generated through invasive arterial catheterization provides a dynamic representation of the pressures in the patient's arterial vasculature due to the action of the left ventricle of the heart during each phase of the cardiac cycle [47]. Invasive blood pressure monitoring is essentially measuring the same physiological phenomenon as noninvasive blood pressure cuffs but does so in a different way. Instead of measuring blood pressure as a function of blood flow through an artery at one point in time, as with a noninvasive blood pressure cuff, invasive blood pressure monitoring uses the transduction of a fluid pressure wave into an electrical signal that is plotted in real time on a cardiac monitor.

When analyzing the arterial pressure waveform, providers must ensure that the transducer has been zeroed and leveled to the patient's right atrium, as stated previously, and that an appropriate scale is selected on the monitor. With a large scale, the wave will appear small on the monitor; with a small scale, the waveform will appear larger. In certain clinical settings, the provider can inspect the arterial pressure waveform in relation to the electrocardiogram and plethysmographic waveform obtained from a pulse oximeter to rule out the possibility of artifacts of the pressure transducer system.

The two phases of the cardiac cycle are reflected in the arterial pressure waveform. The systolic blood pressure (SBP) and diastolic blood pressure (DBP) represent the highest and lowest points on the pressure waveform, respectively (Fig. 13.20a). Systole corresponds to the period of left ventricular contraction, when the aortic valve opens to allow blood to flow from the heart into the aorta and systemic circulation. The *dicrotic notch* is the small, brief increase in blood pressure that appears when the aortic valve closes, due to a small a mount of backward blood flow. As the left ventricle contracts, pressure in the arterial system increases, which correlates to the increasing slope on the pressure waveform. Conversely, diastole is the period after the aortic valve closes and the left ventricle relaxes. In diastole, arterial pressure lowers as blood flows further into the arterial system. Damping of the waveform is associated with the presence of a clot or air collection in the monitoring system, which increases the intrinsic pressure within the system and results in a waveform that may either smooth out or exaggerate certain features of the waveform (Fig. 13.21).

As fluid pressure waves travel through the systemic circulation, the aorta and downstream arteries expand and, to some degree, absorb the pressure generated from left ventricular contraction. The expansion and absorption of these high pressures is a function of the compliance (stiffness) of the arteries. More compliant arteries, as seen in younger patients, are able to expand more than noncompliant arteries, which is common in the aging patient population. As humans age, arteries become stiffer through atherosclerosis or age-related vascular diseases [49]. Arterial compliance can be observed in the arterial pressure waveform through the *pulse pressure*, which is the difference between the SBP and the DBP. A noncompliant arterial system is characterized by a steeper slope of the waveform and a larger pulse pressure.

Another important feature of the arterial pressure waveform is the *dicrotic notch*. The dicrotic notch is seen at the start of diastole and is an artifact of the reflection of the pressure wave from the peripheral vasculature back to the heart. This occurs just following aortic valve closure. The location of the dicrotic notch on the pressure waveform is partially dependent upon the compliance of the arterial system [49]. Less compliant arteries, as in the elderly, will reflect the fluid pressure wave sooner, and the dicrotic notch will be observed closer to the highest point of the pressure waveform. In extreme cases, the dicrotic notch can be superimposed on the peak of the arterial pressure wave and create a prominent spike, giving the false illusion of an elevated SBP. Conversely, more compliant arteries, as seen in children, will reflect the fluid pressure wave later, and the dicrotic notch will be observed later in the down slope of the pressure tracing.

Troubleshooting the Transducer

Inaccurate pressure measurements can result from many common problems [47]. Most problems are due to improper setup of the pressure transducer equipment. If there is no pressure waveform displayed on the cardiac monitor, the provider should inspect the system for disconnection of the cable, improper scaling of the waveform, dislodgement of the cannula, kinking of the cannula, clotting in the cannula, or transducer failure. To test the patency of the cannula, the provider can try to aspirate blood from the stopcock. If there is no blood return, this may suggest an occlusion of the cannula, or the cannula may be dislodged and require replacement. If there is blood return, check the electrical connections of the pressure transducer and confirm that the scale of the monitor has been set appropriately. If there continues to be no signal after these interventions, a new transducer system should be set up, calibrated, and connected to the patient's cannula.

Anything that compromises the transfer of energy of the fluid pressure wave from the arterial system to the pressure transducer can interfere with the accuracy of arterial pressure monitoring. The resulting change in perceived arterial pressure is termed "damping" and is further categorized as either underdamping or overdamping, as illustrated in Fig. 13.20. Underdamping occurs when the fluid pressure wave is transduced too quickly which will cause the SBP to appear to be higher than it truly is and the DBP to be lower than it truly is [46]. Underdamping can occur as an artifact of the catheter, in cases of tachycardia, or with the use of stiff noncompliant tubing. Overdamping creates a slurred waveform, resulting in underestimation of SBP and overestimation of DBP [46]. Overdamping commonly occurs with low blood pressure; air in the tubing; blood clots in the catheter; kinks in the catheter or tubing; narrow, long, or compliant tubing; loose or open connections; and arterial vasospasm.

Considerations for Ultrasound

There is strong evidence to support the use of ultrasound guidance over traditional landmark and palpatory-based techniques for radial artery cannulation in both adult and pediatric populations, as the use of ultrasound increases first-attempt success rate and reduces the total number of attempts [50]. The advantages associated with ultrasound-guided radial artery cannulation include real-time visualization of the vessel, improved pre-procedural planning, increased success rate, reduced complications, and reduced time spent placing the catheter [51]. Ultrasound guidance has also been shown to decrease the risk of vascular complications with femoral artery cannulations [52]. The use of ultrasound has been demonstrated to increase the chances of successful arterial line placement where it is being utilized as a rescue technique after many failed attempts using the palpatory technique [53]. Of course, ultrasound guidance requires available ultrasound equipment and trained practitioners, which may limit its utility in the emergent setting [52].

Considerations for Type of Arterial Catheter

Depending on the targeted artery and expected technical problems, examiners must carefully choose the type of catheter. The length of catheter selected can contribute to the likelihood of failed placement and accidental dislodgment. Longer catheters are recommended for arteries found deeper in the soft tissue (e.g., brachial, femoral, axillary), to reduce the risk of these complications. Catheter length and inner diameter can also affect the accuracy of blood pressure measurement [46]. In adult subjects, for example, 20-gauge catheters provide more accurate blood pressure measurement at the radial site and are associated with fewer complications than larger catheters [54–56]. An 18-gauge catheter (at a minimum of 15 cm in length) is recommended for femoral artery cannulation.

Arterial Blood Sampling

In many cases, providers may wish to sample arterial blood for *arterial blood gas (ABG)* analysis, or other laboratory testing, without placing a catheter in the artery. This requires a simple puncture of the artery, although it is important to consider many of the same anatomic and safety factors explored previously in this chapter. Arterial puncture is often performed at the *radial artery*, due to its superficial location, distance from other vital structures, and anticipated collateral circulation from the ulnar artery. However, the femoral, brachial, and ulnar arteries may also be used for this purpose if the radial artery is not able to be accessed.

While routine blood sampling may be performed with a standard needle and syringe, arterial blood samples for ABG analysis must be collected with a specialized pre-heparinized syringe and handled to minimize exposure to air during the collection process. Clotting or inclusion of air in the sample will alter the results of the ABG analysis and should be avoided. Because arterial blood flow is under greater pressure than venous blood flow, arterial blood sampling does not require significant syringe vacuum pressure to draw the blood into the syringe. In fact, providers should not draw back on the syringe when collecting arterial blood, as this will contribute to hemolysis and may risk arterial injury.

Blood drawn for ABG analysis should be processed quickly after collection to avoid warming of the blood, which will also affect the accuracy of the analysis. For this reason, the syringe should be transported to the lab in a container with crushed ice, if it is not being processed at the point of care.

In general, a 20-, 23-, or 25-gauge needle is used for arterial blood sampling. While providers will want to use higher-gauge needles with smaller arteries, it should be noted that the use of higher-gauge (i.e., smaller-diameter) needles will also increase sample hemolysis, which may compromise the quality of the laboratory results. On the other hand, the use of an excessively large (i.e., low-gauge) needle increases trauma to the vessel. A generic arterial blood gas collection kit is illustrated in Fig. 13.21.

The general procedure [57, 58] for arterial sampling at the radial artery, for example, may be described as follows:

- Position the patient as for arterial cannulation, with the targeted puncture site exposed and in a position comfortable for both the patient and the provider.

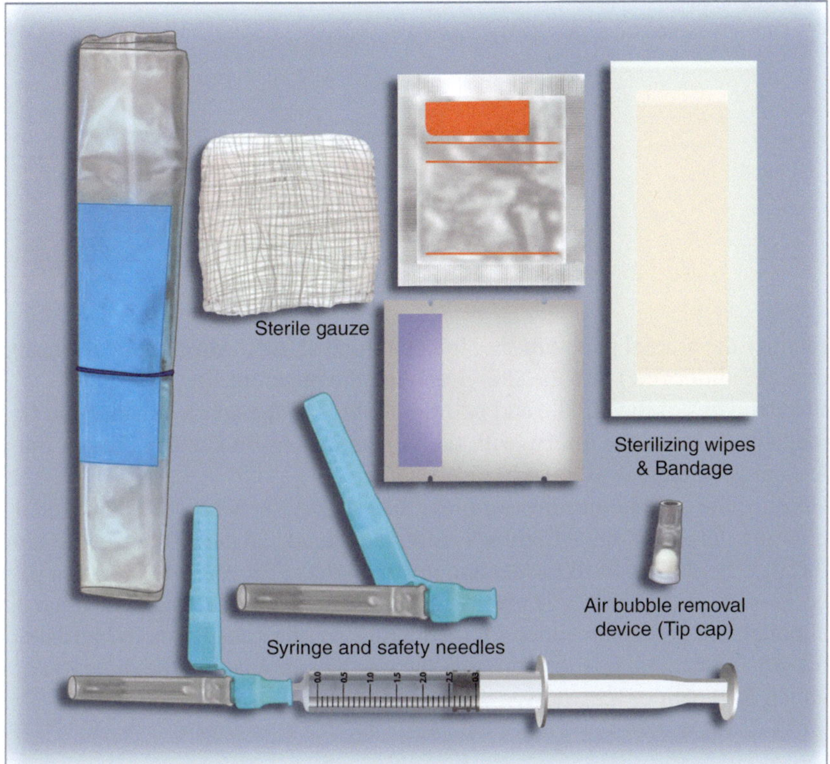

Fig. 13.21 Generic arterial blood gas collection kit

- Assess the artery for evidence of trauma, overlying infection, reduced blood flow, or other contraindications to arterial puncture. In the case of the radial or ulnar arteries, this should include a modified Allen test.
- Don appropriate sterile gloves, impervious gown, and face protection to avoid inadvertent exposure to the patient's blood. Disinfect the puncture site using chlorhexidine or approved sterilizing agent.
- Attach the puncture needle to the syringe. Modern ABG syringes are usually 1 or 3 mL in capacity and made of plastic with lyophilized (i.e., freeze-dried) balanced lithium heparin [59]. If the syringe contains preloaded liquid heparin, you must expel the heparin solution from the syringe through the needle prior to sample collection, leaving only a small amount (e.g., 0.15 mL) of heparin in the chamber. Pull back on the plunger to set the syringe chamber at the recommended volume before arterial puncture.
- If an ultrasound is used to guide insertion, ensure that the portion of the ultrasound probe that will be touching the patient is covered with a sterile surface (e.g., Tegaderm, or sterile probe cover).

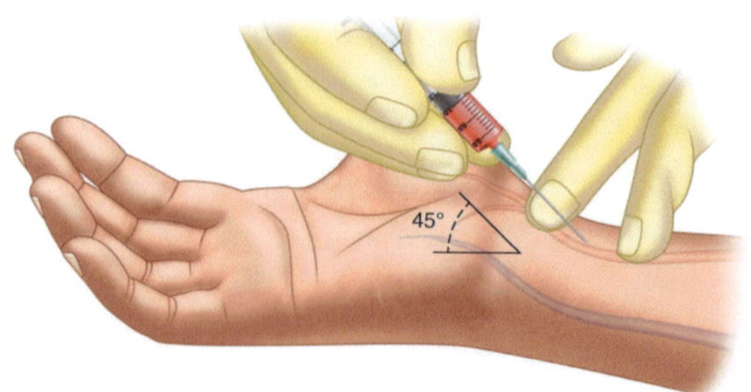

Fig. 13.22 Provider hand positioning for radial arterial puncture

- Identify the arterial puncture site. Inject a small (1-mL) wheal of local anesthetic (e.g., 1% lidocaine) into the skin overlying the puncture site.
- Place the tips of the middle and pointing fingers of the nondominant hand on the palpable pulse of the artery, with the targeted insertion site centered in the gap left between them, as shown in Fig. 13.22.
- Holding the syringe-needle complex "like a dart" between the thumb and the pointing finger of the provider's dominant hand, advance the needle slowly through the skin and soft tissues and into the artery. The angle of puncture should be 30–45° (as in Fig. 13.22) from the skin surface with the radial or ulnar sites, although 90° is recommended for the femoral or other deep sites. When using the 30–45° puncture angle, be sure that the needle is pointed in the direction of the anticipated path of the artery.

- Once a flash of blood is noted to enter the syringe, keep the needle tip at the same position until the needed amount of blood has entered the syringe chamber. Although only a small amount (e.g., 0.2 mL) of blood may be needed, it is recommended to draw at least 1 mL to avoid excessive heparin effect on the sample [59]. Self-filling syringes should be used, which fill with blood after arterial puncture without the need to pull back on the plunger. In fact, pulling back on the plunger is not recommended, as this will cause hemolysis of the specimen. These syringes usually have a vented plunger, which means that air will be able to escape as the syringe chamber fills. After the desired blood volume has been collected, withdraw the needle and apply pressure to the puncture site. Be sure to rapidly invert the syringe to avoid the blood dripping back out of the needle tip.
- Hold direct pressure to the puncture site with a sterile gauze pad to limit hematoma formation at the site. The recommended amount of time is 5 minutes for radial/ulnar artery puncture and 10–15 minutes for deeper sites (e.g., femoral or brachial arteries). An extended duration of time may be required for patients with coagulopathy. A pressure dressing can also be applied to the site with sterile gauze and tape (but avoid circumferential taping).
- With the syringe inverted (i.e., needle pointing to the ceiling), carefully remove the needle from the syringe using a safety device. Place the included tip cap on the syringe. The tip cap serves as an air removal device and prevents the blood in the chamber from directly contacting air in the room. Gently tap the side of the

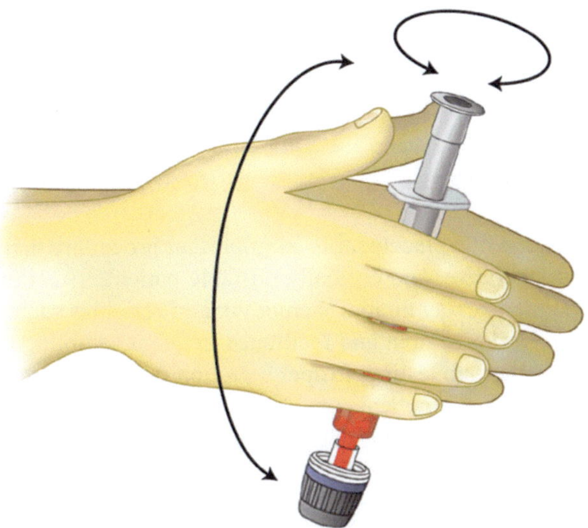

Fig. 13.23 Mixing of the blood sample with residual heparin inside the syringe

syringe to promote air bubbles rising to the surface of the collected blood specimen. Then, expel residual air from the syringe through the tip cap.
- Roll the syringe between your palms, while inverting repeatedly (Fig. 13.23) to mix any residual heparin thoroughly in the sample before placing the sample in the analyzer. Do not aggressively shake the syringe, as this may warm the sample excessively and/or cause hemolysis, which will alter lab results.
- Blood gas analysis should be performed immediately after sample collection. If analysis must be delayed >15 minutes, the sample should be appropriately refrigerated and transported to the lab on ice.

Key Concepts
- Arterial cannulation plays a crucial role in the care of patients in the emergency, perioperative, and critical care settings by allowing continuous hemodynamic monitoring and frequent arterial blood sampling.
- The radial and femoral arteries are the most frequently accessed sites for arterial cannulation.
- Superficial arteries should be considered first to reduce iatrogenic complications. However, site selection should be based on anatomical features, feasibility, provider experience, and the patient's medical condition.
- Arterial vascular access can be accomplished through traditional palpatory techniques, but ultrasound guidance is recommended to increase first-attempt placement success.

Arterial blood specimens may be used to evaluate the partial pressure of oxygen (PaO_2), partial pressure of carbon dioxide ($PaCO_2$), and pH of the arterial blood, as well as other serum tests.

Conclusions

Arterial line placement is an important procedure that can be used in the emergent, perioperative, and critically unstable patient. This invasive procedure allows clinicians to closely monitor hemodynamic variables such as continuous blood pressures and cardiac output and facilitates frequent sampling of arterial blood for blood gas and other lab testing. Proper selection of a target artery depends on myriad factors, including anatomical considerations, feasibility of the site, provider familiarity, and the presence of contraindications.

References

1. McCormack LJ, Cauldwell EW, Anson BJ. Brachial and antebrachial arterial patterns; a study of 750 extremities. Surg Gynecol Obstet. 1953;96(1):43–54.
2. Karacalar S, Ture H, Baris S, et al. Ulnar artery versus radial artery approach for continuous arterial monitoring: a prospective comparative study. J Clin Anesth. 2007;19(3):209–13.
3. Mozersky DJ, Buckley CJ, Hagood CO Jr, et al. Ultrasonic evaluation of the palmar circulation. Am J Surg. 1973;126:810–2.
4. Doscher W, Viswanathan B, Stein T, Margolis IB. Hemodynamic assessment of the circulation in 200 normal hands. Ann Surg. 1983;198:776–9.
5. Doscher W, Viswanathan B, Stein T, Margolis IB. Physiologic anatomy of the palmar circulation in 200 normal hands. J Cardiovasc Surg. 1985;26:171–4.
6. Jarvis MA, Jarvis CL, Jones PR, Spyt TJ. Reliability of Allen's test in selection of patients for radial artery harvest. Ann Thorac Surg. 2000;70(4):1362–5.
7. Brzezinski M, Luisetti T, London MJ. Radial artery cannulation: a comprehensive review of recent anatomic and physiologic investigations. Anesth Analg. 2009;109(6):1763–81.
8. Fernandez R, Zaky F, Ekmejian A, et al. Safety and efficacy of ulnar artery approach for percutaneous cardiac catheterization: systematic review and meta-analysis. Catheter Cardiovasc Interv. 2018;91(7):1273–80.
9. Koutouzis M, Ziakas A, Didagelos M, et al. Ipsilateral radial and ulnar artery cannulation during the same coronary catheterization procedure. Hippokratia. 2016;20(3):249–51.
10. Agostoni P, Zuffi A, Faurie B, et al. Same wrist intervention via the cubital (ulnar) artery in case of radial puncture failure for percutaneous cardiac catheterization or intervention: the multicenter SWITCH registry. Int J Cardiol. 2013;169(1):52–6.
11. Seyahi N, Kahveci A, Altiparmak MR, et al. Ultrasound imaging findings of femoral veins in patients with renal failure and its impact on vascular access. Nephrol Dial Transplant. 2005;20(9):1864–7.
12. Hughes P, Scott C, Bodenham A. Ultrasonography of the femoral vessels in the groin: implications for vascular access. Anaesthesia. 2008;55(12):1198–202.
13. Basmajian JV. Grant's method of anatomy. Baltimore: Williams & Wilkins; 1980.
14. Bangalore S, Bhatt DL. Femoral arterial access and closure. Circulation. 2011;124(5):e147–56.
15. Altin RS, Flicker S, Naidech HJ. Pseudoaneurysm and arteriovenous fistula after femoral artery catheterization: association with low femoral punctures. Am J Roentgenol. 1989;152:629–31.
16. Rapoport S, Sniderman K, Morse S, et al. Pseudoaneurysm: a complication of faulty technique in femoral arterial puncture. Radiology. 1985;154:529–30.

17. Illescas FF, Baker ME, McCann R, et al. CT evaluation of retroperitoneal hemorrhage associated with femoral arteriography. Am J Roentgenol. 1986;146:1289–92.
18. Rupp SB, Vogelzang RL, Nemcek AA Jr, Yungbluth MM. Relationship of the inguinal ligament to pelvic radiographic landmarks: anatomic correlation and its role in femoral arteriography. J Vasc Interv Radiol. 1993;4:409–13.
19. Scheer BV, Perel A, Pfeiffer UJ. Clinical review: complications and risk factors of peripheral arterial catheters used for haemodynamic monitoring in anaesthesia and intensive care medicine. Crit Care. 2002;6(3):199–204.
20. Nuttall G, Burckhardt J, Hadley A, et al. Surgical and patient risk factors for severe arterial line complications in adults. Anesthesiology. 2016;124(3):590–7.
21. Mohr R, Lavee J, Goor DA. Inaccuracy of radial artery pressure measurement after cardiac operations. J Thorac Cardiovasc Surg. 1987;94:286–90.
22. Ahmad RA, Ahmad S, Naveed A, et al. Peripheral arterial blood pressure versus central arterial blood pressure monitoring in critically ill patients after cardiopulmonary bypass. Pak J Med Sci. 2017;33(2):310–4.
23. Dorman T, Brelow MJ, Lipsett PA, et al. Radial artery pressure monitoring underestimates central arterial pressure during vasopressor therapy in critically ill surgical patients. Crit Care Med. 1998;26:1646–9.
24. Soderstrom CA, Wasserman DH, Dunham CM, et al. Superiority of the femoral artery of monitoring. A prospective study. Am J Surg. 1982;144(3):309–12.
25. Greer MR, Carney S, McPheeters RA, et al. Radial arterial lines have a higher failure rate than femoral. West J Emerg Med. 2018;19(2):364–71.
26. Ailon J, Mourad O, Chien V, et al. Videos in clinical medicine. Ultrasound-guided insertion of a radial arterial catheter. N Engl J Med. 2014;371(15):e21.
27. Bur A, Hirschl MM, Herkner H, Oschatz E, Kofler J, Woisetschläger C, Laggner AN. Accuracy of oscillometric blood pressure measurement according to the relation between cuff size and upper-arm circumference in critically ill patients. Crit Care Med. 2000;28(2):371–6.
28. Tiru B, Bloomstone JA, McGee WT. Radial artery cannulation: a review article. J Anesth Clin Res. 2012;3:209.
29. Mandel MA, Dauchot PJ. Radial artery cannulation in 1,000 patients: precautions and complications. J Hand Surg Am. 1977;2(6):482–5.
30. Valentine RJ, Modrall JG, Clagett GP. Hand ischemia after radial artery cannulation. J Am Coll Surg. 2005;201(1):18–22.
31. Lindsay SL, Kerridge R, Collett BJ. Abscess following cannulation of the radial artery. Anaesthesia. 1987;42(6):654–7.
32. Kim JM, Arakawa K, Bliss J. Arterial cannulation: factors in the development of occlusion. Anesth Analg. 1975;54(6):836–41.
33. Hausmann D, Schulte am Esch J, Fischdick G. Radial artery cannulation: a prospective study on its complication rate by clinical and sonographic evaluation [in German]. Anästh Intensivther Notfallmed. 1981;16:269–73.
34. Slogoff S, Keats AS, Arlund C. On the safety of radial artery cannulation. Anesthesiology. 1983;59:42–7.
35. Gurman GM, Kriemermann S. Cannulation of big arteries in critically ill patients. Crit Care Med. 1985;13:217–20.
36. Riker AI, Gamelli RL. Vascular complications and femoral artery catheterization in burn patients. J Trauma. 1996;41:904–5.
37. Fitzpatrick GJ, McDonald NJ, Moriarty DC. Radial artery cannulation: a prospective study. Ir J Med Sci. 1987;156:279–81.
38. Davis FM, Stewart JM. Radial artery cannulation: a prospective study in patients undergoing cardiothoracic surgery. Br J Anaesth. 1980;52:41–7.
39. Russell JA, Joel M, Hudson RJ, Mangano DT, Schlobohm RM. Prospective evaluation of radial and femoral artery catheterization sites in critically ill adults. Crit Care Med. 1983;11:936–9.
40. Bedford RF. Wrist circumference predicts the risk of radial-arterial occlusion after cannulation. Anesthesiology. 1978;48:377–8.

41. Gil RT, Haupt MT, Baharozian MCT, Carlson RW. Arterial catheter complications: are there differences related to the site of insertion? Chest. 1985;88(suppl):39S.
42. Gurman G, Schachar J. Femoral artery cannulation in critically ill patients. Crit Care Med. 1981;9:202–3.
43. Tegtmeyer K, Brady G, Lai S, Hodo R, Braner D. Videos in clinical medicine. Placement of an arterial line. N Engl J Med. 2006;354(15):e13.
44. Mangar D, Thrush DN, Connell GR, Downs JB. Direct or modified Seldinger guide wire-directed technique for arterial catheter insertion. Anesth Analg. 1993;76(4):714–7.
45. Melhuish TM, White LD. Optimal wrist positioning for radial arterial cannulation in adults: a systematic review and meta-analysis. Am J Emerg Med. 2016;34(12):2372–8.
46. Saugel B, Kouz K, Meidert AS, Schulte-Uentrop L, Romagnoli S. How to measure blood pressure using an arterial catheter: a systematic 5-step approach. Crit Care. 2020;24(1):172.
47. Ortega R, Connor C, Kotova F, Deng W, Lacerra C. Use of pressure transducers. N Engl J Med. 2017;376(14):e26.
48. Magder S. Invasive intravascular hemodynamic monitoring: technical issues. Crit Care Clin. 2007;23(3):401–14.
49. van Varik BJ, Rennenberg RJ, Reutelingsperger CP, Kroon AA, de Leeuw PW, Schurgers LJ. Mechanisms of arterial remodeling: lessons from genetic diseases. Front Genet. 2012;3:290.
50. White L, Halpin A, Turner M, Wallace L. Ultrasound-guided radial artery cannulation in adult and paediatric populations: a systematic review and meta-analysis. Br J Anaesth. 2016;116(5):610–7.
51. Miller AG, Bardin AJ. Review of ultrasound-guided radial artery catheter placement. Respir Care. 2016;61(3):383–8.
52. Rashid MK, Sahami N, Singh K, et al. Ultrasound guidance in femoral artery catheterization: a systematic review and a meta-analysis of randomized controlled trials. J Invasive Cardiol. 2019;31(7):e192–8.
53. Sandhu NS, Patel B. Use of ultrasonography as a rescue technique for failed radial artery cannulation. J Clin Anesth. 2006;18(2):138–41.
54. Nuttall G, Burckhardt J, Hadley A, et al. Surgical and patient risk factors for severe arterial line complications in adults. Anesthesiology. 2016;124:590–7.
55. Romagnoli S, Ricci Z, Quattrone D, et al. Accuracy of invasive arterial pressure monitoring in cardiovascular patients: an observational study. Crit Care. 2014;18(6):644.
56. O'Grady NP, Alexander M, Burns LA, et al. Summary of recommendations: guidelines for the prevention of intravascular catheter-related infections. Clin Infect Dis. 2011;52(9):1087–99.
57. Dukic L, Kopcinovic LM, Dorotic A, Barsic I. Blood gas testing and related measurements: national recommendations on behalf of the Croatian Society of Medical Biochemistry and Laboratory Medicine. Biochem Med (Zagreb). 2016;26(3):318–36.
58. Burnett RW, Covington AK, Fogh-Andersen N, et al. Approved IFCC recommendations on whole blood sampling, transport and storage for simultaneous determination of pH, blood gases and electrolytes. Eur J Clin Chem Biochem. 1995;33:247–53.
59. Ordog GJ, Wasserberger J, Balasubramaniam S. Effect of heparin on arterial blood gases. Ann Emerg Med. 1985;14(3):233–8.

Index

© Springer Nature Switzerland AG 2021
J. H. Paxton (ed.), *Emergent Vascular Access*,
https://doi.org/10.1007/978-3-030-77177-5